Teaching psychiatry to undergraduates

Edited by Tom Brown and John Eagles

RCPsych Publications

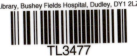

RCPsych Publications is an imprint of the Royal College of Psychiatrists,
17 Belgrave Square, London SW1X 8PG
http://www.rcpsych.ac.uk

British Library Cataloguing-in-Publication Data.
A catalogue record for this book is available from the British Library.

ISBN 978-1-904671-99-2

Distributed in North America by Publishers Storage and Shipping Company.

Printed in the UK by Bell & Bain Limited, Glasgow.

Contents

Figures, tables and boxes

Figures

Tables

Boxes

Contributors

Dr **Benjamin Baig** MBChB MRCPsych MPhil PhD, Clinical Lecturer and Honorary Specialist Registrar, University of Edinburgh

Dr **Vivienne Blackhall** MBChB BSc MedSci (Psychological Medicine), FY1 Doctor, Ayr Hospital, Ayrshire

Dr **Tom Brown** MB ChB BSc MPhil FRCPE FRCPsych, Consultant Psychiatrist, Liaison Psychiatry, Western Infirmary, Glasgow

Dr **Sheila Calder** MBChB FRCPsych, Consultant General Adult Psychiatrist, Royal Cornhill Hospital, Aberdeen

Dr **Madawa Chandratilake** MBBS MMEd, Research Officer, Centre for Medical Education, University of Dundee

Dr **Angela Cogan** MA MBChB MRCPsych, Consultant in General Adult Psychiatry, Glasgow; Hospital Sub Dean for Psychiatry, Greater Glasgow and Clyde; Honorary Clinical Senior Lecturer, University of Glasgow

Professor **Stephen Cooper** MD FRCPI FRCPsych, Professor of Psychiatry, Queen's University Belfast

Dr **Subodh Dave** MBBS MRCPSych MD DPM, Clinical Teaching Fellow and Consultant Psychiatrist, Derby City General Hospital

Dr **Teifion Davies** PhD FRCPsych, Director of Undergraduate Psychiatry Teaching, Institute of Psychiatry, King's College London

Professor **Margery Davis** MD MBChB FRCP, Director, Centre for Medical Education, University of Dundee

Dr **Richard Day** MBChB BSc MRCPsych, Section of Psychiatry, Ninewells Hospital, Dundee

Dr **David Dayson** MBBS FRCPsych, Director of Undergraduate Medical Education, Hampshire Partnership NHS Foundation Trust

Professor **Nisha Dogra** BM DCH FRCPsych MA PhD, Senior Lecturer in Child and Adolescent Psychiatry, Greenwood Institute of Child Health, University of Leicester

Professor **John Eagles** MBCHB MPhil FRCPsych, Consultant General Adult Psychiatrist, Royal Cornhill Hospital, Aberdeen

Dr **Holly Greer** MBBCh BAO DipMH MRCPsych, ST5 Psychiatry of Learning Disability, Belfast

Dr **Elizabeth Hare** MBChB MPhil MRCPsych FRCPsych, General Adult Consultant Psychiatrist, Royal Edinburgh Hospital

Dr **Fiona Hendry** MBChB BSC MedSci (Psychological Medicine), FY1 Doctor, Southern General Hospital, Glasgow

Dr **Faith Hill** BA PGCE MA(Ed) PhD FHEA, Director, Division of Medical Education, School of Medicine, University of Southampton

Miss **Tracey Holley** BA, Mental Health Survivor Educator, Worcester

Professor **Sheila Hollins** MB FRCPsych, Professor of Psychiatry of Learning Disability, St George's Hospital, University of London

Dr **Paul Hopper** MBChB MRCPsych, Consultant Old Age Psychiatrist, Hampshire Partnership Foundation Trust, Southampton

Professor **Robert Howard** MA MD MRCPsych, Dean, Royal College of Psychiatrists

Dr **Lisa Jones**, PhD, Senior Lecturer, Department of Psychiatry, University of Birmingham

Dr **Khalid Karim** BSc MBBS MRCPsych, Senior Lecturer in Child and Adolescent Psychiatry, Greenwood Institute of Child Health, University of Leicester

Dr **Johannes Leuvennink** MBChB MMed(SA) FRCPsych, Consultant General Adult Psychiatrist, Crichton Royal Hospital, Dumfries

Dr **Brian Lunn** MBChB FRCPsych, Clinical Senior Lecturer/Consultant Psychiatrist, School of Medical Sciences Education Development, The Medical School, Newcastle University

Dr **Greg Lydall** MBBCh MRCPsych, Specialty Registrar in General Adult Psychiatry, Barnet, Enfield and Haringey Mental Health Trust, London

Dr **Neil Masson** MBChB BMedSci (Hons) MRCPsych, Specialty Registrar in Psychiatry, Glasgow

Dr **Maggie McGurgan** MBBCh BAO DipMH MRCPsych, ST5 Psychiatry of Learning Disability, Belfast

Dr **Róinin McNally** MBBCh BAO DipMH MRCPsych, ST6, Psychiatry of Old Age, Belfast

Dr **Craig Melville** BSc (Hons) MBChB MRCPsych MD, Senior Lecturer in Learning Disabilities Psychiatry, Centre for Population Health Sciences, College of Medical, Veterinary and Life Sciences, University of Glasgow

Dr **Audrey Morrison** MB CHB MRCPsych, Consultant Psychiatrist and Sub Dean in Psychiatry, Dundee

Dr **Clare Oakley** MB ChB MRCPsych, Clinical Research Worker, St Andrew's Academic Centre, Institute of Psychiatry, King's College London

Professor **Femi Oyebode** MB BS MD PhD FRCPsych, Professor of Psychiatry, University of Birmingham

Dr **Rosalind Ramsay** MA FRCPsych, Maudsley Hospital, London

Dr **Premal Shah** MB ChB BSc MRCPsych MD, Consultant General Adult Psychiatrist, Royal Edinburgh Hospital, Edinburgh

Dr **Peter Sloan** MB BCh BAO DipMH MRCPsych, ST6, General Adult Psychiatry, Belfast

Professor **Lindsay Thomson** MB ChB FRCPsych MPhil MD, University of Edinburgh and Medical Director, State Hospitals Board for Scotland and the Forensic Mental Health Services Managed Care Network.

Dr **Rachel Upthegrove** MB BS MRCPsych MPhil, Consultant Psychiatrist, Birmingham and Solihull Mental Health Foundation Trust, and Clinical Senior Lecturer, University of Birmingham

Dr **Barry Wright** MB BS MRCGP DCH MMedSc FRCPsych MD, Consultant Child, Adolescent and Family Psychiatrist, North Yorkshire and York Primary Care Trust

Preface

In 2003, concern about recruitment into the specialty led to a survey of psychiatrists working in Scotland. Respondents highlighted the link between the quality of undergraduate teaching and the choice of young doctors to pursue a career in psychiatry. Accordingly, the Royal College of Psychiatrists' Scottish Division Undergraduate Student Teaching and Recruitment Group (S-DUSTARG) was constituted. The main aims of the group have been to raise the profile of and enhance the quality of student teaching and, through this and other methods, to increase the numbers of medical graduates entering psychiatry.

The purpose of this book is to further those aims. In particular, we are aware that trainee psychiatrists (just like their senior colleagues) generally receive little in the way of guidance or direction when they undertake student teaching. The earlier chapters address some of the theory and practical aspects of teaching psychiatry to medical students. The later chapters focus more on issues relating to recruitment. We believe that recruiting adequate numbers of the brightest young doctors into psychiatry is a priority if we wish to ensure the longer-term health and credibility of our profession.

As our own interest in this has developed, we have become aware of the work of like-minded colleagues around the country, many of whom have contributed to this book. We thank all of our contributors, but we are even more grateful to Karen Addie, Policy Manager in the Scottish Division of the Royal College of Psychiatrists, for her industry and patience throughout the various stages in the production of this book. Thanks are also due to Lana Hadden for her assistance.

Tom Brown and John Eagles

Foreword

Recruitment of UK medical school graduates into psychiatry is in crisis as I write this. Each year, it seems that we persuade fewer and fewer of our own trainees to follow us into a specialty that we know can offer frustration alongside fascination, but that is, overall, a challenging and rewarding career choice. The College has followed the decline in interest shown by our own medical school graduates through the falling proportion of candidates for the MRCPsych with a primary medical qualification from the UK. This varies between individual examination sittings but is currently running at between 10% and 20%. Where should we look to understand what is going wrong as a first step in trying to reverse the apparent decline? Most of us chose psychiatry on the basis of our undergraduate experience. My own exposure to Ruth Seifert and Anthony Clare at Barts in the early 1980s left me in no doubt that I wanted to become a psychiatrist, despite the counsel and disapproval of the charismatic physicians whom I was subsequently to work for. All the anecdotal evidence that I have been able to glean from undergraduates, foundation and specialist trainees suggests that the medical student experience of psychiatry is currently a dispiriting one. Transient placements with chaotic community teams, where the consultant psychiatrist presents as disengaged and disillusioned rather than inspirational, and poor-quality didactic teaching, delivered by often reluctant teachers, lead unsurprisingly to career choices other than psychiatry.

The material presented in this book represents an important step towards the delivery of high-quality and inspirational undergraduate teaching. Contributions from a hand-picked team of authors cover an imaginative and thought-provoking range of topics. A nucleus of the authors comes from a highly experienced Scottish group who have collected data and written widely about undergraduate psychiatry teaching. The editors have also recruited writers who are distinguished within relevant fields of medical education but find themselves, through accident of birth or employment, on the other side of Hadrian's Wall. The result is a book that carries an international relevance and contains the best ideas and solutions that our profession can provide.

Everyone who teaches undergraduate medical students will have something important to learn from the contributions within this book. If you have read this far and are in a bookshop – I would urge you to proceed to the cash desk to purchase it. If you've bought the book and have read this far and are sitting in your office or at home – do make sure that you finish the whole book before your next encounter with a medical student. As Dean of the Royal College of Psychiatrists and as a psychiatrist who is passionately concerned about the current dire state of undergraduate teaching in our subject and the clear negative effect that this is having upon recruitment, I want to thank the editors and authors for their work in the generation of what I am confident will be regarded as a landmark book.

Professor Robert Howard
Dean
Royal College of Psychiatrists

CHAPTER 1

How do students learn?

Margery Davis & Madawa Chandratilake

Introduction

One definition of teaching is that it is the facilitation of learning. Regardless of whether you teach in a ward, a clinical skills centre, an out-patient clinic or a lecture theatre, it is helpful for you as a teacher to understand how people learn in order to enable you to facilitate their learning.

We shall describe the domains of learning: cognitive (knowledge); psychomotor (skills); and affective (attitudes). For many of you, your teaching will be in all three domains. There are different levels of learning for each domain; for instance, Bloom's taxonomy of learning in the cognitive domain describes six levels of learning (Bloom, 1956). Bloom's taxonomy is not new, but it provides a particularly useful tool to help you to identify whether you are teaching or assessing facts that need to be memorised or the application of facts, or judgement, which require higher-order thinking.

Medical students tackle their learning in different ways and these will be outlined. Many medical students have been called strategic learners (Entwistle & Ramsden, 1982) as there is evidence that they approach their learning in a way that will give them the best chance of passing their examinations. You can help your students learn more effectively by the way that you teach. We shall describe a number of theories about how people learn and present some principles of learning drawn from these theories that you can use in your everyday teaching to facilitate your students' learning. These are called the FAIR principles of effective learning (Hesketh & Laidlaw, 2002*b*).

A good facilitator of learning has certain knowledge, skills, attitudes and personal attributes that we shall identify here to improve your abilities as a facilitator of learning.

Domains of learning

Student learning takes place in three domains: cognitive; psychomotor; and affective (Bloom, 1956). The *cognitive domain* includes intellectual abilities and the learning of content knowledge. You, as a teacher, facilitate the acquisition of knowledge and assess students' ability to memorise facts, apply their learning to clinical situations and make judgements. The *psychomotor domain* encompasses the learning of motor skills such as physical movement and coordination (Gronlund, 1976). Development of these skills requires demonstration by teachers and time and opportunities for students to practise. Usually the psychomotor domain is assessed in terms of speed, precision and performance of procedures or techniques and is less central to psychiatry than to several other medical specialties. Learning of attitudes, feelings, values, appreciations, interests and modes of adjustment constitute the *affective domain* (Gronlund, 1976). Although the areas of learning under this domain can be taught, much of the time they are 'caught': the teaching of attitudes is often implicit as opposed to explicit, and the medical teacher acting as a role-model is particularly important in facilitating learning in this domain. The aspects of this domain are essentially assessed by whether the individual conforms to professional and societal norms, and appropriate attitudes in one culture may be inappropriate in another.

The domains of learning have important implications for assessment. If the examination at the end of the course comprises multiple-choice questions that can be answered by memorising facts, students will learn by rote. If the end-of-course assessment is an objective structured clinical examination, they will focus on learning relevant clinical skills (Malik *et al*, 1988). If it emphasises professional behaviours, as do workplace-based assessment tools such as multi-source feedback or the Professionalism Mini-Evaluation Exercise (PMEX) (Cruess *et al*, 2006), students will ensure that their behaviour is professionally appropriate.

Learning in each of these domains has a hierarchy; that is, it is 'taxonomically tiered'. The taxonomical levels in the cognitive domain will be described below, as they provide a useful framework for educational activities and have been used widely for decades. The taxonomic levels described for the psychomotor and affective domains, however, have been found to be less useful and are infrequently employed.

Levels of learning in the cognitive domain

Bloom (1956) introduced six hierarchical levels, commonly referred to as Bloom's taxonomy, in describing intellectual ability. The levels are recall, comprehension, application, analysis, synthesis and evaluation. The complexity of the thinking process increases across the six levels from recall to evaluation.

The level of your teaching in Bloom's taxonomy conveys a distinct educational message to students. If your teaching is set at the level of *recall* (e.g. 'list the symptoms of depression'), students are encouraged to memorise facts and data. If your teaching is focused on *comprehension*, you expect students to demonstrate their understanding of the meaning of what they have learned (e.g. 'explain the term "depression"'). If you encourage your students to use or apply their learning in new situations, contexts and clinical situations, your teaching and learning is focused at the level of *application* (e.g. relate the genetic basis to bipolar disorders). At the level of *analysis*, the students are expected to categorise, classify or separate the components of a concept (e.g. 'arrive at differential diagnoses of a patient presenting with sleep disturbance'). At the level of *synthesis*, they are expected to formulate a concept or recognise a pattern by assembling diverse elements (e.g. 'arrive at a diagnosis of patients who present with a particular set of symptoms and signs'). If you encourage your students to make argued or evidence-based judgements (e.g. 'decide a particular management plan for a particular patient'), your teaching is at the level of *evaluation.*

These levels need to be considered in your teaching, for example in formulating learning objectives for a course or a session, and can be used to analyse students' answers in written examinations. If the course objectives emphasise higher-order thinking and the examination tests factual recall, then there is a disparity between the teaching and the assessment.

Memorising facts is useful, indeed essential, in medicine, as factual knowledge is a prerequisite for effectively tackling clinical problems (Hager & Gonczi, 1996). However, 'in real professional practice, factual knowledge is mostly not a goal itself, but only a single aspect of solving professional problems' (Schuwrith & van der Vleuten, 2004). Therefore, a focus on the higher levels of Bloom's taxonomy, especially in the assessment of students, is recommended.

Students' approaches to learning

By observing students or reflecting upon your own learning, you may be able to recognise differences in the way that individuals approach their learning. Marton & Saljo (1976) identified three approaches: surface, deep and strategic. The learning approach of an individual is not a fixed personal attribute, but depends on the context and the subject, and may vary over time.

- Surface learners. Certain students like learning words and terms without bothering much about understanding meanings, interconnections, implications or concepts. Their primary intention is the achievement of a minimum standard (in terms of marks, grades or qualifications) for getting through courses, mostly by rote learning the 'most important items' (Biggs, 1987). Surface learning is motivated by external conse-quences, either positive (e.g. progressing through the course by passing examinations) or, more commonly, negative (e.g. dropping out by failing examinations), and not by intrinsic interest in the subject (Biggs, 1987). In the process of learning, surface learners restrict their learning largely to what might be asked in the examinations, in which they expect simply to repeat what they have learned, and they usually fail to distinguish principles from examples (Biggs, 1987).

- *Deep learners*. Other students attempt to understand or explore meaning, relationships, interconnections and concepts behind words and terms in the process of learning rather than memorising words or terms in isolation. These learners are using a 'deep' approach to learning, which is driven by their interest in or curiosity about the subject (Biggs, 1987). In contrast to surface learners, deep learners: interact with the content; read around the topic; use evidence, experience and prior learning to understand the new learning; and attempt to apply what is learned in everyday practice (Biggs, 1987).
- *Strategic learners*. The distinctive feature of strategic learners is that their motivation is to take the approach that delivers the maximum positive outcomes to themselves (Biggs, 1987). Therefore this approach to learning is also referred to as the 'achieving approach'. Strategic learners are not actually mutually exclusive from surface or deep learners. The motivation of strategic learners may be the achievement of the highest grade, as in the surface approach, but, like deep learners, they may be actively involved in the learning process in achieving their goal. In the process of learning, these learners: effectively manage time and effort; carefully select proper conditions and appropriate material for studying; and actively seek past questions and marking criteria before examinations (Biggs, 1987).

The choice of learning approach seems to be largely determined by time allocation, content load and assessments (Biggs, 1987). Time pressure and content overload can be related to either teachers or students, or both. For example, students who postpone studying might struggle with limited time and excessive amounts of work towards the end of the course. On the other hand, students may struggle against time if demands of the curriculum are exhaustive (curriculum overload). In both these situations, students tend to use a surface approach rather than a deep approach to learning. Assessments, however, are designed and conducted by teachers. As 'assessment drives learning' (Schuwrith & van der Vleuten, 2004), it could be regarded as the main determinant of the choice of learning approach. Examinations that assess higher-order thinking inevitably encourage students to choose a deep approach to learning. Where medical education is concerned, strategic learning inclined towards deep learning will result in both the desired intellectual involvement and the achievement of standards with regard to the learning outcomes.

Theories of learning

Learning is not a passive process but requires effort on the part of learners to actively construct meaning from what they are being taught. There are five main theories about how people learn:

1   The *behaviourists* focus on tasks to be learned (Phillips & Soltis, 1985). The basis of this theory is the stimulus–response model of conditioning and the benefits of rewards (Skinner, 1938). *Activity, repetition* and *reinforcement* are thought to help people learn.

2   The *neo-behaviourists* explain learning as a cognitive map, with one thing leading to another and a hierarchy of learning (Bednar *et al*, 1995). Application of learning is emphasised, with 'operant conditioning', where a learner completes a series of tasks. *Activity, repetition* and *motivation* are thought to be important.

3   The *gestaltists* believe that the *pattern* is important (Koffka, 1935; Wallace *et al*, 1998). Understanding is based on insight, the flash of inspiration when the pattern is recognised.

4   The *cognitivists* focus on mental processes. They believe learning takes place through the construction of personal schemes ('conceptual schemata') and that for new information to take its place in the scheme, reflection is necessary (Dewey, 1929). The learning process and learning by discovery are emphasised (Bruner, 1967). The use of advance organisers is advocated to bridge the gap between existing knowledge and what the students need to know (Ausubel, 1960). The advance organiser is somewhat similar to a signpost that points to the possible directions in which learning could go. Learning is seen as cyclical (Kolb & Fry, 1975), and a four-phase cycle for effective learning has been described:

    * concrete experience
    * reflective observation
    * abstract conceptualisation
    * active experimentation.

    Different learners will start at different places in this cycle and will rely more heavily on some phases of the cycle than others. This has led to the description of learning by *experiencing, reflecting, thinking* and *doing*.

5   The *humanists* believe that people have a propensity to learn and will learn when the conditions are appropriate (Rogers & Freiberg, 1994). They emphasise the education of the whole person, of everyone being helped to make the most of themselves. The importance of an environment where all students feel valued is highlighted. Learning as active self-discovery and active learning by doing (experiential learning) are emphasised. Positive emotions will facilitate learning and negative emotions such as stress and anxiety will inhibit it. *Relevance, choice, purposes, goals, anxiety* and *emotion* are seen as important.

Different people learn in different ways and it is not often possible to identify how individual undergraduate medical students learn. Nor is this necessary, as it is not usually possible to provide customised teaching for individual learning styles. Thus, as teachers, we need to cater for different learning styles and provide in our teaching a range of educational experiences that will suit different styles of learning. You can cater for different learning preferences by applying the FAIR principles (Hesketh & Laidlaw, 2002*b*).

Principles of effective learning: the FAIR principles

The FAIR principles for effective learning take key elements of different learning theories and put them together in an easily remembered model that you can use in many different teaching situations: feedback; activities; individualisation/interest; relevance. These principles will help you to provide experiences for your students that encourage 'deep' and more lasting learning than memorising or rote learning facts.

Feedback

Providing feedback to learners regarding their progress allows them to assess their knowledge or proficiency and to identify gaps or strengths; it motivates them to correct any deficiencies or weaknesses. Feedback should be constructive (Hesketh & Laidlaw, 2002*a*); it should be in the form of explanations of how to improve rather than simply telling students that they are poor or incorrect. Feedback should be timely and given immediately after the event, when the student is likely to be avid to learn: the longer the delay is, the less will be the student improvement. Feedback should be *criterion referenced*, that is, it should explain to the student where he or she is situated in relation to the required standard, rather than *norm referenced*, which tells the student where he or she is in relation to fellow students, but does not tell the student how to improve. It is important to remember that students can effectively provide some of their own feedback both for themselves and for their peers (Hesketh & Laidlaw, 2002*a*).

There are many methods of providing feedback. The fact that examination results provide feedback is often forgotten. In recent years there has been a trend to increase the use of formative assessment in medical education, with the specific intention of providing feedback to students on their progress. It should be remembered, however, that summative assessment (the end-of-course examinations, where pass/fail decisions about the students are taken) is also a source of feedback. One of the most successful developments in lecturing in recent years has been the use of audience response systems, which enable the lecturer to set quizzes for the students during delivery (Robertson, 2000). The lecturer is given feedback as to whether the students have understood the messages of the lecture and individual students are given feedback as to whether they have appropriately understood the messages. Workbooks that are submitted by the student for marking (Mires *et al*, 1998), face-to-face discussions with tutors and workplace-based assessment methods (such as multi-source feedback and patient satisfaction questionnaires) also provide students and trainees with feedback.

Activities

Activities encourage learners to engage in the learning process and to internalise their learning. Activities can shift the learning from a low level, such as factual recall and memorisation, to higher-order thinking. Activities can be designed to help learners: to understand the material they have to learn; to apply what they have learned to the clinical situation; and to develop critical thinking and clinical judgement. Activities may include: practical exercises; case studies that set a problem the student has to solve; group discussions about a clinical problem; 'buzz groups' in lectures; reading a relevant section of text; and reflecting on the application of what they are learning to their own practice or to patients seen in the wards or out-patient department.

Individualisation/interest

Sometimes it is possible to individualise learning for different groups of students or trainees (Harden & Laidlaw, 1992). Selection of pertinent examples, dealing with cases at an appropriate level for the group or setting the learning in the context in which the learners work may all help to individualise learning. Whether individualisation is possible or not, arousing the interest of learners is crucial for motivating them to learn (Harden & Laidlaw, 1992). The intrinsic interest of the content matter; the use of an especially fascinating case; and photographic illustrations or other media may all increase interest. Humour can sometimes be used successfully to increase interest and, at the same time, lighten the mood. Care is necessary, however, with the use of humour as it is important not to cause offence or trivialise the material to be learned.

Relevance

Learning will be much more successful if learners see the relevance of what has to be learned to themselves and to their goals (Harden & Laidlaw, 1992). Medical students will be much more engaged in learning psychiatry if they see its relevance to their future career pathway. Pointing out the relevance of learning about psychiatric disorders to those destined for a career in other specialties is an important strategy to encourage learning.

Role-modelling and the personal attributes of a good facilitator of learning

The teacher may have many different roles. Harden & Crosby (2000) have identified 12 roles of the doctor as a teacher. Some of us are teachers in clinical skills centres, wards or out-patient departments, while others may prefer to develop online learning materials for our students or involve ourselves with student assessment or curriculum evaluation. Whatever our teaching role, there are some personal qualities that seem to be important for the facilitation of learning, particularly with small groups of students (Schmidt & Moust, 1995; Harden *et al*, 1999). The ability to communicate with students in an informal way and the skills to express oneself in a language that students understand seem to be important. An empathic attitude and the ability to create an atmosphere in which the open exchange of ideas is facilitated seem to help, as does a willingness to become involved with students in an authentic way.

All those who teach act as role-models for students. A high level of professionalism, both as doctors and as teachers Is important for good role modelling, and we should ask ourselves what sort of example we are providing for our students whether in clinical practice or teaching practice.

As with clinical practice, a good teacher remains abreast of the evidence. BEME (Best Evidence Medical Education) is an organisation devoted to the provision of the best evidence for educational practice; BEME is to medical education what the Cochrane Collaboration is to medicine (Harden *et al*, 1999). From the BEME website (http://www2.warwick.ac.uk/fac/med/beme/) you will be able to access a number of meta-analyses of the literature that will help you decide what works in health professions' education.

Summary

An understanding of how students learn will enable teachers to facilitate their students' learning. It is not usually possible to plan learning for individual students' learning styles and the FAIR principles for effective learning provide a tool that all teachers can use in their teaching in order to facilitate student learning, whatever the student's individual learning style.

It may be possible to provide a wide range of educational opportunities for students and then allow them to select those that best suit their individual learning styles. Some students may find lectures helpful, while others may prefer independent study or study with a group of colleagues. The provision of a study guide that identifies the educational opportunities along with the outcomes of each session will help students to plan their learning to suit their learning preferences.

The professionalism of the individual teacher both as a specialist and as an educator is another area for consideration and the way that teachers interact with students may have a powerful effect on their learning, particularly in a small-group setting.

References

Ausubel, D. (1960) The use of advanced organisers in the learning and retention of meaningful verbal material. *Journal of Educational Psychology*, **51**, 267–272.

Bednar, A. K., Cunningham, D., Duffy, T. M., *et al* (1995) Theory into practice: how do we link? In *Instructional Technology: Past, Present and Future* (2nd edn) (ed. G. Anglin), pp. 100–111. Libraries Unlimited.

Biggs, J. (1987) *Student Approaches to Learning and Studying*. Australian Council for Educational Research.

Bloom, B. S. (1956) *Taxonomy of Educational Objectives: The Classification of Educational Goals*. David McKay.

Bruner, J. S. (1967) *On Knowing: Essays for the Left Hand*. Harvard University Press.

Cruess, R., McIlroy, J. H., Cruess, S., *et al* (2006) The Professionalism Mini-Evaluation Exercise: a preliminary investigation. *Academic Medicine*, **81**, s74–s78.

Dewey, J. (1929) *The Quest for Certainty*. Minton.

Entwistle, N. J. & Ramsden, P. (1982) *Understanding Student Learning*. Croom Helm.

Gronlund, N. E. (1976) *Reliability and Other Desired Characteristics: Measuring and Evaluating in Teaching*. Collier Macmillan.

Hager, P. & Gonczi, A. (1996) What is competence? *Medical Teacher*, **18**, 15–18.

Harden, R. M. & Crosby, J. (2000) AMEE Education Guide No. 20: The good teacher is more than a lecturer – the twelve roles of the teacher. *Medical Teacher*, **22**, 334–347.

Harden, R. M. & Laidlaw, J. M. (1992) Effective continuing education: the CRISIS criteria. *Medical Education*, **26**, 408–422.

Harden, R. M., Grant, J., Buckle, G., *et al* (1999) BEME Guide No. 1: Best Evidence Medical Education. *Medical Teacher*, **21**, 553–562.

Hesketh, E. A. & Laidlaw, J. M. (2002a) Developing teaching instinct: feedback. *Medical Teacher*, **24**, 245–248.

Hesketh, E. A. & Laidlaw, J. M. (2002b) Developing the teaching instinct: facilitating learning. *Medical Teacher*, **24**, 479–482.

Koffka, K. (1935) *Principles of Gestalt Psychology*. Harcourt, Brace.

Kolb, D. A. & Fry, R. (1975) Towards the applied theory of experimental learning. In *Theories of Group Process* (ed. L. Cooper), pp. 33–57. John Wiley.

Malik, S. L., Manchandra, S. K., Deepak, K. K., *et al* (1988) The attitudes of medical students to the objective structured practical examination. *Medical Education*, **22**, 40–46.

Marton, F. & Saljo, R. (1976) On qualitative differences in learning. *British Journal of Educational Psychology*, **46**, 4–11, 115–127.

Mires, G. J., Howie, P. W. & Harden, R. M. (1998) A 'topical' approach to planned teaching and using a topic-based study guide. *Medical Teacher*, **20**, 438–441.

Phillips, D. S. & Soltis, J. F. (1985) *Behaviourism in Perspectives in Learning*. Teachers College Press.

Robertson, L. J. (2000) Twelve tips for using a computerised interactive audience response system. *Medical Teacher*, **22**, 237–239.

Rogers, C. & Freiberg, H. J. (1994) *Freedom to Learn*. Macmillan.

Schmidt, H. G. & Moust, J. H. C. (1995) What makes a tutor effective? A structural-equations modelling approach to learning in problem-based curricula. *Academic Medicine*, **70**, 708–714.

Schuwrith, L. & van der Vleuten, C. E. M. (2004) Changing education, changing assessment, changing research? *Medical Education*, **38**, 805–812.

Skinner, B. F. (1938) *The Behaviour of Organisms*. D. Appleton-Century.

Wallace, D., West, S., Ware, A., *et al* (1998) The effect of knowledge maps that incorporate gestalt principles on learning. *Journal of Experimental Education*, **67**, 5–16.

CHAPTER 2

Recent developments in undergraduate medical education

Margery Davis & Madawa Chandratilake

Introduction

The curriculum is a dynamic process. A static curriculum is a sick curriculum (Abrahamson, 1996). The constant remodelling of the educational programme in response to educational developments, local needs and national policy is an ongoing necessity. In this chapter we shall look at five areas of undergraduate medical education where dramatic change has taken place in recent years – curriculum design, teaching and learning, student assessment, student selection and staff development – and we shall explore the reasons behind these changes.

Curriculum design

In this section we explain: (a) the introduction of newer educational strategies (developed in response to societal pressures and problems) within the undergraduate medical educational programme itself; (b) the recent move to outcome-based education; (c) how models of curriculum design have changed, adapted and developed over the past decades; and (d) how educational theory has influenced the structure of the undergraduate medical curriculum.

(a) Educational strategies

An educational strategy is the approach taken to teaching and learning in the curriculum. At the end of the Second World War, when the world had changed in so many ways, it seemed inappropriate to young doctors returning from the fighting to Case Western Reserve University in the USA that medical education should continue as before. They wanted to train better doctors and to train doctors better. The innovations produced by that group signalled the start of 'ROME' (World Health Organization, 1989), the Reorientation Of Medical Education, which spread throughout the world.

There were many different educational strategies involved in ROME and the SPICES model of educational strategies (Harden *et al*, 1984) was developed to classify them. SPICES is an acronym for: Student centred; Problem based; Integrated; Community based; Electives and core; and Systematic. These aspects of educational strategy will be described below.

Student centred

In a traditional curriculum, the teacher and the institution are the focus for the teaching and learning; formal lectures and laboratory sessions dominate delivery. Involvement of students in the educational process within this model is minimal, leading to somewhat passive learning. In contrast, in a student-centred approach, the focus is on the student. The emphasis is on what and how students learn. In this strategy, the active involvement of students in the learning process is expected and encouraged and the teacher's role is to facilitate learning. Small-group learning, simulated learning environments, study guides and virtual learning environments are some of the approaches used in the facilitation process. The adaptive curriculum (Davis & Karunathilake, 2004) is a highly sophisticated student-centred approach that allows quicker learners to fast track through the curriculum but also gives slower learners more time to achieve the required standard.

Problem based (see Chapter 9)

Students learn theories, concepts and principles in a traditional curriculum in what is called an 'information-gathering' approach, which may occur with minimal understanding of the relevance and utility of what they learn. In contrast, in problem-based learning (PBL), groups of students learn the underpinning theories, concepts and principles through examples. The problem is usually a written case scenario or a real-life situation encountered by professionals. Students are actively engaged in tackling the problem and, in doing so, learn about the related topics. Because they can see the relevance and understand the utility of what they are learning, the efficiency and effectiveness of the learning process are thought to be enhanced.

Integrated

In a traditional curriculum, the content is covered by individual disciplines as discrete entities at different times (e.g. anatomy in year 2, pharmacology in year 3 and psychiatry in year 4). This is therefore referred to as a discipline-based educational strategy. Some students may have difficulty integrating their learning from different disciplines at different times and applying it to patient care. In contrast, different disciplines can be brought together under themes and delivered at the same time in an integrated course. These themes could be based on organ systems (e.g. cardiovascular, respiratory, neurological), stages of the life cycle (e.g. birth, childhood, adolescence, adulthood, the elderly, death and dying), or clinical presentations or tasks (e.g. unconsciousness, abdominal pain, head ache) (Harden *et al*, 2000).

Community based

Students are taught in secondary or tertiary referral centres in the traditional curriculum, but this does not reflect the high proportion of medical students who identify general practice or other community-based specialties as their career of choice on graduation (Goldacre *et al*, 2004). Consequently, many medical schools have introduced community-based teaching and learning, to provide students with first-hand experience of: the work of the general practitioner; work in local health centres; the healthcare needs of local communities; how patients present in primary care; and the continuity and context of care in the community. Community-based teaching is one way of ensuring the community orientation of a curriculum.

Electives and core

In the traditional model, all students follow the same curriculum, but different students have different interests and career aspirations and so a better model would offer students different 'blends' of components of a curriculum (e.g. scientific knowledge, clinical skills, laboratory skills, research skills). The core curriculum with options was one of the most important notions introduced by *Tomorrow's Doctors* in 1993 to counteract curriculum overload and to cater for the individual interests and needs of students (General Medical Council, 1993). Study of the core is required for all students, but students can also select particular topics in the optional and elective parts of the course that they wish to study in more depth.

Systematic

Student learning in the clinical years of a traditional curriculum depends on the patients who are admitted to the wards or who present to the clinics. Thus the learning can be opportunistic and somewhat piecemeal. During their clinical attachments, students may not see essential clinical cases, leaving gaps in their knowledge, or they may encounter the same cases repeatedly, making their educational experience inefficient. These potential problems can be offset through the use of simulated patients (see Chapter 19). In creating a systematic course, the educational experience is made explicit and learning opportunities are arranged to meet the students' requirements. Identifying key clinical cases, setting up outcomes and objectives with communication of these to students, and the use of logbooks and study guides are some of the measures used to make the educational experience explicit. Learning opportunities are provided by means of clinical rotations, clinical skills centres and virtual learning environments.

Summary

The move away from traditional approaches towards newer educational strategies has been a feature of curriculum development in recent decades. Identification of the educational strategies to be employed in a curriculum is an important first step in the selection of appropriate teaching and learning methods. The educational strategies give the curriculum its flavour, or 'spice'. Each medical school is unique and the way that the 'spices' are blended contributes to the creation of a unique educational environment.

(b) Outcome-based medical education

Overload of the undergraduate medical curriculum in the UK was identified by Huxley in 1876 and continued unchecked, in spite of regular exhortations by the General Medical Council to reduce factual overload and allow time for the medical students to think (most recently General Medical Council, 1993). It became apparent that there was a need to focus the curriculum on the essence of being a doctor and the outcome-based education (OBE) movement in medicine was born (Harden *et al*, 1999). OBE enables educators to be explicit about what it is to be a doctor and to identify appropriate learning outcomes for medical education, thus reducing the amount of irrelevant material that had crept into undergraduate medical programmes and had contributed to curriculum overload. Educators focus on 12 'exit learning outcomes', which are classified into three groups (Harden *et al*, 1999):

- what doctors are able to do (e.g. clinical skills and practical procedures)
- how they should do it (e.g. with appropriate attitudes and ethical approaches)
- their professionalism (e.g. a commitment to lifelong learning).

The curriculum is then planned to ensure that students have achieved the exit learning outcomes by the time they graduate. There are many outcome models for different medical schools in different countries but they are based on the above three-circle model (activities, approach and professionalism). This model of curriculum design is transformationally different from the 'building block' approach of the past, when students went through a discipline-based curriculum process and were assumed to have achieved the outcomes by virtue of having passed discipline-based examinations. OBE emphasises product, not process. How the outcomes are achieved is less important than the demonstration of achievement of the outcomes by the end of the course. This shift from process to product is one of the most important recent developments in medical education.

(c) Models of curriculum design

There have been ongoing developments in the design of the undergraduate medical curriculum since the introduction of medical education into higher education. These developments were summarised by Papa & Harasym (1999) as:

- the apprenticeship model of the early 19th century and before
- the discipline-based approach of the early 20th century
- the move to systems-based teaching following the Second World War
- the advent of problem-based learning (PBL) in the late 1960s
- the most advanced of today's curricula, based on the complaints with which patients present.

Each model has its strengths and weaknesses and most medical schools have retained elements of previous models when introducing successive revisions.

The apprenticeship model

The apprenticeship model consisted of a period of training with an individual medical practitioner of the student's choosing. This doctor was the master of the apprentice. The student saw the patients his master treated and learned to practise medicine in the fashion of his master. This is an important model for learning the practice of medicine and it continues to be used today, particularly in the form of clinical rotations and postgraduate training. When it is the only model used, however, it is problematic, in that the quality of student learning depends on the master's resources, knowledge and expertise. It restricts the student's learning to what the master is able to offer. Basic science may not be emphasised if it is considered to have little clinical utility. The quality of the doctors produced by this system up to the 19th century was variable, as there was no assessment of the student's ability at the end of training.

The discipline-based curriculum

By the 20th century, basic medical education had moved into institutions of higher education. Each individual medical school identified a discipline-based curriculum that instructed the student what to study and an examination system tested the student's learning. Learning of basic sciences was emphasised and students were taught the hypothetico-deductive reasoning process to prepare them to tackle clinical problems. This was a strong model, in that standardisation of learning was introduced, at least within individual institutions, and there was some attempt to ensure the standard of graduates. Notwithstanding these strengths, disadvantages of the discipline-based model became apparent. There was usually a divide between the preclinical, basic and laboratory science disciplines and the clinical disciplines, with some students unable to integrate their learning across disciplines when dealing with patients. Sequencing learning to create a cohesive and coherent experience for students was difficult. Also, curriculum overload became rife as specialties struggled to teach all of their discipline and not just what was relevant for students at their specific stage of learning.

The systems-based curriculum

Case Western Reserve University introduced its organ-system based curriculum in the 1950s to help students to integrate their learning around the organ systems of the body. The systems-based curriculum sought to eliminate the preclinical/clinical divide and help students to construct a clinically relevant knowledge base. Curriculum overload was reduced by removing control of the curriculum from departments and placing it in the hands of 'system teaching' teams or a centralised curriculum committee. Integrated teaching, however, did not necessarily result in integrated learning and some students continued to have difficulty in making use of what they had learned to reach a differential diagnosis. Attention turned to cognitive psychology to resolve these issues and PBL was introduced in McMaster Medical School in the 1960s.

Problem-based learning (PBL) (see Chapter 9)

In PBL, groups of students working in a classroom study a clinical or basic science or a community scenario that requires elucidation. The approach involves group discussion, independent study and sufficient mastery of the study topic to explain it to fellow students. The approach has the following advantages:

- student learning takes place within a clinical scenario, which makes learning more understandable and clinically useful
- it is active and encourages a deep approach to learning
- it is fun
- the process mimics clinical reasoning.

By the 21st century, however, many medical schools moved away from the exclusive use of PBL to a hybrid model that utilised PBL as one of multiple teaching methods. The reasons for the move included the finding by Elstein *et al* (1978) that problem solving is unlikely to be a generic skill and that clinical diagnostic ability is heavily dependent on the development of knowledge specific to each clinical presentation. Studying chest pain in relation to angina, for example, does not necessarily help students to diagnose chest pain related to pulmonary embolism. There were other issues, too, that led to disenchantment with PBL and many medical schools moved towards a curriculum model based on clinical presentation as the best model yet to help students develop the knowledge base and cognitive processes of experts.

The curriculum model based on clinical presentation

This model was developed at the University of Calgary Faculty of Medicine in 1991. Student learning is focused on the complaints with which patients present. Students structure their learning around chest pain, wheezing, abdominal pain and so on. Approximately 120 clinical presentations have been found to be sufficient to cover what students need to learn (Mandin *et al*, 1995). A modification of the clinical presentation model is the task-based learning curriculum developed at the University of Dundee Centre for Medical Education (Harden *et al*, 2000), where theory and on-the-job experience are integrated through the use of a study guide. Task-based learning is particularly relevant in clinical rotations and postgraduate training, where the task is the clinical management of the 120 or so clinical presentations. Task-based learning is independent learning for the clinical situation. Students learn about the 12 exit learning outcomes in relation to each of the 120 or so tasks. It is too early to identify the disadvantages of the clinical presentation model or of task-based learning, but the latter has been described by Race (2000) as 'a very useful approach to integration of the medical curriculum and, not least, a time-efficient and cost-effective approach to developing highly relevant skills, attitudes and competence for the profession'.

Summary

As each new curriculum model is introduced, previous models usually do not simply disappear. Some or all of the five curriculum models may coexist within one institution, for example, with apprenticeship learning used particularly in postgraduate training, systems-based teaching in the early years of the undergraduate course and discipline-based teaching and learning in the clinical rotations. PBL may be used as a small-group teaching and learning method in places throughout the curriculum, with task-based learning employed in the clinical rotations for independent learning.

(d) Educational theory and the structure of the curriculum

Utilising learning theory in the design of the curriculum can benefit student learning. Some learning theorists (the behaviourists and neo-behaviourists) emphasise the importance of repetition (Phillips & Soltis, 1985), and several types of curricula include repetition in their structure. The iterative curriculum (Rittle-Johnson et al, 2001), where students repeatedly rotate round courses at increasing levels of sophistication, is a popular curriculum design (Fig. 2.1). The courses may be discipline based, system based, or based on aspects of the life cycle. The first iteration may deal with the basic sciences, the second with the pathological sciences and the third with clinical practice.

The constructivists believe that the construction of cognitive schemata (Dewey, 1929) is important for learning and that reactivation of these schemata will help new learning to take place in the scheme. The spiral curriculum (Dowding, 1985; Harden & Stamper, 1999) is a particularly sophisticated version of the iterative curriculum, as it also makes use of constructivism in its design. As well as the benefits of repetition, this curriculum design emphasises the reactivation of prior learning (conceptual schemata) and then building and elaborating on those conceptual schemata as new learning takes place (Fig. 2.2). Reactivation, building and elaboration distinguish the spiral from the iterative curriculum, where these features are not explicit or may indeed be absent.

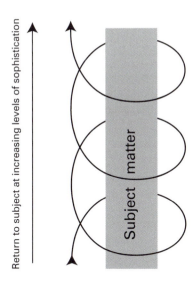

Fig. 2.1 The iterative curriculum: students repeatedly rotate round courses at increasing levels of sophistication.

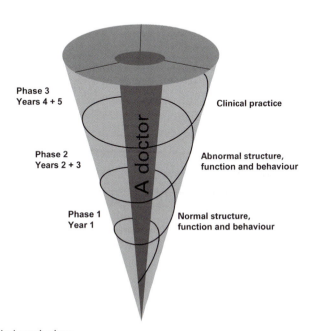

Fig. 2.2 The spiral curriculum.

Teaching and learning

The recent developments in teaching and learning in undergraduate medical education include:

- the early introduction to clinical practice
- the introduction of simulation
- the use of ambulatory care and general practice for student teaching
- an emphasis on reflective practice
- consideration of multi-professional or inter-professional learning.

These topics will be discussed in turn.

Early introduction of clinical practice

Early clinical contact is part of the strategy to integrate the curriculum and Schmidt *et al* (1996) showed that medical students who had studied integrated curricula developed better diagnostic competence than students from a traditional, discipline-based curriculum. There are two types of integration: horizontal and vertical. In horizontal integration, disciplines usually taught at the same curriculum stage are taught and learned together, for example maternal and child health or normal structure and function. In vertical integration, there is early clinical contact and continuation of basic science teaching into the later years of the undergraduate medical curriculum. Early clinical contact can motivate student learning of basic sciences and provide relevance for it. Basic science teaching in the later years of the curriculum may occur when, for example, reproductive physiology is taught within a course on assisted conception, when students are more likely to appreciate its relevance. Contact with patients with, for instance, neurological disorders when students are learning about the nervous system enables them to set their basic science study in the context of patients they have seen personally. Early clinical contact also enables students to begin the development of clinical and communication skills.

Introduction of simulation (see Chapter 19)

The UK government's emphasis on care in the community has resulted in patients spending less time in hospital. When patients are admitted to secondary and tertiary care hospitals they are often too ill to be able to see medical students and the short time they spend in hospital tends to be busy with investigations and treatment, leaving little time to interact with medical students. Attitudes, too, have changed and some patients may not wish to see medical students, let alone to be 'practised on' by them. For all these reasons, clinical skills centres have been introduced by most UK medical schools to provide a protected environment for students to master the technicalities of clinical and communication skills before encountering real patients in hospitals and community settings. Clinical skills centres may make use of plastic models or simulations, like those for teaching cardiopulmonary resuscitations. Simulated patients, such as volunteers from the local community, can be trained to give feedback to the students on their empathy or communication skills. 'Standardised' patients are real patients who volunteer for medical student teaching and are trained to give standardised histories or responses. The planned nature of the teaching in clinical skills centres enables staff to sequence the progression of learning in a way that is not often possible in the real world.

Use of ambulatory care and general practice

For the reasons identified above, the search for educational settings for student learning outwith the in-patient wards of teaching hospitals led to increased use of out-patient departments and community settings. Out-patient departments (often called ambulatory care settings) provide opportunities for students to interact with patients who are somewhat less ill than in-patients and to learn about ongoing care, although it may be less easy to learn about postoperative complications (Davis & Dent, 1994). Community settings provide opportunities to learn about:

- the patient experience of illness, as opposed to disease processes
- the challenges created by the social circumstances of patients
- medical conditions not usually seen in hospitals.

About 25% of medical students aspire to become general practitioners (Goldacre *et al*, 2004) and it seems appropriate, therefore, that at least some of their teaching should take place in health centres or general practice surgeries. The general practitioner has much to offer students in developing their consultation skills and the one-to-one relationship often provided between student and general practitioner trainer can bring benefits to student learning in terms of mentorship.

Emphasis on reflective practice

The need to keep up to date in medicine is accepted everywhere, and has led to a medical school emphasis on a commitment to lifelong learning. Identification of one's own learning needs is crucial for improving and updating practice, but ensuring that medical students systematically reflect on their own practice is an ongoing challenge. The work of Schon (1983) has identified two types of reflection: reflection *in* practice, the type of reflection that occurs during the patient consultation, for example, and leads the direction of the consultation; and reflection *on* practice, which occurs following a practice event and stimulates the identification of further learning needs. Tools to encourage reflection within practice include videotaping of consultations. Tools to encourage reflection on practice include consultation videos, logbooks and portfolios.

Multi-professional and inter-professional learning

Traditionally, healthcare professionals have been taught in separate schools for different careers. In the delivery of healthcare, however, doctors, nurses and the professions allied to medicine are expected to work together for the benefit of patients. Some of what each healthcare profession needs to learn has a common core and there has been interest in teaching this common core to multi-professional groups. While the economic advantages of multi-professional learning may be behind some of these innovations, if improved learning and improved collaborative working result, then multi-professional learning will be worthwhile. Inter-professional learning goes further than the teaching of multi-professional groups and involves the different professional groups learning from each other.

Multi-professional learning can be implemented using a range of teaching methods, including lectures, small-group seminars and sessions in clinical skills centres. Inter-professional learning is more difficult to implement, but simulated ward or theatre exercises, PBL or joint study of case scenarios may all be successful. At undergraduate level, timetabling is one of the main barriers to the implementation of multi-professional and inter-professional learning.

Student assessment (see Chapter 5)

Substantial changes to student assessment in recent years have been aimed at producing assessment systems tailored to curriculum needs. The need for accountability, patient safety and a greater educational understanding of measurement as a science has driven these changes, which have led in turn to the development of assessment systems and the burgeoning of new assessment tools at all levels of medical education.

The move from testing to assessment

The greatest change has been the move away from testing towards assessment. 'Assessment is undergoing a paradigm shift', suggested Gipps (1994), 'from psychometrics to a broader model of educational assessment, from a testing and examination culture to an assessment culture'. The assessment culture includes: establishing closer links between learning and assessment; using assessment to support learning, particularly through the provision of feedback; and extending assessment from the testing of factual knowledge to the assessment of all the outcomes of undergraduate medical education.

There has been a greater understanding of the ability of examinations to drive student learning (Wass *et al*, 2001; McLachlan, 2006), to the extent that assessment has been called 'the tail that wags the dog' (Lowry,

1993). 'A distinct advantage of introducing OSPE [the objective structured practical examination]', indicated Malik *et al* (1988), 'was in the change in students' learning behaviour'. If we assess clinical skills with the objective structured clinical examination (OSCE, as the OSPE is now more commonly known), students will make certain they attend clinical skills teaching and focus on learning clinical skills. We can go even further, by using the portfolio assessment process, which has been shown to improve student understanding of the outcomes of medical education (Davis *et al*, 2009), truly using assessment to support learning. The use of assessment for feedback purposes is also increasing, with the introduction of assessments for the sole purpose of providing feedback regarding progress (formative assessment). Summative assessment is the type of assessment from which pass/fail decisions are made, but there is also potential for this type of assessment to provide feedback to students. Profiling students in terms of their strengths and weaknesses is one way in which student feedback may be provided. Remedial courses or supplemental instruction may be provided to support students in the areas in which they have been found to have weaknesses.

Assessment systems

There is no single test or instrument that can assess everything necessary to enable us to decide whether someone is fit to become a doctor. The introduction of outcome-based education (OBE) has focused attention on assessment of outcomes and the need to assess not only what the doctor does, but also attitudes and professionalism. An assessment toolkit or an assessment system is required that comprises different assessment instruments and methods that together are capable of assessing all the outcomes. For example, single best-answer multiple-choice questions may be used to assess knowledge; the OSCE may be used to assess clinical and communication skills; workplace-based assessments (WPBAs) such as 360-degree assessment or multi-source feedback may be used to assess team working and attitudes; and the Professionalism Mini-Evaluation Exercise (PMEX) may be used to assess professionalism. It is only through utilising an assessment toolkit that all outcomes can be assessed.

The utility of assessment instruments

A greater understanding of the psychometric properties of assessment instruments and the realisation that the way that many traditional tests were used in medical education was incapable of providing trustworthy results (van der Vleuten, 1996) have led to greater interest in the utility of assessment instruments. In his utility formula, van der Vleuten (1996) has provided us with a tool to look at the utility of examinations or assessment instruments. We would express the utility formula as follows:

the utility of an examination = reliability × validity × practicability × acceptability × educational impact × cost-effectiveness

We have altered his formula to tease apart his original 'feasibility' into practicability (a measure of whether we can run the examination properly) and acceptability (to the stakeholders within our culture). Multipliers are used in the formula to emphasise that, if any component is zero, then the utility of the examination is zero.

Levels of assessment

George Miller was the founding father of medical education in the USA and in 1990 he advanced our thinking about assessment with the introduction of Miller's pyramid. He identified the need to assess medical students at four different levels: knowledge; its application; demonstration of ability in a simulated (examination) situation; and what the student does in real life (see also Fig. 16.2, p. 195). This pyramid can help us assemble our examiners' toolkit, since we have to include at least one assessment instrument for each level at which we need to test the medical students, although not all courses need to test their students at all four levels.

Student selection

Tests of academic achievement (examinations sat in secondary education such as A-levels and Scottish Highers) have been the mainstay of selection procedures for UK medical schools and remain the best predictor of success that we have available. High academic ability is necessary to cope with the study and practice of medicine. However, doctors removed from the UK medical register for misconduct suggest that a small number of medical students are graduating and practising with inappropriate attitudes and professional behaviours. Changing attitudes and the personal attributes that comprise professionalism, such as altruism, honesty and trustworthiness, is notoriously difficult (Stern, 2006) and so the trend is to try to avoid selecting those with inappropriate attitudes and unsuitable personal attributes for the study and practice of medicine. Selection processes thus had to be changed and this has led to the introduction of additional new tests for the selection of medical students. Aptitude tests such as the UKCAT (United Kingdom Clinical Aptitude Test), the UK equivalent of the long-standing Medical College Admission Test (MCAT) in the USA, have been introduced to assess cognition in areas such as problem solving, critical thinking, general intelligence and reflective ability (see http://www.ukcat.ac.uk). Combined personality and aptitude tests such as the Personal Qualities Assessment (PQA; Lumsden et al, 2005) have also been trialled to assess professionalism, communication skills, personal qualities (such as openness, conscientiousness, empathy, anxiety and lack of neuroticism) and areas such as ethical sensitivity, moral framework, teamwork and integrity. The challenge with these newly introduced tests is to establish their predictive validity (Ponnamperuma, 2008). It will take many years to follow up cohorts of applicants and find out whether the tests have appropriately identified those suitable for medicine.

Among the most promising of such new admission tests are the selection OSCE (Ponnamperuma, 2008) and the Multiple Mini Interview (MMI; Eva *et al*, 2004). In the selection OSCE, appropriate exit learning outcomes are used to design a series of OSCE stations, capable of providing reliable results. Examples of stations include role-play with a simulated friend with an ethical dilemma and numerous tests of communication skills and honesty (Ponnamperuma, 2008). While such selection OSCEs are capable of producing reliable results, their predictive validity will also take some time to establish.

Staff development

One of the greatest challenges facing medical schools is that of staff development for teaching. In the past it was assumed that gaining a medical qualification also equipped the doctor to teach. This assumption may have been unwarranted in some instances; education funders such as the Postgraduate Medical Education and Training Board, which have responsibility for postgraduate training and the teaching provided to undergraduate medical students by National Health Service doctors, and the Higher Education Funding Councils, which have responsibility for teaching provided to undergraduate medical students by university-employed staff, are driving a quality assurance agenda for the delivery of teaching. While universities can and do insist that new lecturing staff undertake some teacher training, the approach towards staff who may have been teaching for many years remains an issue. The Higher Education Academy (HEA) is the body set up for all those who teach in the higher education sector and it accredits training courses for university teachers. Such accredited courses give their graduates automatic entitlement to either associate or full membership of the HEA. It seems likely that the trend will be for all doctors who teach to have basic teacher training and for those who have a significant role in teaching or training to have a postgraduate certificate, diploma or master's degree in medical education.

Summary

We have identified five recent and not so recent developments in undergraduate medical education. These developments have had a fundamental impact on the learning experiences of our students and our roles as teachers and trainers. They affect what we do, how we do it, the professionalism with which we carry out teaching roles, the type of students that we teach and the educational environment in our medical schools. The intention is that the quality of the graduates of undergraduate medical education will improve through these developments, but clear proof of that will remain elusive until we can answer the question 'what is a good doctor?' and measure the quality of a doctor reliably and validly.

References

Abrahamson, S. (1996) *Essay on Medical Education.* University Press of America.

Davis, M. H. & Dent, J. A. (1994) Comparison of student learning in the outpatient clinic and ward round. *Medical Education,* **28,** 208–212.

Davis, M. H. & Karunathilake, I. (2004) The adaptive curriculum. *Medical Teacher,* **26,** 501–503.

Davis, M. H., Ponnamperuma, G. G. & Ker, J. S. (2009) Student perceptions of a portfolio assessment process. *Medical Education,* **43,** 89–98.

Dewey, J. (1929) *The Quest for Certainty.* Minton.

Dowding, T. (1985) The application of a spiral curriculum model to technical training curricula. *Educational Technology,* **33,** 18–28.

Elstein, A., Schulman, L. & Sprafka, S. (1978) *Medical Problem Solving: An Analysis of Clinical Reasoning.* Harvard University Press.

Eva, K. W., Rosenfeld, J., Reiter, H. I., *et al* (2004) An admissions OSCE: the multiple mini-interview. *Medical Education,* **38,** 314–326.

General Medical Council (1993) *Recommendations on Undergraduate Medical Education. Tomorrow's Doctors.* GMC.

Gipps, C. (1994) *Beyond testing.* Falmer.

Goldacre, M. J., Turner, G. & Lambert, T. W. (2004) Variation by medical school in career choices of UK graduates of 1999 and 2000. *Medical Education,* **38,** 249–258.

Harden, R. & Stamper, N. (1999) What is a spiral curriculum? *Medical Teacher,* **21,** 317–322.

Harden, R., Sowden, S. & Dunn, W. (1984) Some educational strategies in curriculum development: the SPICES model. *Medical Education,* **18,** 284–297.

Harden, R., Crosby, J. & Davis, M. H. (1999) An introduction to outcome based education. *Medical Teacher,* **21,** 7–14.

Harden, R. M., Crosby, J., Davis, M. H., *et al* (2000) Task-based learning: the answer to integration and problem-based learning in the clinical years. *Medical Education,* **34,** 391–397.

Lowry, S. (1993) *Medical Education,* pp. 25–26. BMJ Publishing Group.

Lumsden, M. A., Bore, M., Millar, K., *et al* (2005) Assessment of personal qualities in relation to admission to medical school. *Medical Education,* **39,** 258–265.

McLachlan, J. C. (2006) The relationship between assessment and learning. *Medical Education,* **40,** 716–717.

Malik, S. L., Manchandra, S. K., Deepak, K. K., *et al* (1988) The attitudes of medical students to the objective structured practical examination. *Medical Education,* **22,** 40–46.

Mandin, H., Harasym, P., Eagle, C., *et al* (1995) Developing a 'clinical presentation' curriculum at the University of Calgary. *Academic Medicine,* **70,** 186–193.

Miller, G. (1990) The assessment of clinical skills/competence/performance. *Academic Medicine,* **65,** S63–S67.

Papa, F. & Harasym, P. (1999) Medical curriculum reform in North America 1765 to the present: a cognitive perspective. *Academic Medicine,* **74,** 154–164.

Phillips, D. & Soltis, J. (1985) *Behaviourism in Perspectives in Learning*. Teachers College Press.

Ponnamperuma, G. G. (2008) Development, implementation and evaluation of a medical school selection test: the objective structured selection examination (OSSE). Unpublished PhD thesis, University of Dundee.

Race, P. (2000) Task-based learning. *Medical Education*, **34**, 335–336.

Rittle-Johnson, B., Siegler, R. S. & Alibali, M. W. (2001) Developing conceptual understanding and procedural skills in mathematics: an iterative process. *Journal of Educational Psychology*, **93**, 346–362.

Schmidt, H. G., Machiels-Bongaerts, M., Hermans, H., *et al* (1996) The development of diagnostic competence: comparison of a problem-based, an integrated, and a conventional medical curriculum. *Academic Medicine*, **71**, 658–664.

Schon, D. A. (1983) *The Reflective Practitioner: How Professionals Think in Action*. Temple Smith.

Stern, D. T. (2006) A framework for measuring professionalism. In *Measuring Medical Professionalism* (ed. D. T. Stern), pp. 3–13. Oxford University Press.

van der Vleuten, C. P. M. (1996) The assessment of professional competence: developments, research and practical implications. *Advances in Health Science Education*, **1**, 41–67.

Wass, V., van der Vleuten, C. E. M., Shatzer, J., *et al* (2001) Assessment of clinical competence. *Lancet*, **357**, 945–949.

World Health Organization (1989) *Rationale and Vision. Reorientation of Medical Education*. WHO.

CHAPTER 3

Undergraduate psychiatry teaching – the core curriculum

Stephen Cooper, Nisha Dogra, Brian Lunn & Barry Wright

Introduction

The word 'curriculum' derives from a Latin word meaning *a running,* and can be translated as a *contest in running*; the Latin *curro* means to run or hasten. Thus, there is the implication that a curriculum is to hasten individuals to a particular endpoint. Whereas a century ago some students may have taken a leisurely period of years to reach qualification, in this century there is a definite sense of purpose among teachers and students alike to reach the conclusion of the undergraduate medical course with the production of a well rounded medical graduate. It is important that the teaching in our medical schools assists this process, encourages the learning of relevant knowledge and clinical skills and encourages appropriate attitudes. A well-designed curriculum provides the framework upon which this may be achieved.

We should distinguish between syllabus and curriculum. In current educational taxonomy, the term syllabus relates to the content of what is taught on a particular course. The term curriculum has a wider meaning and encompasses not only course content but also methods of learning and assessment, as well as the organisation and integration of these. Often, however, the term is used more loosely. To some extent, therefore, the word curriculum could be applied to describe the entire content of this book.

A curriculum relating solely to the teaching of psychiatry to undergraduate medical students could also be seen as a contradiction in terms, as a true curriculum will integrate psychiatry with all the other medical disciplines to be mastered. However, this must be the province of each individual medical school, as the approach to integration within curricula depends very much on the ethos and resources available within each school.

Drivers of the development of medical school curricula (see also Chapter 2)

The development of more formal curricula in medical schools seems to have begun in the early 19th century. For example, the website of the University of Glasgow, in describing the history of the Glasgow medical school, states that:

In 1801, the University Senate appointed a committee to inquire into the existing regulations for medical degrees and the first definite curriculum was established in 1802. This required three years of medical study and evidence of attendance at courses in anatomy, surgery, chemistry, the theory and practice of medicine and botany. There were three examinations: on chemistry, materia medica, pharmacy and botany; on anatomy and physiology; and on the theory and practice of medicine. If these were passed successfully, the Latin papers on a medical case and an aphorism of Hippocrates followed. (From http://www.gla.ac.uk/faculties/medicine/history/19thcentury)

Histories of other medical schools established at the time suggest similar developments.

Another important driver in the development of medical education was the formation of the General Medical Council (GMC) by the Medical Act of 1858. The GMC was responsible to the Privy Council for establishing a register of qualified practitioners and defining their qualifications. This helped to drive medical schools to develop curricula that would lead their students towards the required standards. The four main functions of the GMC are: keeping an up-to-date register of qualified doctors; fostering good medical practice; dealing with doctors whose fitness to practise is in doubt; and promoting high standards of medical education. The last of these has been a particular focus over the past 20 years, and led to the publication of the first version of *Tomorrow's Doctors* in 1993 (GMC, 1993) and a revised version in 2003 (GMC, 2003). This was under review at the time of writing. The 2003 version stated that 'the core curriculum must set out the essential knowledge, skills and attitudes students must have by the time they graduate'. In order to maintain standards, the GMC also runs the Quality Assurance of Basic Medical Education Programme (QUABME), the main quality assurance programme for medical education in the UK.

In addition to the GMC, the Quality Assurance Agency for Higher Education (QAA; http://www.qaa.ac.uk) also reviews various aspects of all courses in institutions of higher education. The QAA was established in 1997 to safeguard quality and standards in higher education in the UK. The primary responsibility for academic standards and quality in UK higher education, though, rests with individual universities and colleges, each of which is autonomous. The QAA checks how well they meet their responsibilities, identifies good practice, makes recommendations for improvement and publishes guidelines to help institutions develop effective systems to ensure students have a high-quality experience.

While the focus for the GMC is particularly on the content of the curriculum, the focus for the QAA is mainly on the means by which institutions maintain academic standards, how these standards are set and how they are communicated to students. Assessment of this will, in part, involve review of the 'programme specification' for a course. A programme specification is a concise description of the intended learning outcomes from a higher-education programme, and how these outcomes can be achieved and demonstrated. Thus, for any course, the determination of learning outcomes and the description of how these will be assessed is seen as an important aspect of the curriculum. The QAA has published guidelines on the development of programme specifications (QAA, 2006).

Models of curriculum delivery

Leinster (2005) succinctly describes the full scope of what should be involved in curriculum planning, which he suggests should cover content, delivery, assessment, structure, resources and evaluation. Full discussion of all of these aspects is beyond the scope of this chapter, which is focused on the content of the psychiatry curriculum. However, some general recommendations are made in Appendices 7 and 8 of this chapter regarding delivery and assessment. Issues relating to the detail of delivery, assessment and resources are discussed in Chapters 2 and 5.

However, at this point it is perhaps worthwhile considering different models for the structure of a curriculum. Peyton & Peyton (1998) and Leinster (2005) give accounts of the main types employed: horizontal, vertical, spiral, web and core plus options. Taking the last two of these, the core plus options approach has become a part of all medical curricula over the past 15 years, although future GMC guidance is likely to reduce the proportion of time (currently 25–33%) to be spent on 'options' or 'student-selected components' (SSCs). Core plus options can be a useful approach in academic disciplines where the 'core' is relatively narrow. It may have less utility for medical curricula, where the core is considerable and where good integration of the many component parts is an important consideration. Thus, it needs to be used judiciously in medicine to ensure that core subjects receive sufficient attention. However, SSCs are an excellent way of enabling students to build upon particular areas of interest from the core curriculum or as opportunities to learn about specialist areas not included in the core curriculum (see Chapter 15).

In the web model (nothing to do with the worldwide web!) many subject areas are available for study simultaneously and it is up to the student to decide which to tackle and in what order to tackle them. This can be a good approach for more mature and well-motivated learners and in part reflects how some problem-based courses may operate. However, it requires considerable flexibility of the available teaching resources, something increasingly difficult in the complex relationships between medical schools and National Health Service trusts, and requires that students have a very clear idea of how best to organise the assimilation of a very large and complex body of information.

Most courses at medical school tend to be a mixture of horizontal, vertical and spiral models. In the horizontal model, links are established between different subjects being taught concurrently. This applies to the commonly employed 'systems based' approach to teaching basic sciences, such as anatomy, physiology and biochemistry. The vertical approach implies a curriculum where subjects studied sequentially have more tenuous links with each other but where each new area requires good knowledge of the previous one and in which there may be loose themes running throughout the course. The spiral approach (see Fig. 2.2, p. 17) involves elements of both of the above. Subjects will be taught concurrently, with integration of some clinical science with basic sciences, but with evolution towards increased complexity and a gradual shift from understanding normality to learning about abnormality.

As indicated in the Introduction to this chapter, we do not recommend any specific approach in relation to how psychiatry is integrated within the curriculum. It would seem reasonable that there should be some integration with other aspects of the overall curriculum, an issue discussed in the *Report of the Royal College of Psychiatrists' Scoping Group on Undergraduate Education in Psychiatry* (Royal College of Psychiatrists, 2009), but the precise model for this must be determined locally. It would also seem appropriate that SSCs on topics related to mental health are available for students with a particular interest.

Development of the College core curriculum

The development of this core curriculum was carried out by a subgroup within the Royal College of Psychiatrists' Scoping Group on Undergraduate Education in Psychiatry, which met during 2007 and 2008, the report from which is now available on the College website (Royal College of Psychiatrists, 2009). A draft version of this curriculum was written and discussed within the Scoping Group. It was also sent for consultation specifically to the educational leads for psychiatry in each medical school, to key academic general practitioners with expertise in teaching mental health issues and to key members of the Royal College of Psychiatrists. In addition, members of the College were invited to comment via the College e-bulletin. The core curriculum subgroup then integrated many of the comments received into the final version, which is reproduced in Appendices 1–6 of the present chapter. Unfortunately, funding was not available to allow any detailed consultation with service users, carers or medical students themselves.

In formulating this core curriculum, those involved recognised that there are variations between medical schools in the amount of time allocated to, and integration between, 'core' theoretical and clinical teaching within psychiatry (usually in the third or fourth year of the undergraduate programme) and what is taught on related topics, often in other years, such as psychology (including health psychology and neuropsychology), sociology, psychopharmacology and communication skills. Some schools have considerable 'vertical integration' of aspects of psychiatry throughout the curriculum but for others psychiatry appears mainly in one block.

The purpose of the proposed core curriculum is to outline the key aspects of knowledge, skills and attitudes related specifically to psychiatry that medical students require for basic competence and to meet the standards of *Tomorrow's Doctors*.

This will then form the basis for subsequent training through the foundation programme and into specialty training in whatever area. It is important to remember that undergraduate teaching is intended not just to produce foundation doctors but is also the basis for their future learning and clinical development. It is sometimes necessary to counter the argument that all they need to know is how to deal with the clinical challenges they may meet as F1 doctors. Students must also be taught to recognise that medical assessment of patients includes their entire health – physical and mental health and social functioning.

We must also be aware that high-quality teaching, relevant to the future needs of our students, is one of the most influential factors in promoting psychiatry as an exciting medical discipline. The core curriculum presented here is relevant to all doctors but should be supplemented by other components, such as SSCs, to meet the needs of those with a greater interest in psychiatry; support for appropriate electives and the development of undergraduate psychiatry societies can supplement these. The Royal College of Psychiatrists' website (http://www.rcpsych.ac.uk) provides further information that can be shared with students.

In constructing this curriculum for undergraduate psychiatry teaching we have followed the model of knowledge, skills and attitudes and have set these out in terms of learning outcomes. This approach derives originally from Bloom's taxonomy of educational objectives (Bloom, 1956) where he proposed classifying educational objectives into three principal domains: cognitive (knowledge and intellectual abilities), affective (attitudes and values) and psychomotor (motor skills). We acknowledge that the three areas are linked and that there may be overlap. However, in developing curricula it is helpful to think about the three domains to ensure comprehensive cover.

Thus, the final section of this chapter outlines the curriculum in terms of aims and objectives, objectives being described in terms of learning outcomes. Appendices 1–6 give greater detail regarding what might reasonably be included within the knowledge, skills and attitudes required; Appendices 7 and 8 provide brief statements regarding delivery and assessment of the curriculum, again with suggestions for what may be an ideal approach.

The College core curriculum

Overall aims

Specific to teaching in clinical psychiatry, the principal **aims** of the undergraduate medical course should be:

- to provide students with knowledge of the main psychiatric disorders, the principles underlying modern psychiatric theory, commonly used treatments and a basis on which to continue to develop this knowledge
- to assist students to develop the necessary skills to apply this knowledge in clinical situations
- to encourage students to develop the appropriate attitudes necessary to respond empathically to psychological distress in all medical settings.

Learning outcomes

There are three sets of learning outcomes, relating to knowledge, skills and attitudes.

Knowledge

On completion of undergraduate training the successful student will be able to:

- describe the prevalence and clinical presentation of common psychiatric conditions and how these may differ according to age and developmental stage
- summarise the major categories of psychiatric disorders, for example using ICD–10
- explain the biological, psychological and sociocultural factors which may predispose people to, precipitate or maintain psychiatric illness and describe multifactorial aetiology
- describe the current, common psychological and physical treatments for psychiatric conditions, including the indications for their use, their method of action and any unwanted effects
- state the doctor's duties and the patient's rights under the appropriate mental health legislation and mental capacity legislation
- describe what may constitute risk to self (suicide, self-harm, self-neglect, engaging in high-risk behaviour) and risk to and from others (including knowledge of the protection requirements relating to children, adults with intellectual disabilities and older people)
- describe how to assess and manage psychiatric emergencies, which may occur in psychiatric, general medical or other settings, and, in particular, be able to describe the elements of a risk assessment and the management of behavioural disturbance
- describe the basic range of services and professionals involved in the care of people with mental illness and the role of self-help, as well as service user and carer groups in providing support to them (as part of this students should be able to describe when psychiatrists should intervene and when other clinicians should retain responsibility).

Skills

On completion of the course the successful student will be able to:

- take a full psychiatric history, assess the mental state (including a cognitive assessment) and write up a case, which will include being able to describe symptoms and mental state features, aetiological factors, differential diagnoses, a plan of management and assessment of prognosis
- screen empathically for common mental health problems in non-psychiatric settings and recognise where medically unexplained physical symptoms may have psychological origins
- evaluate and describe patients presenting with abnormal fears/anxieties, pathological mood states and problematic, challenging or unusual behaviours
- summarise and present a psychiatric case in an organised and coherent way to another professional and be able to discuss management with doctors or other staff involved in a patient's care
- recognise the differences between mental health problems and the range of normal responses to stress and life events
- evaluate information about family relationships and their impact on an individual patient, which may involve gaining information from other sources
- assess patients' potential risks to themselves and others, at any stage of their illness, and in particular be able to assess a patient following an episode of self-harm
- evaluate the impact of psychiatric illness on individuals and families, and those around them
- find, appraise and apply information and evidence gained from in-depth reading relating to a specific clinical case
- discuss with patients and relatives the nature of their illness, management options and prognosis.

Attitudes

On completion of the course the successful student will be able to:

- utilise an empathic interviewing style, one that is suitable for eliciting information from disturbed and distressed patients
- recognise the importance of the development of a therapeutic relationship with patients, including the need for their active involvement in decisions about their care
- demonstrate sensitivity to the concerns of patients and their families about the stigmatisation of psychiatric illness
- recognise the importance of multidisciplinary teamwork in the field of mental illness in psychiatric, community and general medical settings, primary care settings and some non-medical settings
- demonstrate awareness of capacity, consent and confidentiality issues as they apply in psychiatry

- reflect on their own attitudes to patients with mental health problems and how these might influence their approach to such patients
- reflect on how working in mental health settings may affect their own health and that of colleagues.

Summary

In this chapter we have covered the purpose of a curriculum, models for delivery and how the psychiatric core curriculum has been developed. The College core can be adopted by individual medical schools as it is, although some adaptation may be required to suit local circumstances. It is key in any curriculum that there should be clarity about the main outcomes, methods of delivery and means of assessment for the educational experience to deliver on expectations, and the following Appendices set these out.

Appendices

These outline in more detail specific aspects of the knowledge and skills that are referred to above and also to wider areas of knowledge and skills that should ideally be taught across the curriculum.

Appendix 1. Brain function

This will include aspects of neuroanatomy, physiology and psychology:

- physiology of neuronal function
- mechanisms underlying attention, perception, executive function, memory and learning
- mechanisms relevant to the experience of emotion
- mechanisms related to psychological function
- human development and life cycle.

Appendix 2. Sociological issues

This will encompass:

- the meaning of 'illness' to individuals and society
- awareness that different models of illness – bio-psychosocial, multi-axial, medical, developmental and attributional – as they relate to mental health problems (and the competing claims made for each of the models promoted by various groups) are important to the understanding of psychiatric illness, its symptoms and associated behaviours
- ethics and the values that underpin core ethical principles
- the law and mental health and issues relating to 'capacity'

- relevance of family, culture and society and the individual's relationship with these
- the importance of life events
- stigma
- understanding of the public health importance of mental health nationally and internationally in terms of personal economic and social functioning, including a knowledge of prevalence, disability, chronicity, carer burden, cultural attitudes and differences, suicide and service provision.

Appendix 3. Psychiatric disorders and related topics

Knowledge of the following is a minimum:

- simple classification of psychiatric disorders
- anxiety disorders
- mood disorders
- psychosis (specifically schizophrenia)
- substance misuse, especially alcohol and cannabis (acute and chronic effects)
- delirium
- dementia
- somatoform disorders
- acute reactions to stress and post-traumatic stress disorder
- eating disorders
- disorders of personality
- effects of organic brain disease
- patients who harm themselves
- major disorders in childhood and differences in assessment
- differences in presentation in older people
- problems of those with intellectual disability
- comorbidity.

The degree to which a student may have clinical exposure to individual disorders will depend on the time allocated within the curriculum and the nature of the clinical experience available. It will not always be the case that exposure takes place in the setting of the psychiatric clinical attachment.

Appendix 4. Psychopharmacology

This will cover:

- function of the main neurotransmitter systems in the central nervous system
- basic neurochemical theories of depression, schizophrenia and dementia
- mechanism of action and clinical pharmacology of commonly used psychotropic drugs – anxiolytics, antidepressants, antipsychotics, mood stabilisers, drugs for dementia

- mechanism of action of common psychoactive drugs used recreationally, such as alcohol, cannabis and stimulants.

Appendix 5. Psychological treatments

Students should have an understanding of:

- the principles of psychological management of common psychiatric disorders, especially those that are likely to be seen in primary care, such as depression and anxiety
- cognitive–behavioural therapy, counselling and motivational interviewing
- the importance of lifestyle on mental health and its impact on treatments, for example factors such as sleep hygiene, nutrition, social interaction, physical activity, education, occupation and family and community involvement.

Appendix 6. Communication skills

The following aspects of interview skills are important:

- active listening
- empathic communication and building rapport
- understanding non-verbal communication
- skills in opening, containing and closing an interview.

These skills are often difficult for undergraduate students to attain fully. Observation and feedback on assessments is recommended.

Appendix 7. Delivery of the curriculum

Delivery of the curriculum will depend on local resources, support and history and should involve a variety of teaching methods. During the clinical attachment it is important to ensure that contact time with consultants is effectively used, as sometimes there may be very little of this. It is also important that consultant psychiatrists are a visible component of the student experience. Students need any teaching to be made relevant to practice (Dogra, 2004) and there are benefits from seeing senior clinicians interested in their educational experience (especially for recruitment to psychiatry). Attention needs to be paid to consideration of which learning outcomes are expected to be achieved in different parts of the attachment. It is important to note that observation (where used as a learning experience) is of little value without adequate follow-up. A ward round or clinic in which observation alone is used is unlikely to help meet the learning outcomes outlined. Teaching should, where possible and appropriate, be delivered in the clinical settings where patients present and include professionals involved in their care.

Appendix 8. Assessment

'Assessment drives learning' is a frequently quoted aphorism. It should also be recognised that assessment confers value to a course. For psychiatry to receive recognition as a valuable element of undergraduate medicine, assessment has to be robust and be an element of the overall terminal assessment of the undergraduate medical course.

Two elements are key to the assessment of undergraduate students in psychiatry:

- *Formative assessment* provides information for students about where they are in their learning process and what they need to do to reach their learning objectives. Ideally, students should be directly observed interviewing patients and feedback should be given on their clinical skills. Additionally, through case presentations, students' progress in attaining the required knowledge outcomes can be assessed. Further, by employing a continuing process of assessment, attitudes can be assessed and, if required, challenged.
- *Summative assessment* needs to be related directly to the specified learning outcomes for each medical school's course. It should be at the end-point of a student's learning in psychiatry. Each assessment should include components that address knowledge, skills and attitudes. For each of these areas, differing assessment methods are indicated and assessors need to be clear about what objectives they are assessing in each component.

Clinical skills may be assessed using real patients or role-players in a variety of objectively driven examination formats. It is important that the complexity of the cases is appropriate for the students' level of experience. Direct observation of students is the best means to assess clinical skills. The use of clinical cases for students at the end of their courses should allow them to demonstrate higher-level skills, such as synthesis of multiple sources and types of information and clinical application of knowledge.

References

Bloom, B. (1956) *Taxonomy of Educational Objectives: The Classification of Educational Goals, Handbook One: Cognitive Domain.* McKay.

Dogra, N. (2004) *The Learning and Teaching of Cultural Diversity in Undergraduate Medical Education in the UK.* Doctoral thesis, University of Leicester.

General Medical Council (1993) *Tomorrow's Doctors* (1st edn). GMC.

General Medical Council (2003) *Tomorrow's Doctors* (2nd edn). GMC.

Leinster, S. (2005) The undergraduate curriculum. In *A Practical Guide for Medical Teachers* (2nd edn) (eds J. A. Dent & R. M. Harden), pp. 19–27. Elsevier/Churchill Livingstone.

Peyton, L. & Peyton, R. (1998) Curriculum and course development. In *Teaching and Learning in Medical Practice* (ed. J. W. R. Peyton), pp. 14–39. Manticore.

Quality Assurance Agency for Higher Education (2006) *Guidelines for preparing programme specifications*. QAA. Available at http://www.qaa.ac.uk/academicinfrastructure/ programSpec/default.asp

Royal College of Psychiatrists (2009) *Report of the Royal College of Psychiatrists' Scoping Group on Undergraduate Education in Psychiatry*. Available at http://www.rcpsych.ac.uk/ pdf/Final%20Education%20in%20Psychiatry%20Scoping%20group%20report%20 May%202009.pdf

CHAPTER 4

The organisation of undergraduate teaching

Lindsay Thomson & Subodh Dave

Introduction

The organisation of undergraduate teaching is the province of individual universities, but since the publication of *Tomorrow's Doctors* in 1993 (General Medical Council, 1993, with subsequent editions in 2003 and 2009), the emphasis has shifted from the acquisition of factual knowledge to that of relevant attitudes and skills, with a core curriculum and self-directed learning. Clear roles were defined and guidance issued for all the key players, including universities, National Health Service (NHS) trusts, individual trainers and medical students. This has led to a broad redesign in many universities, with 'vertical' themes (see Chapter 2) running throughout the course and the development of new methods of assessment to reflect the new emphasis in training.

Concurrently, there has been a major change in psychiatric practice. Community-based care has become the norm and the creation of specialist services such as crisis teams has led to a significant reduction in psychiatric in-patient facilities, where, traditionally, most of undergraduate medical education was delivered (see Chapter 15 for a medical student view of some of the problems this can create). The problem has been compounded by the significant increase in the number of medical students (Department of Health, 2004). In some parts of the UK, it is now not unusual to see 12 students posted on an in-patient unit with 30 beds, jostling for precious patient contact with nursing and occupational therapy students, while other universities send their students over a large geographical area to find suitable placements .

Change has also occurred within the universities. The research assessment exercise, which dictates the academic standing and funding of universities and departments, has placed a major emphasis on the production of high-quality research papers. At times, this has led to the withdrawal from teaching of those extremely well placed to carry it out. Financial pressures in the NHS have also led to a reduction in the number of clinical academic posts (House of Commons Health Select Committee, 2006). Universities are also expected to demonstrate robust educational governance, with greater accountability in their educational spending (NHS Executive, 1995). Some universities (e.g. Edinburgh) have made an attempt to redress the imbalance between the emphasis on research as opposed to teaching by the creation of specific organisations or structures to deliver medical teaching; some (e.g. Liverpool, Manchester and Glasgow) have chosen to implement problem-based learning (PBL) to deliver most of their curriculum, while others (e.g. Cardiff and Nottingham) have incorporated PBL only within some specific modules.

Most universities have moved away from reliance solely on didactic teaching to more interactive methods of teaching and the organisation of teaching has evolved to reflect this. There has also been a greater awareness of the importance of NHS institutions in structuring and delivering medical student education. However, this does require closer collaboration between universities and the NHS, with a transparent quality assurance structure to ensure accountability of educational funding (Dave *et al*, 2010). Examples of excellent practice in this area reveal joined-up working between the NHS and universities, with clear academic leadership, a well-defined position within the university hierarchy and structures, and apprenticeship training in consultant-led psychiatric teams. NHS Education in Scotland is a good example of this joined up process (Eagles, 2005). Considerable sums of money are given by government to the NHS for undergraduate teaching through the service increment for teaching (SIFT, in England and Wales) or Additional Costs of Teaching (ACT, in Scotland). Universities collect data on quality of teaching but do not control the finance. It is important that money follows good teaching, with a clearly defined chain of responsibility and an educational governance structure (see Chapter 22).

However, it is not only the structures delivering teaching that need to change. The advent of evidence-based medicine (Sackett, 1996) and advances in technology have significantly changed the content and method of delivery of medical education. On the one hand, students are exposed to highly technical displays of science in some branches of medicine. This can reinforce the impression of psychiatry not being a scientific subject (Neilsen & Eaton, 1981). On the other hand, the sheer volume of knowledge, attitudes and skills to be taught in the medical school makes pruning the curriculum a necessity. This inevitably places pressure on psychiatry, large parts of which may be perceived as being 'desirable but not essential' learning.

The General Medical Council (GMC) does not provide a standardised national curriculum but does provide guidelines on the core competencies. Unfortunately, most of them relate to non-psychiatric skills, such as the ability to perform a venepuncture. The Royal College of Psychiatrists provides a curriculum for postgraduate training but none for undergraduate medical students, although its Scoping Group on Undergraduate Medical Education has produced a core curriculum theme (see Chapter 3). Similar guide curricula have been produced by the World Psychiatric Association

(Walton & Gelder, 1999) and individuals such as Thornhill & Tong (2006), Crisp (1994) and Nasser (1996). Yet others have explored the impact on student learning and attitudes of teaching undergraduate psychiatry in primary care (Walters *et al*, 2007) and the effect of 'bashing' medical specialties (Holmes *et al*, 2008). This latter phenomenon is not exclusive to psychiatry but does impinge on its perception by medical students. The issue of psychiatry education research as a new field is addressed by Hodges (2008).

The main aim of undergraduate teaching in psychiatry is to equip future doctors with the knowledge, skills and competencies to assess and manage mental disorders to a standard appropriate to foundation year 1. However, an equally important aim is to recruit future psychiatrists (see Chapter 20). Psychiatry is in crisis in terms of its recruitment, with only 6% of candidates for a recent Part I examination for membership of the Royal College of Psychiatrists being UK trainees (Royal College of Psychiatrists, 2009a). Goldacre *et al* (2005) studied career choices for psychiatry in national surveys of students who graduated between 1974 and 2000 from UK medical schools. There were over 21 000 doctors involved and a 75% response rate. Three factors in particular were found to influence career choice: experience of the subject; the doctors' personal assessment of their own aptitudes and skills; and working conditions. There was little change between 1974 and 2000 in the 4.9% of doctors who chose psychiatry 1–3 years after qualification but there was significant variation by medical school, from 7.2% of graduates from the University of Edinburgh to 3.2% from Imperial College London. Experience of the subject, identified as a key indicator by Goldacre *et al*, reflected more students' experience of the placement than 'sweeping curricular changes' (Kelly *et al*, 1991), suggesting that the impact of *Tomorrow's Doctors* is likely to be limited unless we address the organisation of teaching. This is of particular relevance, as a recent survey by Karim *et al* (2009) of the structure and delivery of teaching in 35 medical schools across the UK and Ireland showed significant variations in the organisation of psychiatric teaching. Wilson & Eagles (2008) reported the findings of a similar survey carried out by the Scottish Divisional Undergraduate Student Teaching and Recruitment Group (S-DUSTARG) of the Royal College of Psychiatrists; they found significant variation in the length of training and course content, as well as in course structure and methods of delivery. Such variations, alongside the variable rates of recruitment into psychiatry, suggest that altering the organisation of undergraduate teaching in psychiatry may influence later recruitment. A recent survey of clinical teachers in psychiatry identified improved organisation of teaching as the most frequently cited solution to improving clinical teaching in undergraduate psychiatry (Dogra *et al*, 2008). In this chapter, we examine the organisation of psychiatry teaching in British universities and provide recommendations for future improvements in the structure and delivery of undergraduate psychiatric teaching.

Course structure

Length of placement

The timing and length of the course have been shown to affect end-of-placement performance on standardised examinations (Case *et al*, 1997). The length of psychiatry placements in British universities varies from 4 to 11 weeks. Internationally, even shorter rotations (as short as 2 weeks) have been reported (Case *et al*, 1997). While it is clear that the quality of teaching is more important than quantity (Singh *et al*, 1998), it is difficult to achieve the learning objectives of psychiatry in a brief placement, especially as there is little likelihood of medical students acquiring psychiatry-related knowledge or skills in previous placements. There is some evidence that shorter placements are more likely to provide knowledge-related competencies than skills-related competencies or appropriate attitudes (Rosenthal *et al*, 2005). The Association of Directors of Medical Student Education in Psychiatry (2006), recognising the time required to teach complex skills of psychiatric assessment and diagnosis and the need to teach these skills to medical students in view of the general burden of psychiatric illness in society, especially in primary care, has advocated a minimum placement of 8 weeks. This is actually the average length of placements in British medical schools.

Timing of placement

Traditionally, undergraduate medical training has been structured longitudinally along preclinical and clinical tracks, with psychiatric teaching usually in the clinical years (3–5) of the undergraduate course. Newer medical schools, however, especially those following a PBL curriculum, tend to have much greater vertical integration, with blurring or in some cases even obliteration of the preclinical–clinical divide. Integration was first suggested some decades ago (Rezler, 1974). It improves students' attitudes to psychiatry and their confidence in dealing with psychological disorders in medical settings (Williams *et al*, 1997). Nevertheless, despite some form of integration now being seen in nearly half of UK medical schools, a significant minority remain unhappy with the level of integration with other branches of medicine (Karim *et al*, 2009). The high rates of recruitment in Edinburgh have been linked to the presence of an introductory 10-week basic year 3 course, comprising lectures and tutorials, aimed at exposing students to major mental disorder and giving them the opportunity to learn to take a psychiatric history and to carry out a mental state examination *before* their 6-week clinical placements in year 4 (comprising 4 weeks in general adult psychiatry and 2 weeks in a subspecialty). Even relatively brief exposure to subspecialties has been shown to stimulate career interest (Thomson *et al*, 1999).

While integration is generally lauded, it is difficult to implement, especially between clinical specialties (Oakley & Oyebode, 2008). A quarter of the medical schools in the UK have some joint neurology–psychiatry teaching, although, worryingly, psychiatrists were keener than neurologists to establish such links (Schon *et al*, 2006). The model of integrating primary care experience during a psychiatry placement suggested by Walters *et al* (2007) led to improvements in attitudes towards mental illness and a better understanding of patients' and general practitioners' perspective – a crucial learning objective considering that the majority of mental illnesses are likely to present in primary care (Goldberg & Huxley, 1992).

Course content

Historically, course curricula have been based on listing subject topics in a detailed syllabus. The broad principles of *Tomorrow's Doctors* have been adopted in the design of the course curriculum but these are meant to influence medical education in general rather than psychiatric education specifically. As a result, despite some similarities, large differences remain between the curricula of the universities (Table 4.1), as shown by Wilson & Eagles (2008). From a medical education perspective, it is vital that the curriculum reflects not what students should be taught but what they should learn (Harden, 1986), a subtle but important distinction often ignored by curriculum designers. From this perspective, it is clear that an identical curriculum cannot meet the learning needs of different cohorts of students.

Most medical schools have a defined 'core curriculum' around which the teaching is structured. Karim *et al* (2009) found that most British universities cover core subjects such as history taking, mental state examination, risk assessment and 'common mental disorders', including schizophrenia and mood disorders. Variation was seen in the inclusion of subspecialties such as child psychiatry or less common conditions such as psychosexual disorders, which were not included in the psychiatric curriculum in nearly 25% of the medical schools. Curriculum planners have to make hard choices in deciding what to leave out, as more and more subjects compete for limited curricular space and skills and attitudes objectives make the older knowledge objectives less applicable.

Many medical schools have adopted a curriculum based around a set of core competencies, in line with the revised curriculum for postgraduate training in psychiatry (Royal College of Psychiatrists, 2009b). When applied appropriately, a competency-based curriculum can improve flexibility and accountability of learning but can encourage a downward drift to minimum learning standards and professional demotivation (Leung, 2002). Students are usually not involved in designing the curriculum (Oakley & Oyebode, 2008) and the expectations of general physicians of a psychiatry curriculum may differ from those of psychiatrists (Wilson *et al*, 2007). It is, therefore, important to have the input of key stakeholders, including students, primary

Table 4.1 Similarities and differences in university undergraduate curricula

Similarities	Differences
Adoption of the GMC's *Tomorrow's Doctors* principles	Educational approach
Defined syllabus	Length of exposure
Clinical attachments	Assessments
	Varying vertical themes

care and general hospital physicians, along with service users and carers, in designing the curriculum. This ensures that there is widespread ownership of it. Underpinning the curriculum with prioritised learning objectives, embedding those objectives in the practical clinical world and mapping the psychiatric curriculum beyond the psychiatry placement to the entire medical curriculum seems to be broadly acceptable and effective (Brodkey *et al*, 2006) and can offer a model or otherwise guide curriculum development.

Teaching staff

Increasingly, there is greater involvement of non-medical NHS staff such as nurses and psychologists in psychiatric teaching in medical schools (Karim *et al*, 2009), which promotes interprofessional learning, a key objective in *Tomorrow's Doctors*. However, the bulk of formal psychiatric teaching in medical schools is carried out by NHS psychiatrists and clinical academic staff. There is a general perception that teaching is poorly supported by research-heavy academic departments and in general has a poor profile and low status. Clinical psychiatrists interested in teaching find themselves battling for protected teaching time in their job plans (Dogra *et al*, 2008). Delivering good-quality education requires quality teaching staff skilled in medical education, with the ability not merely to deliver but also to design, coordinate and assess psychiatric teaching. This is a task that requires defined ownership and dedicated time. Traditionally, it has been the role of clinical academics. Some centres have reported positive results by creating new posts, termed academic psychiatrists or clinical teaching fellows in psychiatry, with a dedicated medical education job portfolio (Dave *et al*, 2010).

The course lead needs to provide clinical educational leadership and to liaise with all the key stakeholders, including the university hierarchy, the teaching leads at different placement sites, the clinical teaching staff, the placement consultants and, above all, the students. A good understanding of medical education is vital and formal qualification in clinical education is desirable. The lead tutor at each site needs to have a similar understanding of educational issues, including the core curriculum objectives, and should be able to communicate these to the placement consultants.

Health Service policy (Department of Health, 2001) emphasises the importance of involving service users and carers in the planning and delivery of mental healthcare, and patients are increasingly involved in teaching (see Chapter 12), but, to our knowledge, there are no users of psychiatric services employed as teaching staff in any medical school, although they are playing an increasing role in delivering and designing teaching, for example in Aberdeen, Derby and Birmingham. Simulated or standardised patients can also bring the experience of service users to the fore. Most universities use simulated patients for assessment in objective structured clinical examinations (OSCEs) but their use in teaching is limited (for an exception see Chapter 19).

The more recent edition of *Tomorrow's Doctors* (General Medical Council, 2003) explicitly recommends training in teaching for all those involved in it. All teaching staff, including patients, carers and simulated patients, need training in teaching and must be fully aware and signed up to the core curriculum. After the initial training, teaching must be regularly monitored and reviewed through staff appraisals, student feedback and peer review. Appropriate supervisory structures need to be in place, with clear lines of management within an educational governance framework to support teaching staff and to maintain accountability.

Behind every successful undergraduate course lies a competent under-graduate administrator. Although not directly involved in teaching, the administrator plays a crucial role in liaising with students, teachers and placement consultants, running the placement and teaching timetables, organising examinations and, most importantly, anticipating and dealing with problems from students or consultants.

Teaching methods

Lectures

It is clear that despite advances in e-learning (Hare, 2009; see also Chapter 6) and a culture of self-directed learning, lectures and the clinical placement remain the universally employed methods of teaching in British universities (Karim *et al*, 2009). Large-group lectures are being replaced with more interactive and less didactic methods of teaching, but they remain a cost-effective method of introducing a topic and of providing a structure to material being learnt elsewhere. Audience response systems can add more interactivity, as they allow ongoing assessment and feedback, while the use of multimedia, including commercial film clips, makes lectures more engaging. Purely knowledge-based lectures can quite successfully be delivered as web-lectures or as audio or video podcasts (Agrawal, 2007).

Small-group teaching

This is a very common method of teaching, in both clinical and non-clinical environments, and includes tutorials, seminars and case discussions. It is covered in detail in Chapter 8. Usually involving 6–10 participants, small-group teaching is an effective format that supports active learning but it is resource intensive and highly dependent on the quality of the presenter/facilitator. PBL is a specific type of small-group teaching, one that emphasises self-directed learning. Role-play is especially useful for teaching skills and attitudes but requires a confident facilitator to engage and involve the students, who are often hesitant to role-play. Clear instructions to the role-players with brief pre-role coaching, explanation of the learning objectives and nomination of an observer with a task or a checklist enhances the educational effectiveness of role-plays.

Teaching in clinical settings

For most students, teaching in ward rounds or out-patient clinics forms the bulk of their teaching. However, crowded ward rounds and busy out-patient clinics do not make for good learning environments without some prior preparation. Booking lighter clinics or creating longer time slots for each patient allows for extra teaching time. Providing students with specific tasks (observing mental state examination, noting examples of reflective statements or questions related to mood assessment, etc.) encourages active rather than passive learning. Similarly, on in-patient units, it is better to assign an individual student responsibility for one or two patients. The student can then be tasked with summarising case notes, taking a detailed history and conducting a mental state examination, interviewing carers, interviewing the named nurse, care coordinator and occupational therapist, and so on. Assigning such responsibility has been found to encourage in-depth learning (Scher *et al*, 1988) and allows for an appreciation of the different perspectives patients, carers, psychiatrists and other professionals may have on mental illness and its management. The student can then have an active role on ward rounds in presenting the mental state, discussing differential diagnosis or presenting the carer's viewpoint, for example.

Dispersed care in the community has meant that in-patients are fewer in number and more likely to be too ill to participate in the teaching of medical students. Furthermore, for many students a chaotic acute in-patient unit may appear intimidating and present a negative image of psychiatry. Establishing a bank of trained volunteer patients can provide a safe and contained environment for medical students to acquire the basic skills of history taking, mental state examination and establishing a therapeutic relationship. In our experience, medical students particularly value the feedback they receive from volunteer patients. Similar patient-centred teaching clinics can be set up in in-patient units with carefully identified patients willing to volunteer to help medical students. Trainee psychiatrists can be a useful resource in delivering these (see Chapter 10) but the effectiveness of such clinics can be maximised if the learning objectives are to do with relatively discrete tasks, such as eliciting delusions or assessing mood.

Teaching in the community setting can provide a good model for patient-centred collaborative learning (Valsraj & Lygo-Baker, 2006) but, again, this does need preparation, with prior involvement of other professionals such as community psychiatric nurses and social workers. Working in multiple settings can be disorientating and may convey to some students a feeling of chaos, which may appear very different to the relatively contained environments of general hospital medicine. Each placement must develop a weekly timetable and a list of activities to be completed, which fits in with the overall aims and objectives of the course. This must take into account the likely clinical exposure in each placement, particularly where the placement is with a highly specialised team, such as assertive outreach or early intervention. An induction session orienting students to local services and placing them in the context of national practice is useful to provide students with an overview of the structure and function of mental health services.

Teaching materials

Most universities have a study guide setting out the aims and learning objectives of the course, relevant timetables, a checklist of tasks to be completed, and information on methods of assessment and feedback. Others have a course workbook with sections on core cases, resources and course materials, history taking, the logbook, lecture notes and a glossary of terms, as well as notes for clinical teachers. Most schools have a web-based course management system such Web-CT or NLE (National Learning Environment) that provides access to all study guides, workbooks and lecture notes. It is important for course organisers to be familiar with these systems and able to use them effectively to further the key learning objectives.

Teaching resources vary but should include access to teaching videos or DVDs, the ability to make a video of a patient interview, computerised assessment learning packages (Hare *et al*, 2007) and use of simulated patients or actors.

Assessment

Timing and setting

The major difference in assessments is whether they are part of a wider assessment with other subjects or whether psychiatry is assessed separately. Arguments are made that the integration of psychiatry into medicine is helped by cumulative assessments and sharing knowledge. Learning, however, is improved by examining at the end of a course rather than many months or even years later, and this may make integration more difficult. In addition, if the overall contribution of one subject to the content of an examination is small, there may be a tendency to study less for that topic. It remains the case that medical students are driven by assessment. It is important, therefore, that even where psychiatric assessment is part of the final examinations, there is no compromise in the breadth and depth of assessment.

Methods

Summative assessment

The commonest form of summative assessment is now OSCEs, with assessment of key skills and attitudes incorporated into different stations. Some universities have adopted a portfolio of case reports and projects, which account for a proportion of the summative pass mark. This may be collated (often online) through the entire medical course, with the inclusion of one or two psychiatric cases, or may be confined to the psychiatry placement. Written assessments are largely based on multiple-choice questions, although some centres still resort to essays and short-answer questions, while others have moved on to extended matching questions (EMQs).

Formative assessment

Assessment drives learning and it is important to provide regular feedback to students during their placement. Medical schools tend to rely on high-stakes summative assessments and to ignore continuous assessment; in contrast, workplace-based assessments and 360-degree feedback are becoming the norm in postgraduate medical training. Some centres use weekly case-based tasks involving demonstration of key skills and attitudes such as the ability to communicate with carers or communication with a colleague who has a mental illness.

Logbooks can provide a useful mechanism for conducting and recording formative assessments and providing students with in-placement feedback. They can play a critical role in documenting students' progress, as well as the degree and range of exposure to clinical cases;they may also be used to log any concerns about clinical competency or professionalism issues. However, logbooks can work well only where clinical teachers use them meaningfully. Reflective logs followed by discussions with experienced clinical staff can be very helpful in unearthing key attitudinal learning points.

In some centres, the feedback is formalised, for example through mid-placement appraisal, which allows identification of training deficits and the institution of remedial teaching where indicated. Equally, the appraisal may identify those students who are performing well above the average, whose interest may be channelled through self-selected special study modules (SSMs). Finally, it is important to make available post-assessment feedback to all students, irrespective of whether they have passed or failed. The importance of prizes and merits in psychiatry to encourage a specific interest in and recruitment into the specialty should be recognised.

Feedback and evaluation

Feedback is essential to the delivery of any course. Some care needs to be taken to tailor the questions to the individual institution or site, as they ought to cover course content, teaching methods and delivery, placement experience and general facilities. This varies from formalised and standardised university feedback on all placements, perhaps gathered electronically, to individual reports at the end of lectures. Audience response systems may allow such feedback to be collected and collated relatively effortlessly. All feedback must be conveyed to lecturers and clinical teachers alongside averages for similar placements. This can then form a part of the teaching staff's appraisal portfolio. It is not unusual for a few students to be negative about placements; it is the combined picture over several placements that matters.

Quite often, institutions collect feedback but fail to evaluate it. All feedback and especially information listing problematic placements must therefore be collated and a mechanism must be in place for such information to be regularly reviewed.

Summary

The past decade has seen increasing public scrutiny of medical professionals and revalidation of fitness to practise has become a reality for all medical staff. Similar scrutiny is being extended to the quality of education provided in medical schools. Universities and NHS trusts, as providers and facilitators of education, are not only accountable to their funding bodies but also, more importantly, to the students who are the doctors of the future. This political context along with the current recruitment crisis provides the perfect opportunity for clinical teachers in psychiatry to influence universities to reorganise their teaching to make it fit for purpose in the 21st century. For such a change to materialise, appropriate educational governance structures need to be in place. Having clinical teachers in psychiatry as leaders in university structures is vital to ensure that psychiatry modules are of optimum duration and, more importantly, structurally integrated both with basic sciences and with other clinical specialties. There has to be an acceptance of the maxim that 'less is more' so far as the core curriculum is concerned. It needs to be acknowledged that students are adult learners and need to take responsibility for their own learning. However, a well-planned, learner-focused curriculum based on key principles delivered in a clinical context can foster long-term interest in the specialty, and thereby ultimately improve patient care.

Table 4.2 The gold standard

Key factors	Course structure
Leadership to influence university structures	Clarity of learning objectives
	Study materials – paper and web based
Exposure to psychiatry in other clinical disciplines, especially primary care	Formal teaching programme with lectures and tutorials
	Preclinical attachment preparation
Resources to support teaching	Clinical attachments – 'apprenticeships'
Ongoing innovation	Standardised assessments – 'both summative and formative
	Formalised feedback mechanisms to staff and students

Table 4.2 summarises the key factors in the organisation and delivery of a successful psychiatry placement.

The best of curricula can fail miserably unless there is effective delivery and this requires a range of diverse, well-trained teaching staff who can own and deliver the curriculum in a variety of clinical settings. Delivering this in the modern world needs ongoing innovation, using information technology solutions combined with modern educational methods of teaching and assessment. The challenge for today's educators is to organise the various components of teaching to deliver tomorrow's doctors.

References

Agrawal, V. (2007) Podcasts for psychiatrists: a new way of learning. *Psychiatric Bulletin*, **31**, 270–271.

Association of Directors of Medical Student Education in Psychiatry (2006) The psychiatry clerkship: a position statement on the length of the psychiatry clerkship. *Academic Psychiatry*, **30**, March–April. Available at http://ap.psychiatryonline.org/cgi/reprint/30/2/103.pdf

Brodkey, A. C., Sierles, F. S. & Woodard, J. L. (2006) Use of clerkship learning objectives by members of the Association of Directors of Medical Student Education in Psychiatry. *Academic Psychiatry*, **30**, 150–157.

Case, S. M., Ripkey, D. R. & Swanson, D. B. (1997) The effect of psychiatry clerkship timing and length on measures of performance. *Academic Medicine*, **72**, S34–S36.

Crisp, A. (1994) Psychiatric contributions to the undergraduate medical curriculum. *Psychiatric Bulletin*, **18**, 257–259.

Dave, S., Dogra, N. & Leask, S. (2010) Current role of service increment for teaching funding in psychiatry. *Psychiatric Bulletin*, **34**, 31–35.

Department of Health (2001) *Involving Patients and the Public in Healthcare: A Discussion Document.* Department of Health.

Department of Health (2004) *Medical Schools: Delivering Doctors of the Future.* Available at http://www.dh.gov.uk/prod_consum_dh/groups/dh_digitalassets/@dh/@en/documents/digitalasset/dh_4075406.pdf

Dogra, N., Edwards, R., Karim, K., *et al* (2008) Current issues in undergraduate psychiatry education: the findings of a qualitative study. *Advances in Health Sciences Education*, **13**, 309–323.

Eagles, J. (2005) Should the NHS revise its role in medical student education? *Scottish Medical Journal*, **50**, 144–147.

General Medical Council (1993) *Tomorrow's Doctors* (1st edn). GMC.

General Medical Council (2003) *Tomorrow's Doctors* (2nd edn). GMC.

General Medical Council (2009) *Tomorrow's Doctors* (3rd edn). GMC.

Goldacre, M. J., Turner, G., Fazel, S., *et al* (2005) Career choices for psychiatry: national surveys of graduates of 1974–2000 from UK medical schools. *British Journal of Psychiatry*, **186**, 158–164.

Goldberg, D. & Huxley, P. (1992) *Common Mental Disorders: A Bio-social Model*. Routledge.

Hare, E. E. (2009) E-learning for psychiatrists. *Psychiatric Bulletin*, **33**, 81–83.

Hare, E., Evans, P., McIntosh, C., *et al* (2007) Case-based online learning for medical undergraduates. *Psychiatric Bulletin*, **31**, 73–75.

Harden, R. M. (1986) Approaches to curriculum planning. *Medical Education*, **20**, 458–466.

Hodges, B. D. (2008) Psychiatry education research: the birth and development of a new field. *Canadian Journal of Psychiatry*, **53**, 75–76.

Holmes, D., Tumiel-Berhalter, L. M., Zayas, L. E., *et al* (2008) 'Bashing' of medical specialties: students' experiences and recommendations. *Family Medicine*, **40**, 400–406.

House of Commons Health Select Committee (2006) *NHS Deficits – First Report of Session 2006–07*. Vol. 1, 13 December. Available at http://www.publications.parliament.uk/pa/cm200607/cmselect/cmhealth/73/73i.pdf

Karim, K., Edwards, R., Dogra, N., *et al* (2009) A survey of the teaching and assessment of undergraduate psychiatry in the medical schools of the United Kingdom and Ireland. *Medical Teacher*, **31**, 1024–1029.

Kelly, B., Raphael, B. & Byrne, G. (1991) The evaluation of teaching in undergraduate psychiatric education: students' attitudes to psychiatry and the evaluation of clinical competency. *Medical Teacher*, **13**, 77–87.

Leung, W. C. (2002) Competency based medical training: review. *BMJ*, **325**, 693–696.

Nasser, M. (1996) Psychiatry in the medical curriculum. *Canadian Journal of Psychiatry*, **30**, 586–592

Neilsen, A. C. & Eaton, J. S. (1981) Medical students' attitudes about psychiatry. *Archives of General Psychiatry*, **38**, 1144–1154.

NHS Executive (1995) *SIFT into the Future: Future Arrangements for Allocating Funds and Contracting for NHS Service Support and Facilities for Teaching Undergraduate Medical Students* (Winyard report). NHS Executive.

Oakley, C. & Oyebode, F. (2008) Medical students' views about an undergraduate curriculum in psychiatry before and after clinical placements. *BMC Medical Education*, **8**, 26.

Rezler, A. G. (1974) Attitude change during medical school: a review of the literature. *Journal of Medical Education*, **49**, 1023–1030.

Royal College of Psychiatrists (2009a) *Dean's Newsletter*, May. RCPsych.

Royal College of Psychiatrists (2009b) *A Competency Based Curriculum for Specialist Training in Psychiatry*. RCPsych. Available at http://www.rcpsych.ac.uk/training/curriculum2010/curriculum2009.aspx

Rosenthal, R. H., Levine, R. E., Carlson, D. L., *et al* (2005) The 'shrinking' clerkship: characteristics and length of clerkships in psychiatry undergraduate education. *Academic Psychiatry*, **29**, 47–51.

Sackett, D. L. (1996) Evidence based medicine: what it is and what it isn't. *BMJ*, **312**, 71–72.

Scher, M., Hartford, J. F., Khan, A., *et al* (1988) Comparison of two formats for a psychiatry clerkship. *Journal of Medical Education*, **63**, 140–143.

Schon, F., MacKay, A. & Fernandez, C. (2006) Is shared learning the way to bring UK neurology and psychiatry closer: what teachers, trainers and trainees think. *Journal of Neurology, Neurosurgery, and Psychiatry*, **77**, 943–946.

Singh, S. P., Baxter, H., Standen, P., *et al* (1998) Changing the attitudes of 'Tomorrow's Doctors' towards mental illness and psychiatry: a comparison of two teaching methods. *Medical Education*, **32,** 115–120.

Thomson, L. D. G., Gray, C. & Humphreys, M. S. (1999) Medical students' perspective of maximum security psychiatric care. *Psychiatric Bulletin*, **23**, 230–232.

Thornhill, J. T. & Tong, L. (2006) From Yoda to Sackett: the future of psychiatry medical education. *Academic Psychiatry*, **30**, 23–28.

Valsraj, K. M. & Lygo-Baker, S. (2006) A balancing act: developing curricula for balanced care within community psychiatry. *Advances in Psychiatric Treatment*, **12**, 69–79.

Walters, K., Raven, P., Rosenthal, J., *et al* (2007) Teaching undergraduate psychiatry in primary care: the impact on student learning and attitudes. *Medical Education*, **41**, 100–108.

Walton, H. & Gelder, M. (1999) Core curriculum in psychiatry for medical students. *Medical Education*, **33**, 204–211.

Williams, C., Milton, J. & Strickland, P. (1997) Impact of medical school teaching on pre-registration house officers' confidence in assessing and managing common psychological morbidity: three centre study. *BMJ*, **315**, 917–918.

Wilson, S. & Eagles, J. M. (2008) Changes in undergraduate clinical psychiatry teaching in Scotland since 'Tomorrow's Doctors'. *Scottish Medical Journal*, **52**(4), 22–25.

Wilson, S., Eagles, J. M., Platt, J. E., *et al* (2007) Core undergraduate psychiatry: what do non-specialists need to know? *Medical Education*, **41**, 698–702.

CHAPTER 5

Assessment of undergraduates in psychiatry

Brian Lunn

Introduction

Most, if not all, of those involved in teaching medicine have probably encountered a variant on the question 'Will this be in the exam?' It is understandable that with students facing a high-stakes examination, which influences progress through a career path, they will choose to focus their energies on those aspects of the course that will be assessed. There can be no more accurate truism in medicine than 'assessment drives learning'. With this in mind, it is evident that, whatever the focus of a course, if assessment is not at the centre of planning the curriculum, efforts to direct student learning will fail. Newble & Kaeger (1983) describe how laudable aims for a curriculum can fail to be met when assessment is not structured to direct student learning down a desired route.

It is easy to become nihilistic when faced with an awareness that students will choose to focus on what is examined. Yet if all of us were honest, we would realise that they are only repeating our own patterns of behaviour. It is therefore our duty to see this not as an impediment but as an opportunity. With appropriately shaped assessment built into a curriculum, students will be directed down a chosen learning path and appropriate attributes developed. Assessment then becomes central to any curriculum, not as an end in itself but as a signpost and driver to excellence.

Despite reflective educators recognising similarities between current students' views and their own student experience, another common experience for those who have been involved in 'new' implementations of assessment is hearing that familiar plaintive cry of clinicians, 'But it was good enough for me ...'. Changes in assessment methods can induce mistrust and alarm in those who deliver teaching and unless they can be encouraged to see the point of the chosen method of assessment these, usually, well meaning teachers can derail the process and purpose of assessment by communicating their views, consciously or unconsciously, to students. Concern is usually about standards purportedly falling, along with the bar for success. With the media and politicians constantly playing such a populist card, it should be no surprise to find this concern among colleagues in medicine. However, it is not always the case that what is believed to be examined in a particular assessment is what is actually tested. For example, the traditional 'long case' is thought to assess candidates' history taking and examination skills when in fact it is the candidates' presentation skills that are assessed, with the former elements assessed only by inference. This chapter will cover several key theoretical areas in the design of an assessment and will also give examples of how what we believe is examined and what is actually examined can differ.

Purpose

As in any endeavour, the first questions in designing an assessment must be 'Why am I doing this?' and 'What do I hope to measure?' With the various iterations of *Tomorrow's Doctors*, the General Medical Council has given us a steer on what it expects to be assessed (General Medical Council, 2009). The recent suggestion for a national curriculum in undergraduate psychiatry (see Chapter 3) fleshes this out in some detail and has the advantage of having been derived from the actual practice and priorities of psychiatrists who deliver curricula in UK medical schools.

The main purposes of assessment include the following:

- measuring academic achievement
- setting standards
- identifying student problems
- allowing self-assessment
- demonstrating the effectiveness of the course and teachers
- driving approaches to learning
- predicting the future.

Measuring academic achievement

When seeking to measure academic achievements of any individual or group, those designing a curriculum will need to consider covering three main domains: knowledge, skills and attitudes (sometimes called professionalism). It has long been the case that knowledge assessment has been at the core of undergraduate assessment in psychiatry, even in clinical examinations. Historically, inferences were made about skills, generally from the presentation of information; skills were rarely assessed by direct observation. Even when observation occurred, the assessment of skills was highly subjective and rarely operationalised. The last of these domains was rarely assessed at all.

Assessment of academic achievement is core to any course. It tends to be summative assessment that defines end-points. These can be passing a stage of the course or the course itself. It is therefore precisely this high-stakes assessment that will be any medical student's primary focus. With changes in recruitment and the need for UK medical schools to rank students, these examinations have, to a certain extent, attained a higher priority for students.

Setting standards

Tomorrow's Doctors has already been mentioned. This is an example of one standard-setting document that pertains in medical education, and for medical students it is the primary focus, for it sets out the minimum standard that must be achieved for an individual to be regarded as suitable to progress in a medical career. Later on in doctors' careers, the Postgraduate Medical Education and Training Board (PMETB; now subsumed by the GMC) and the various medical Royal Colleges set out the standards at which doctors can be regarded as safe to practise independently and at what level (Howard, 2007). It is important that such standards are 'absolute', and are not a measure of performance relative to that of other medical students or doctors.

Identifying student problems and allowing self-assessment

Traditionally, summative assessment has tended to be used and students in difficulty are identified only when they fail at the end of a course or module. In recent years there has been a trend to introduce formative assessment within medical curricula. These interim assessments are designed to enable a student to identify difficulties and formulate a remedial plan to address any problems. It is important that such assessments do not rely on a final score or mark as a marker of achievement but are structured to give feedback in appropriate areas. In knowledge assessments this may be simply a matter of providing students with the correct answers and/or appropriate references, or in assessments of skill or attitudes more detailed narrative feedback and, if required, counselling.

It is important that formative assessments remain just that and are not used to contribute to a final summative assessment. A student who performs at a lower level early in a course may make significant efforts and achieve a final high summative grade; in contrast, some of those who start with a better performance may 'rest on their laurels' and not reach as high a final grade. Clearly, it would be wrong for the former student to be penalised for early problems that had been addressed.

Demonstrating the effectiveness of the course and teachers

Both formative and summative assessments can be used to identify whether the courses are achieving desired aims, but also to identify good or poor practice in teachers, either as individuals or as groups. This can be particularly useful when new teaching approaches are introduced or when teaching is delivered in a new clinical base. Individual teachers may be able to use such data in a reflective way to modify their own practice or indeed in their appraisal process.

Driving approaches to learning

As covered in the Introduction, assessment drives learning. A properly designed assessment process can encourage students to approach their learning in the manner the curriculum designers intended. If a summative examination is focused on knowledge assessment, then it is inevitable that students will focus their energies on book learning, at the expense of developing clinical skills. If that emphasis is shifted to a direct assessment of clinical skills, such as history taking and the mental state examination, then they will clamour to have access to patients and to be observed assessing them.

Predicting the future

Increasingly, as with ranking medical students at qualification, there is a desire to use assessments to predict future performance. The problem with this is that current assessment practices are designed to identify academic achievement and whether core competencies have been achieved. As such, these tests have little or no predictive value beyond the early years. Furthermore, in the UK at least, most of those who qualify from medical school still do so at a relatively young age, when there remains a substantial period of personality development ahead of them. It is therefore all the harder to predict the future performance of graduates.

In the selection of medical students, the UK Clinical Aptitude Test (UKCAT) has been developed 'to assist in creating a "level playing field" for applicants from diverse educational and cultural backgrounds' (see http://www.ukcat.ac.uk/pages/details.aspx?page=ValidityReliability). Here, standardised computer assessment is used in the hope of developing a reliable and valid tool to predict which applicants will make good medical students. Such a tool should ensure that the advantage accrued by those students who attend secondary schools that are experienced at coaching candidates for medical school does not exempt equally able candidates who have not been in such a privileged position. To date, such a coordinated approach has not been attempted for those leaving medical school and entering the job market.

A note on recruitment

There is one further possible purpose for assessment in psychiatry for medical students, and that is later recruitment into the profession. Since assessment drives learning, it is clear that if psychiatry does not contribute substantially to the overall examination process in medical school, particularly finals, there will be no incentive for students to gain knowledge and skill in psychiatry. Active engagement therefore of psychiatrists in the general examination process in medical schools is essential if our specialty is to maintain or achieve prominence in students' learning.

Domains

As mentioned above, the three key domains in assessment are knowledge, skills and attitudes; traditional assessments have focused on the first of these and latterly the second has gained more prominence. More recently attention has shifted to attitudes. In the lead-up to the 2009 review of *Tomorrow's Doctors*, the Academy of Medical Royal Colleges & NHS Institute of Innovation and Improvement (2009) published a document entitled *Medical Leadership Competency Framework*, which set out competencies in discrete domains: personal qualities; working with others; managing services; improving services; and setting direction. There will now be a drive to include focused assessment in these domains within medical school assessments. The challenge is to ensure that this strand, which will pervade all elements of the curriculum, is appropriately assessed with respect to psychiatry.

The modes of assessment in all three domains have seen substantial development in the past few years. While the focus is now shifting to assessment of the 'professionalism' strand, there remains a need to address assessment frameworks in all three domains.

Knowledge

Assessment of knowledge has long been at the core of medical student examinations. Even so, there has been considerable revision of how knowledge has been assessed over the past couple of decades. In particular, the previous core methods of essays and short answers have been largely dropped from examinations. These methods present both logistical and pedagogical problems. Logistical problems include the need for human marking (with the attendant problem of resource provision, double marking to improve reliability and additional marking/arbitration where there is disagreement over marks). Even the same examiner re-marking the same essay after a 6-month gap has been shown in one study to have a correlation of only 0.35. This (logistical) reliability issue is compounded by a pedagogical question of validity: it is difficult to formulate questions that are not open to a variety of reasonable interpretations, which means, in essays in particular, that there may be perfectly reasonable essays that diverge significantly from that which the examiners intended. While short-answer questions (SAQs) are theoretically easier to focus on a specific area, there remains the enduring problem of students' interpretation of what is asked. This results in the SAQ being not only an assessment of knowledge but also of the candidate's ability to infer accurately what the examiner desired. It is therefore the case that students may come up with varieties of answers beyond those envisaged by the question writer. Improving validity and reliability in SAQs is easier than with essays but carries significant costs (Milton, 1979). (Validity and reliability are considered in general terms below.)

The validity issues have led to the rejection of essays and SAQs in favour of other assessments of knowledge. With the loss of essays there has had to be a move to other assessments of writing skills. This will be picked up on in the discussion below on the 'skills' domain.

Multiple-choice questions (MCQs) have been used for many years to assess medical students, but over recent years theories relating to their design have led to several changes in their format (see Table 5.1). One reason for this is that question design influences the validity of MCQs (Shively, 1978). Currently, the shift has been to single-item questions with an adjusted mark to take guessing into account. Previously, negative marking was used to facilitate this, but it can reward examination technique as opposed to knowledge.

It must, however, be acknowledged that a move to MCQs exclusively would not be viewed without trepidation. SAQs and other 'free response' formats are often said to test higher-order skills than MCQs (McGuire, 1987). Additionally, MCQs can reward good guessing and thus reward 'recognition' rather than 'knowing' (Newble et al, 1979).

Extended matching items/questions (EMIs or EMQs) allow testing of application of knowledge in a superior way to MCQs and with a greater reliability than with SAQs or essays (Case & Swanson, 1993). In EMIs a number of questions can be asked; the candidate is required to select one or more answers from a large, provided, list of potential options. One option can be the correct answer for more than one question, so the number of

Table 5.1 Influence of format on the validity of multiple-choice questions

Format	Associated problems and disadvantages
Stem with one correct choice from 4 or 5	There are usually only two realistic choices, which increases the chance of guessing correctly
Single stem with multiple true/false options	Difficulty in creating enough options for one stem, which results in the value of all options not being equal. It also rewards guessing unless the pass mark is adjusted for guessing or negative marking is used
Single item true/false	Rewards guessing unless the pass mark is adjusted for guessing or negative marking is used

Table 5.2 The four elements of a well-constructed extended matching item (EMI) assessment

Element	Content
The theme	This is the topic that will be addressed by the stems and is the unifying element of the option list. Examples might be psychopathological terms, laboratory investigations or results, drugs from a class, diagnostic terms, etc.
The option list	This provides the various possible answer for the stems. While the number of options can vary, it is important that there is uniformity of theme as covered above and that there are sufficient options to allow testing of knowledge. Questions can be made 'more difficult' by increasing the number of options or decreasing the degree of difference between options. Options can be single words, phrases or numerical 'results'. It is important that there is a common structure as well as a common theme.
The lead statement	A single lead statement should be used for all the stems in each individual EMI to provide direction and identify the relationship between the stems and the option list. The lead statement can require the candidate to select more than one option or to order the options in some way. It is vital to give explicit directions as EMIs with non-specific lead statements can lead to ambiguity.
The stems	In psychiatry perhaps the most useful form of item is a clinical vignette, which describes a patient in a clinical situation. If carefully constructed these can be used to draw relationships between basic and clinical sciences and test understanding of topics such as descriptive psychopathology or application of diagnoses. In common with the other components of EMIs stems in each EMI should be similar in structure to minimise guessing.

options is not reduced by each successive question. In higher-order examinations, the candidates may be asked to rank choices or to select the 'single best' option. The candidates have less chance to guess correctly than in MCQs and 'recognition' cueing is less likely too. The larger the list of options the more like a 'free response' question an EMI becomes (Veloski *et al*, 1988), but it is vital that there is commonality between the options. That is, if the question is about investigation, the answer options should all be similar sorts of investigation, not an *ad hoc* mix, as that would allow the candidate to select only from blood tests for one answer or from imaging investigations for another. This is important, as candidates of poorer ability benefit from shorter lists of options. This may be because options are limited due to lack of commonality or simply because too few options are supplied.

The theoretical model for the design of EMIs is shown in Table 5.2.

Skills

In the mind of the public, media and clinicians, the final clinical examination has been synonymous with a 'long case'. Unfortunately, some assumptions made about the traditional long case do not hold up to scrutiny. The traditional model has been for the student to spend a period (usually around an hour) with a patient unobserved and then report findings and conclusions to examiners, sometimes with a requirement to carry out a portion of the physical, or in psychiatry mental state, examination. The examination is usually concluded by a *viva voce* examination around the subject matter of the case.

The long case has a high face validity (see 'Validity', below), as it simulates the clinical encounter. With the emphasis on candidates assessing a real patient with no prior knowledge of that individual, the examination mimics the real world in which the candidate will work. Additionally, as the candidate is required to integrate clinical findings and knowledge to produce a diagnostic formulation and (usually) a management plan, this examination can test high-order skills. The potential problems are, unfortunately, so many, however, that there are concerns regarding validity of the examination and more emphatically the reliability.

In the majority of set-ups, candidates are not observed for the whole of the clinical examination. How they conduct themselves when they assess the patient, in terms of both their professionalism and their clinical skill, is often an unknown variable, but one of great significance. There can be a significant component of luck (good or bad) in the allocation of the patient. Not all patients are equal. The case may just happen to play to a candidate's strengths or weaknesses; the patient may be helpful or hostile, regardless of the candidate's performance; signs may be more difficult or more unusual in some patients than others; and choice of cases may depend on local clinical services. Finally, the skill set and prejudices/preferences of the examiners can play a significant role. The *viva voce* component is a particularly vulnerable area unless structured and the risk is that assessment of knowledge assumes primacy.

Issues concerning the reliability and validity of the long case have led to a drive to develop examinations that are more reliable. Approaches have included examinations designed to focus on skills, observed long cases (Newble, 1991) and more substantial modifications of long cases (Wright *et al*, 2009). In the desire to focus on objective assessment of skills, Harden & Gleeson (1979) described the use of what was then a new form of examination, the objective structured clinical examination (OSCE). This was described in undergraduate psychiatric education relatively late (Famuyiwa *et al*, 1991) but has grown in use, including its use in the previous MRCPsych Part I examination and in a modified form as the clinical examination in the new MRCPsych examination process ('Clinical Assessment of Skills and Competencies').

Typically, OSCE stations will have a simulated patient interacting with a candidate. A variety of skills can then be assessed in a structured format with a differing focus between stations to allow a breadth and depth not readily organised with real patients. As with other examination formats, if quality is adequate it is the quantity of stations that influences reliability. A very real concern often expressed with respect to the use of simulated patients, however, is that there is a lack of verisimilitude in the clinical encounter. There is, though, evidence that medical students make similar empathic responses to simulated patients as they do in real clinical encounters (Sanson-Fisher & Poole, 1980) and that in comparison with more traditional examinations the long case is 'no worse and no better than OSCEs in assessing clinical competence' (Wass et al, 2001). Importantly, the assessment of clinical skills in an OSCE has been shown to correlate with assessments of skills 'on the job' (Melding et al, 2002).

Ultimately, as with other assessments, the value of OSCEs comes down to their design, principally the number of stations, the number of examiners, the design of the stations, the quality of the 'cases' (whether simulated patients or otherwise) and, finally, the marking schedule. While in testing less experienced candidates a checklist approach to marking can have validity, as one moves to testing higher-order skills and more senior candidates this becomes less true. A more global marking schedule has been shown to have value in psychiatry (Hodges et al, 1999). An interesting feature of OSCEs (as examinations of skill) is that awareness of what will be assessed does not apparently alter the assessed level of competence, as was serendipitously shown by Wilkinson et al (2003).

The desire to evaluate higher-order skills in medical students by combining their assessment of 'real' patients in the long case with the benefits of the structure and specified objectives of OSCEs has resulted in the development of a hybrid of the two formats at Newcastle University (Wright et al, 2009). Previously, candidates had been assessed using a variant of the long case, termed the objective structured long examination record (OSLER; Gleeson, 1997), which had been shown to be superior to the traditional long case. But, owing to concerns about validity and reliability, a modified version was introduced, the modified OSLER (MOSLER). Candidates complete a circuit of four stations, three populated with real patients, one with a simulated patient, and are asked to carry out specified tasks in front of examiners before engaging in a structured discussion of their findings and specified clinical topic. Each station lasts 20 minutes. A psychiatric example of this might be seeing a patient with treated depression to clarify what, if any, depressive symptoms/cognitions are present, presenting the findings and then discussing a management plan based on the presumption that the patient's mental state meets specific criteria. Initial data suggest that not only does this produce reliable results but it does so with greater validity than the OSLER.

While writing skills typically tend to be assessed in relation to pieces of written work submitted for summative assessment, there have been recent attempts to assess particular skills such as the writing of discharge summaries and other focused clinical pieces. Assessment here benefits from structure and typically assessments focus on information included, accuracy and clarity. Even then, owing to the individuality of candidates' writing (the same data can be presented in different ways) dual marking and clear marking schemes are important to ensure consistency and appropriate reward of marks .

Attitudes

Assessing attitudes, or professionalism, has become one of the biggest challenges in modern medical education. Both politically and at the behest of patient groups and the GMC, it has moved to the forefront of the assessment of potential doctors. Approaches to this could merit an entire chapter on its own. One of the most useful tools is assessment in the workplace. Multi-source feedback can be used formatively to identify issues and to highlight the need to address 'failing' students. It is when challenges to dysfunctional attitudes do not effect change that 'failing' a student becomes an issue. Despite the clear need to identify potential doctors with problematic attitudes, many medical teachers still feel ill equipped to discriminate objectively. In this respect, forthcoming work, building on the 2009 edition of *Tomorrow's Doctors*, by the Academy of Medical Royal Colleges and the NHS Institute of Innovation and Improvement (mentioned above) may be useful in providing a framework around which educators can work.

Establishing the pass mark

What determines the pass mark in an examination is a frequent bone of contention. Unsurprisingly, there is greatest agreement between examiners with respect to those candidates who obtain grades that are a clear pass or fail. The area of contention tends to be around the borderline and it is here, therefore, that educationalists have focused efforts to establish methods to define a pass mark. It is beyond the scope of this chapter to cover this in any detail. It is perhaps sufficient to highlight two approaches: the borderline groups method and the contrasting groups method.

The borderline groups method is used in the OSCE run by the Professional and Linguistic Assessments Board (PLAB). Here, each candidate obtains two marks. One is a percentage mark; the other is a decision on a global basis as to whether the candidate has achieved a 'pass' a 'fail' or whether performance is 'borderline'. The percentage marks for all those deemed 'borderline' are reviewed and the mean of those candidates graded at the 'borderline' is used to determine the pass mark for that station.

In the contrasting groups method, again the examiner makes a global judgement as well as giving a percentage mark. This time the decision is dichotomous, with a decision simply being whether a candidate has passed or failed. The marks for the 'pass' group and the 'fail' group are then plotted and the point where the two curves intersect becomes the pass mark for that station.

From this point, in both examples given above, the results can be handled in a variety of ways. All the individual station pass marks could be summed and that then gives the pass mark for the examination. Alternatively, a threshold can be chosen such that candidates have to pass an agreed number of stations. The potential problem with the former approach is that it is possible for a candidate to pass a minority of stations but still pass the examination. The latter method can be seen as arbitrary, even if it does have some face validity.

Finally, it is obvious that when global decisions alone are made, neither of these methods would be of use. In such circumstances the Angoff method is frequently used (Zieky, 2001). This requires an expert group to evaluate each station in a clinical examination, or question from a written paper, to estimate what proportion of 'minimally competent' candidates would succeed at the specific task or answer the question correctly. The individual 'expert' ratings are averaged to set the pass mark for that station/question. These are then usually summed to obtain the pass mark for the overall examination. It is important to realise that this equates with the level of a 'minimally competent' candidate.

Test quality

At several points above, the quality of testing has been highlighted as the key to any examination, regardless of examination format or what domain is being tested. Ultimately, decisions about what tests are used depend on a number of variables, which can include practicality, cost, resources and whether the examination tests what it sets out to. Judgement about whether an examination is any good requires measuring whether it is valid and reliable. Validity is a measure of whether it assesses what it purports to assess and reliability is a measure of whether it does so consistently and in a reproducible manner.

Validity

Validity can be separated into four main types:

- content or face validity – whether the examination actually tests the objectives chosen
- construct validity – whether the test shows correlation with what might be considered a 'gold standard'
- criterion validity – whether the test result has predictive value (an example might be whether a final medical examination can predict the competence of a Foundation Year 1 doctor)
- constraints on learning – whether the assessment changes what candidates do in preparation for the examination.

Content validity

This is usually the first priority of any examination board, as it will want to ensure that the full range of syllabus material is included in an examination.

Here, blueprints have particular value (Lunn, 2005). While there is no quantitative statistical test that can ascertain whether content validity has been achieved, qualitative methods are increasingly used to assess this. A blueprint in psychiatry may result in a grid that has disorders or subject areas along one axis and skills along the other, ensuring that sufficient core skills are assessed and over enough of the subjects covered in the curriculum so as to give confidence in the examination. Equally, this method can be used for knowledge assessments.

Construct validity

In attempting to assess a new examination format it can be useful to compare the new format with previous methods. This construct validity can give confidence that the new approach to assessment matches expectations and experience with the previous examination.

Criterion validity

Perhaps the most important question any examination can answer is whether a successful candidate will perform in an intended role to the standard expected. There is remarkably little evidence to answer this in medicine, yet there is increasing dependence on it in recruitment within the National Health Service. Equally important is whether those who fail an examination would not have succeeded in the intended role.

Constraints on learning

The aphorism that assessment drives learning applies here again (Newble & Kaeger, 1983). It is important that this form of validity be considered in any assessment decision, whether an examination format is taken 'off the shelf' or a new format is designed.

Reliability

Reliability is a way of expressing, statistically, how consistent and how generalisable the results of an examination are. Several factors affecting the reliability of tests have already been mentioned. Key factors are variability in marking (or subject matter in the case of non-standardised clinical examinations), the number of items assessed, the distribution of results and the difficulty of the examination. In general, moderately hard examinations with more items, statistically normal results and agreement in the assessment will prove to be more reliable.

Types of reliability include:

- test–retest reliability
- inter- and intra-rater reliability
- equivalent test forms
- internal consistency.

Broadly speaking, values above 0.8 are considered acceptable for assessments. Below 0.7 there is a clear need to improve the assessment method. In assessments where examiners have a degree of discretion, they become the variable that can most significantly affect the reliability of an examination. Tactics such as increasing the number of examiners, providing unequivocal guidance on what constitutes satisfactory candidate performance, examiner training and double marking can address this. The most efficient way, however, to improve reliability is to increase the number of test items.

Generalisability theory has allowed more comprehensive assessment of the reliability of clinical examinations in particular and across the board has shown that poor inter-station (for OSCEs, etc.) or inter-item correlation is a significant factor. This does not mean that the individual stations are poorly designed but rather that a candidate's score on one station does not necessarily have predictive value for other stations. This observation adds to the argument that a broad range of skills should be assessed over enough stations, with the total examination taking a much longer time than would otherwise be the case.

Summary

The place of assessment in psychiatry in undergraduate medical education is important, to ensure not only that medical students learn psychiatry but also that the appropriate learning methods are adopted and curricula are supported by the assessment structure. Psychiatry's place among other medical specialties can be reinforced by engagement of psychiatrists in general medical school examination boards and by delivering high-quality examination components.

References

Academy of Medical Royal Colleges & NHS Institute of Innovation and Improvement (2009) *Medical Leadership Competency Framework: Enhancing Engagement in Medical Leadership*, (2nd edn). NHS Institute for Innovation and Improvement.

Case, S. M. & Swanson, D. B. (1993) Extended matching items: a practical alternative to free-response questions. *Teaching and Learning in Medicine*, **5**, 107–115.

Famuyiwa, O. O., Zachariah, M. P. & Ilechukwu, S. T. (1991) The objective structured clinical examination in undergraduate psychiatry. *Medical Education*, **25**, 45–50.

General Medical Council (2009) *Tomorrows' Doctors* (3rd edn). GMC. Available at http://www.gmc-uk.org/education/undergraduate/undergraduate_policy/tomorrows_doctors/tomorrows_doctors_2009.asp

Gleeson, F. (1997) AMEE Medical Education Guide No. 9: Assessment of clinical competence using the Objective Structured Long Examination Record (OSLER). *Medical Teacher*, **19**, 7–14.

Harden, R. M. & Gleeson, F. A. (1979) Assessment of clinical competencies using an objective structured clinical examination (OSCE). *Medical Education*, **13**, 39–45.

Hodges, B., Regeher, G., McNaughton, N., *et al* (1999) OSCE checklists do not capture increasing levels of expertise. *Academic Medicine*, **74**, 1129–1134.

Howard, R. (2007) The Postgraduate Medical Education and Training Board and quality assurance of training standards. *Psychiatric Bulletin*, **31**, 41–43.

Lunn, B. (2005) The OSCE blueprint and station development. In *OSCEs in Psychiatry* (ed. R. Rao), pp. 24–32. Gaskell.

McGuire, C. (1987) Written methods for assessing clinical competence. In *Further Developments in Assessing Clinical Competence* (eds I. Hart & R. Harden), pp. 46–58. Can-Heal Publications.

Melding, P., Coverdale, J. & Robinson, E. (2002) A 'fair play?' Comparison of an objective structured clinical examination of final year medical students training in psychiatry and their supervisors' appraisals. *Australian Psychiatry*, **10**, 344–347.

Milton, O. (1979) Improving achievement via essay exams. *Journal of Veterinary Medical Education*, **6**, 108–112.

Newble, D. I. (1991) The observed long case in clinical assessment. *Medical Education*, **25**, 369–373.

Newble, D. I. & Kaeger, K. (1983) The effect of assessments and examinations on the learning of medical students. *Medical Education*, **17**, 165–171.

Newble, D., Baxter, A. & Elmslie, R. (1979) A comparison of multiple-choice and free-response tests in examinations of clinical competence. *Medical Education*, **13**, 263–268.

Sanson-Fisher, R. W. & Poole, A. D. (1980) Simulated patients and the assessment of medical students' interpersonal skills. *Medical Education*, **14**, 249–253.

Shively, M. J. (1978) Improving the quality of multiple-choice examinations. *Journal of Veterinary Medical Education*, **5**, 71–76.

Veloski, J., Robinowitz, H. & Robeson, M. (1988) Cueing in multiple-choice questions: a reliable, valid and economical solution. *Research in Medical Education*, **27**, 195–200.

Wass, V., Jones, R. & van der Vleuten, C. (2001) Standardized or real patients to test clinical competence? The long case revisited. *Medical Education*, **35**, 321–325.

Wilkinson, T., Fontaine, S. & Egan, T. (2003) Was a breach of examination security unfair in an objective structured clinical examination? A critical incident. *Medical Teacher*, **25**, 42–46.

Wright, S., Bradley, P. M., Jones, S., *et al* (2009) Generalisability study of a new Finals examination component – the MOSLER. AMEE Conference 2009, 29 August–2 September, Málaga, Spain (http://www.amee.org/documents/AMEE%202009%20 FINAL%20ABSTRACT%20BOOK.pdf).

Zieky, M. J. (2001) So much has changed: how the setting of cutscores has evolved since the 1980s. In *Setting Performance Standards* (eds G. J. Cizek & N. J. Mahwah), pp. 19–52. Lawrence Erlbaum Associates.

CHAPTER 6

Using computers to teach undergraduate psychiatry

Elizabeth Hare & Paul Hopper

Introduction

Medical students' time is precious; they have a lot to learn. As psychiatrists, we are inclined to think psychiatry is a crucial part of the undergraduate course. We also have an important role to play in helping students to develop communication skills with vulnerable people – a key task identified by the General Medical Council in *Tomorrow's Doctors* (2003). Many of the 'facts' will change in the course of their careers, so as well as providing training in specific skills, and providing positive role models as clinicians, our role as medical teachers should include laying down strategies for knowledge to sustain the capacity for new learning. This chapter will address the areas in which information technology can assist, and where it might be an irrelevance, or even a costly distraction.

We realise that many medical teachers will come to this topic with an appropriately sceptical eye. We have all seen computer projects start out promising to change everything, but then failing miserably. E-learning can be as simple or as complex as you need it to be – the key is to ask yourself and your colleagues the right questions before getting stuck in.

Why bother with e-learning?

The 'e' in e-Learning stands for education – we too often forget that – it is not about bandwidth, servers, and cables. It is about education – first and foremost (Gaines, 2004).

Information technology (IT) is only an educational medium, namely a means of delivering an experience which can encourage learning. Its success is predicated on the use of established teaching methods: taking students from the known to the unknown, clearly delivering the relevant content, and checking their understanding (Chan & Robbins, 2006). Consider first what you want the students to be able to do after the activity or, from the learner's perspective, consider how any one particular lesson will help them accomplish their goal of being a good doctor. One of the long-established principles of e-learning is that however much work the developer puts in, the only real value lies in users performing their role better afterwards (Kirkpatrick, 1998).

It is interesting to consider how much of a difference there is between the processes of being taught by and with a human being, as opposed to by electronic means. These differences are highlighted in Table 6.1.

There may be other reasons for teachers to consider using IT, apart from its educational value. These include the following:

- other people are doing it
- a personal interest in using it
- using new software tools might inspire the teachers
- money is available for these projects
- students might judge a subject in part by how IT embraces it
- in hospital there are fewer 'real' patients for students to see
- it might be seen by the unwary as an opportunistic and cheaper way of delivering an educational 'product' (even though creating high-quality systems and products takes expertise, time and effort).

Whatever the motives, an appreciation of what IT can and cannot do and the costs and benefits of such endeavours is necessary. When considering whether IT has a role in your teaching, ask 'Can it substitute, or enhance, current methods of delivery and assessment?' As with clinical services, making changes where there are gaps, or deciding what can be done away with to fund new developments, is a useful exercise in seeing if costs might be balanced or even recouped.

From the general to the specific: how can technology enhance a psychiatry course?

Good teachers take learners from the known to the unknown, repeat key messages and test what has been learned. E-learning programmes can take the student beyond passive observation by building in checks for

Table 6.1 Comparison of being taught by and with a person, and by electronic means

Person	E-learning
Spontaneous, flexible	Consistent, thorough
Subject to demands of clinical work	Available round the clock
Complexity of typical in-patients	Simplified to begin learning
Clinician's feedback open to bias	Computers disinterested
Thrill of patient encounter	Safe place to practise repeatedly

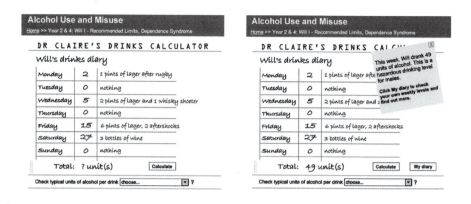

Fig. 6.1 An interactive diary used to monitor alcohol use.

understanding, and opportunities for reflection and practising of skills (albeit limited). Moreover, the repetition of key messages ('telling three times') can be extended to telling at increasing levels of complexity, and telling using text, sound, diagrams, animation and video to address different learning styles. For example, rather than listing the recommendations for 'safe drinking', one of the present authors has provided students with an interactive diary (Fig. 6.1) in which they can log different quantities of alcohol intake over a week and get relevant feedback for their patients or themselves.

When technology promotes interaction, the students learn further by telling one another. Ideally, each lesson should be quickly repeated in practice so the student can apply rather than recount the content.

Medical undergraduates, particularly those who enrol straight from school, straddle the transition between child and adult learners (Brookfield, 1986) in that though they may be choosing a medical course, much of the content, other than the student-selected components, is prescribed. Often, students' expectations are that learning outcomes should be explicit and that any call on their time should focus on their goal of obtaining a degree. If that is how it seems to many students, we as teachers need to work with that reality. Some students will love psychiatry as we do, but most will see it as a means to an end. We need to pass on our passion for our subject while at the same time showing, over and over again, how what we teach is useful and relevant. This is most likely to happen if we concentrate on developing skills and attitudes, while at the same time imparting knowledge.

Imparting knowledge, building on what students already know, is the bread and butter of clinical teaching. E-learning can help to present information in a variety of ways:

- *Narrated slide presentations.* Tutors can use one of a number of off-the-shelf programs to record their speech while moving through a slide show.

Students can then access the recording as an alternative to attending the event or as an aid to revision later (Martin & Bennet, 2004).

- *Lecture notes with embedded attachments.* Electronic lecture notes can be more useful than paper notes if they are sent out with embedded links to documents, images and websites that had been used during the lecture.
- *Topic web pages.* Most universities have a website to support students, and these sites often contain pages covering specialty topics (e.g. Newcastle University's medical student teaching resource, http://www.ncl.ac.uk/nnp/teaching/disorders/liaison). These pages can be very useful to students if they focus tightly on what is relevant to that institution's curriculum. Core details can be presented in a fresh way without trying to make the web pages be all things to all people. A good example of such learning material has been provided by the University of Southampton (https://www.som.soton.ac.uk/learn/mentalhealth/bmyr3yr5/curriculum). Authors should bear in mind the 'so what?' question: why should a student bother to come to this web page rather than go to a wiki or a textbook?
- *Podcast.* Audio files are being produced by a number of clinical teachers and are well received by students (Agrawal, 2007). Capturing audio is a relatively straightforward technical process and once the audio file is uploaded to a site almost all students will be able to use it via their ubiquitous MP3 players and mobile phones. There are a number of factors to consider when planning podcasts. While it is desirable to have a local expert talking about a topic, it is probably even more important that whoever delivers the talk does so in an enthusiastic and engaging way, as if speaking to an audience in the room. Interviews may provide a more interesting product (Wilson *et al*, 2009). The content itself should cover the topic area succinctly; students are likely to be looking for concentrated information which will hold their attention in spite of the distractions around them as they listen.

The role of technology in assessment

Some say that knowledge is power, but for medical students knowledge is only one step on the path to success. It becomes useful when it allows them to do things, and to think about things in a different way. Once technology has been used to deliver information, students must be given the opportunity to check that they have understood it, to make use of it and to reflect on it – that is, to develop skills and attitudes. Clinical teachers are thoroughly used to testing and giving feedback in a formative way, for example by setting a task of clerking and presenting a case, and then grading students on their performance. In the same way, technology can help teachers to build testing within tasks in such a way that the testing seems natural, unintrusive and encouraging.

Specifying which bits of learning content are essential could appear to be a reductionist approach, but it is nevertheless essential for our patients, who will encounter many non-psychiatrist doctors in the course of their lives. If we are up-front about what is optional but interesting, we can still attract potential recruits to psychiatry while helping the majority to stay focused on core material. Specifying which part of the content is to be assessed is only fair, although you have to be sure this information is shared and agreed upon by those setting and undertaking assessments. Using computers to do the assessing should help ensure consistency.

Testing in this context is most likely to meet student needs if consideration is given to the following questions:

- Should each topic have an associated pre-test or post-test? Pre-tests reinforce the key learning outcomes for that topic as well as helping to expose the student's gaps in understanding. Where there are potentially many learning objectives to work through, students particularly value being allowed to 'skip' a topic if their performance on pre-testing is good enough.
- How are marks allocated? Students need to know in advance what each question is 'worth'. Since the assessment of a worthwhile e-learning module will contain different types of questions (it is important to avoid endless true/false lists, for example) and some questions will require careful judgements, it may be fairer to award scores of 1, 2 or 3 rather than the all-or-nothing score of 0 or 1. Where some questions are weighted more heavily than others, this should be made clear. It should also be stated at the outset whether a module can be retaken so as to improve the score.
- How do the test scores fit into the overall course assessment? Students think strategically – they are likely to approach each task differently depending on who will see their results and how they will be used.

Virtual cases and tutor-allocated tasks

E-learning tasks can take many forms. Your imagination is the only limit. The most common can be divided into two broad categories: virtual cases and tutor-allocated tasks. Table 6.2 lists some of the similarities and differences. Tutor-allocated tasks include the following kinds of activity.

- The tutor presenting a video-clip and instructing each student to work through associated questions. Once answers are submitted, the tutor may respond with further questions to clarify their answers, or with questions that elicit student attitudes.
- The tutor presents a media file or a document and give questions about the material to a number of small groups. Once all answers have been submitted, every group's questions and answers are published by the tutor for all groups to see.

Table 6.2 Virtual cases and tutor-allocated tasks: similarities and differences

	Virtual case	Tutor-allocated task
What is it?	A complex simulation of a clinical case which typically takes students 30 minutes or more to work through on their own. Once implemented, it remains in use for some years	The tutor presents clinical material which students use to answer set questions on their own or in groups. The material or the questions are changed for each subsequent student group
How does it work?	It leads the student through a case that has been designed to present specific clinical situations and to require clinical decisions to be made. The situation can change over time	It presents one or more clinical items for students to access and then requires them to submit a response by a specific deadline
Type of clinical material shown	Can include any combination of items that feature in everyday clinical experience, for example images, video of people interacting, reports to be read, or realistic documents to be completed	Can include any combination of items that feature in everyday clinical experience, for example images, video of people interacting, reports to be read, or realistic documents to be completed
Testing	Interspersed throughout the case, with a final score and summary comments displayed at the end	The quality of the student's final submission is scored by the tutor
Links to other sites	Can be technically difficult to 'pause' the virtual case so as to cross-link to other sites and then return the student to the case	Can be extensive. The tutor can present both clinical material and web links that students need to access in order to answer set questions

- The tutor asks students to produce a complex submission such as a patient information leaflet. The tutor presents relevant files or web addresses and sets tasks for small groups of students. Each group submits its work to a single coordinating group of students, which is tasked with putting the submissions together into a comprehensive final product.

What is happening around the UK and Ireland?

Medical schools should take advantage of new technologies to deliver teaching. (*Tomorrow's Doctors*, General Medical Council, 2003)

Different centres have come up with different approaches, often pioneering e-learning separately from the host institution, some now breaking out of password-protected environments to embody constructionist models of learning. This individualism of medical schools has in part been necessitated by the singular nature of medical courses, where much of the content is obligatory and, student-selected components aside, the student's progress has to be planned and evaluated over an entire 5-year course, in contrast to a standard degree, which can be constructed from discrete courses delivered by completely separate university faculties. Some examples from the UK and Ireland follow.

Sheffield

A pioneering unit and an energetic clinician produced a series of films on differential diagnosis in psychiatry showing a variety of 'patients' being interviewed. Still available through Athens, Educational Media Online (EDINA, 2011), the series was successful in generating income for other projects, but as they lack interaction such films are likely to be soporific if used for individual study.

Nottingham

In 2005, a course of 22 lectures was put online by taking existing Power-Point presentations and/or handouts and getting the lecturers to record voice-overs. This 'low-tech' option was chosen for pragmatic reasons and the programme only took 6 months to get up and running.

The online material is used as the 'core knowledge content' for the psychiatry course, which the students are expected to watch. This has made time for lecturers, senior lecturers and specialist registrars to run weekly teaching seminars to address the core skills of psychiatric history taking, the mental state examination and risk management, using summary lectures, patients, simulated patients, role-play and small-group work. Current developments include adding options for 'Keepad' interactive responses (via keypads) to the teaching to enhance the interactivity. The keypads can collect feedback on the course and generate a record of attendance.

The course is delivered through a password-protected learning management system (LMS), that is, software which both delivers materials and tracks its use by the students. Nottingham's so-called Network Learning Environment (NLE) was developed by faculty staff in 1999, making it one of the first medical schools in the country to have such a system. The university has suggested that the medical school move its material onto the commercial system called 'WebCT', as the university now has a site licence for this, but no one has come up with the money for the necessary conversion of the content. The NLE site contains a variety of materials for students in all their modules, psychiatry featuring the lecture course, information about the module, examinations and placements (contacts, joining instructions), formative knowledge tests and links to other resources. Interestingly, the medical school has also produced an online course to train examiners (specifically those for the observed structured clinical examinations), which has the useful by-product of generating kappa scores for each examiner cohort from their performance on test examples.

Newcastle

This pioneering department worked on projects under the Joint Information Systems Committee (JISC) of the Higher Education Academy (HEA) and more recently with funding from Open Educational Resources, to develop reusable e-learning objects. The basic content of the psychiatry course, hosted on the Newcastle University website (http://www.ncl.ac.uk/nnp/teaching/), is thus available to the public. It was developed under a 'creative commons' licence agreement, and so is free to all to use or modify, the only 'price' being acknowledgement and giving feedback on content together with information on its use.

Additional clinical material features video interviews of 'patients' provided by Role Play North, a professional organisation with pre-existing links to the whole university for teaching and examinations, and also using some staff members. A DVD featuring such 'long cases', and aspects of the mental state examination, have been given to the Malawi project (see Chapter 17) and have been used by both the Australian police and the US federal government for staff training.

The university recommends making materials free of conditions with open access as opposed to behind firewalls with password protection, in part because contributors can see what is already there and appreciate how widely their efforts might be used. As National Health Service computers usually block streaming of videos from the internet, the university plans to move away from fixed PC to mobile solutions in different formats (e.g. Real Media) with podcasts downloadable to smart phones, MP3 players and e-books. It has begun to host video-clips on the YouTube site (http://www.youtube.com/user/psychiatryteacher/) and plans to include pedagogical aspects by directing students to areas to observe and asking for responses.

Leeds

This psychiatric department took an early role in developing multimedia computer modules for students and has published guidelines on rating such packages (Williams & Harkin, 1999).

More recently, third-year projects offering student-selected compon-ents (SSCs) have involved various e-learning activities for and by the students – initially podcasts on psychopharmacology, materials on mental health competencies, and a training video on the use of electroconvulsive therapy (ECT). Students have also used the Articulate software program to add narration to a PowerPoint presentation on designing and running an observed structured clinical examination (OSCE), and produced a video on how to make podcasts, as a resource for future students to make their own e-learning materials.

The Higher Education Funding Council for England (HEFCE) has provided funding for centres for excellence in teaching and learning (CETL), one such CETL being Assessment and Learning in Practice Settings (ALPS; http://www.alps-cetl.ac.uk), a multidisciplinary education project. ALPS is piloting the use of mobile technology in clinical settings, for learning and assessment, and the University of Leeds is an ALPS partner.

With funding from the strategic health authority and assistance from the local ALPS team, documents and podcasts on psychiatry have been available to download to 'smart phones' for 'just-in-time' learning. Fourth-year undergraduate psychiatry students are issued with a device during their attachment. Using these machines in clinical settings makes information governance an important consideration, and so students are required to sign a specific contract regarding confidentiality. The mobile device project is run through its own website, which has other psychiatry resources. A section for multi-source feedback is password protected. All basic slides for the psychiatry course are available online, and there are plans to add voice-overs, and more podcasts, such as a guide to history taking. There are also plans to use the e-portfolio and site for collecting multi-source feedback for students.

Edinburgh

A password-protected website, the Edinburgh Electronic Curriculum (EEMec), has been developed for medical students, which has timetables, course outlines, academic discussion forums for specific courses, and sites for individual students' portfolio cases for storage; it also allows staff access to students' online submissions (for marking) and has links to resources within (e.g. a student drug formulary) and outwith the site. The specific psychiatric content consists of the course study guide, including summaries and multiple-choice questions (MCQs) for the lecture programme, and case-based multimedia modules on the topic of alcohol use and misuse, used to integrate basic science, diagnosis, pharmacology and the use of mental health legislation (Hare et al, 2007). These modules are not available to the public but three examples of the interactive elements are (see http://www.lts.mvm.ed.ac.uk/article/04_10_2010/labyrinth). The virtual learning platform has also been used internationally, joining students from the Gifu medical school in Japan to collaborate in a problem-based learning project on the genetics of phenylketonuria (Evans et al, 2008). There are plans to use Labyrinth, a web-based e-learning content creation tool developed by the e-learning Technology Section in the College of Medicine and Veterinary Medicine at Edinburgh, whereby students together with IT and clinical staff can produce simulated psychiatry cases with multiple assessment and treatment paths with different outcomes.

Dublin

University College Dublin has evaluated the use of IT to enhance e-learning, by making the text of lectures available online for students to access before they are delivered. Guerandel *et al* (2003) found this was popular with the students and attendance did not appear to be affected.

Trinity College has produced an unique online video-system, Virtual Interviews for Students Interacting Online (VISIOn), where students can ask questions from a list of options; because differing responses are elicited, students can explore the history and mental state (Fitzmaurice *et al*, 2007). This project was made possible by funding from a pharmaceutical company, which uses the material for its staff training. Access is password protected. Current topics include depression, mania, schizophrenia, medication concordance and smoking cessation. Trinity College has allowed the University of Stellenbosch to use the system to write its own interviews, and the two institutions share one another's products. Trinity College has sold the intellectual property of the system to a campus company, called Aspire. This enables other practitioners to use the Aspire software for writing, integrating and editing content and to personalise the interviews for other healthcare professions, a recent example being to create video answers to 'frequently asked questions' for a website aimed at reducing student examination stress.

Southampton

Teaching clinicians wanted to change of the university's psychiatry web pages fundamentally. Content had grown organically over the years, with the result that material was difficult to find and sometimes out of date. The new concept was of a 'mental health portal', through which all students would enter and be able to find material easily. The e-learning materials would be designed to cater for a variety of learning styles and would be accessible to students in all years of the course. Funding was obtained from the International Virtual Medical School Project (IVIMEDS) and from the local strategic health authority.

The most significant components within the portal include virtual cases (see for example http://www.som.soton.ac.uk/learn/virtualpatient/no_ database/depression), a compendium of video-clips illustrating symptoms and signs, core curriculum topic material presenting the scientific knowledge base of psychiatry in a visually appealing form, and a forum for staff–student interaction.

The unique value of the portal is that there is strong interlinking and cross-referencing between the components, which allows students to experience clinical topics from a variety of perspectives and in a range of complementary styles.

How to get an e-learning project started

Many clinical teachers will have been involved in service developments and will therefore be familiar with the basic processes (often common sense) of project management. In addition to those familiar processes, it is worth investing some time and effort in the following activities.

Work through your initial ideas

- Look at what other universities and institutions are providing. Have a go with their modules and get a feel for what works well and what does not.
- Take a critical look at your own institution's e-learning modules. How successful are they? Are students using them? Does the material reflect the preferences of your local developers? (Are some topics covered in detail, while others are not covered at all?)
- Review your own students' curriculum. Your e-learning project stands the best chance of success if it prioritises core subjects which students know they have to master.
- Find some allies. One clinical teacher on his or her own is unlikely to make much headway, but a small group is likely to reach a sensible consensus on what is needed and will more likely be listened to by management.

Whom should I speak to?

- There will be people who can help you to develop and evaluate e-learning materials. You will need the advice and support of academics to help keep you focused on the educational principles that should underpin everything you develop. Your institution's librarian can be an extremely helpful (and often overlooked) ally.
- Students tend to have clear ideas about what they want from e-learning and what they dislike. You will need their help at various points, for example as performers when you record video-clips and later on when you are testing your materials.
- Course organisers should be able to help you to align learning materials as closely as possible with the curriculum. You will need their agreement at the outset regarding how e-learning is to fit into the course timetable.
- Your project will go nowhere unless the local IT department is willing to program the material you devise, and host that material on servers that students can access. It will shape from the outset what your

learning materials will look like, by estimating how easy or difficult (i.e. expensive) your ideas will be to implement.

- University and National Health Service legal advisers will clarify what needs to be included in your recording consent forms. They can also provide useful advice on how to acknowledge rights and protect the confidentiality of volunteers and patients.
- Having done some reading and looked at other people's e-learning projects, you will quickly get a sense of who is already involved in e-learning. You might approach them for some down-to-earth advice and encouragement.
- Finally, you should make every effort to enthuse university authorities. When they have to make hard decisions about academic resources, you do not want them to be pulling staff and funding away. Similarly, clinical teachers should make their trust's medical director and senior management aware of the project.

Open or restricted access?

You will need to agree on this important principle at an early stage in your project because it will have major implications for how the university can help you. Most universities will expect to host material on their password-protected site, which obviously restricts your ability to show colleagues elsewhere what you are constructing. They may also have agreements in place to share completed learning materials with partners. You should at least agree with your institution how non-members can be given limited access to see and comment on the work in progress, and you need to establish who will own the intellectual property rights to the e-learning materials you are constructing.

Drafting a proposal or bid

Many clinical teachers will already have experience of this. There will be at least two important considerations: whom to approach for funding, and what to write.

- *Sources of funding*. The local head of department of psychiatry may be a helpful source of advice on sources of funding. Failing this, it is worth approaching the school of medicine or even the university, as either may have dedicated e-learning development budgets, and be looking for suitable bidders. If local resources are not available, consider national bodies. In the UK you might consider approaching the Higher Education Academy (or its Joint Information Systems Committee – JISC) or educational charities.
- *Writing the proposal*. As with any proposal, you will need to be clear about what you are going to deliver, when and why it has to be done in this particular way. Given the general air of scepticism about IT

projects, you will need to work even harder to ensure the proposal is credible. You will need funding both for staff time and for equipment. Most e-learning projects consume much more time than had been anticipated, so do not underestimate staffing costs but be prepared to account for those hours very closely. A project end date will have to be stated and a timeline drafted. The proposal will be particularly impressive if you include your analysis of potential risks to the project and how you will manage those risks. If you are submitting a bid using a prescribed form, stick to the bid instructions: it is like an examination, so answer the question, stick to the word limit and make it easy to read.

Assemble a project oversight group

As a minimum, you will need a project lead, one or more clinicians who will produce clinical material, and a representative from the institution's IT department. If at all possible, you should also look to recruit a student representative and a service user representative.

Decide which formats will deliver the e-learning outcomes

With the curriculum as your starting point, you will be able to identify the most important learning outcomes to be achieved. Only then should you start to think about what specific computerised learning materials should be created. One of the best-known in medicine is the virtual case. A good virtual case can achieve a wide range of outcomes, such as knowledge about a clinical condition, the clinical skills of assessing it, and making sense of the emotions evoked.

However, virtual cases can be difficult and time-consuming to develop. It may be possible to achieve the e-learning outcomes you need through a simpler format. Skills in assessment could be developed by showing footage of a patient and asking students to complete an online form, which could be scored or a model answer displayed. Empathy and professionalism can be developed by displaying a clinical situation and asking students to post their response to a forum, which the tutor can then moderate.

Storyboarding

If a module is going to consist of more than one or two web pages, it will need to be sketched out in a draft format that displays both the text and the images that should appear on screen. The purpose of doing this is to allow the rest of the project team, including academics and programmers, to understand what you want the student to experience and then to advise you on how to implement it in practice.

This is the stage at which you will decide on the style of the more complex learning materials, for example how the story in a virtual case will be told – some virtual cases are presented as character-driven stories (Hare *et al*, 2007), while some are presented as first person experiences told directly by the patient to the student (D'Alessandro *et al*, 2004).

Including self-assessment material in learning programmes

A real benefit of computerised learning is that students can check their understanding repeatedly, without it being anxiety provoking to themselves or the tutor. Effective e-learning materials are designed to ensure that wherever information is presented, there will be an opportunity to apply it, through testing or tasking. Questions that encourage reflection provide useful variety.

The following factors will need to be considered:

- Will the assessment be formative or summative? If formative, the model answer (or at least an explanation of why an answer was wrong) should be provided every time. If summative, ask only questions that can be answered from the content.
- What types of question should be used? True/false questions and 'one best answer' questions are fairly easy to devise and implement, but other types of question will provide variety and may provoke deeper thinking. Examples include 'Match the items in list A with the items in list B', 'Click on relevant objects in the still image' and 'Move the following features into the correct cluster'.
- Could an off-the-shelf or a bespoke quiz engine be used? There are many quiz software packages which can be plugged into an e-learning module. There will be a trade-off between the convenience they offer and the limitations they set on how you can present questions.

Keeping to production targets

Like it or not, management speak such as 'timelines' and 'deliverables' is going to crop up. As soon as the clinicians, programmers and advisers are in place, there must be an agreed project plan, even though it will inevitably be adjusted along the way. A Gantt chart, a type of histogram modified to include a timeline, may be helpful. In essence, you need to clarify who will complete what, and by when.

If you do not have the luxury of a project manager, the best way to keep the plan on track is to ensure that production targets are on the agenda for every meeting of the project oversight group. As with any worthwhile meeting, the combined expertise will throw up quick solutions for some of the problems.

Managing relationships

Any project reliant on technology and programming is capable of making the teaching clinician feel helpless at some point. And in turn, the technical team may think of clinicians as being slow and indecisive. It will be a very wise investment if you create opportunities for the various collaborators to meet and get to like each other before targets start to loom. It can be easy for programming teams to say 'no' for 'technical reasons'; you are more likely to hear 'we'll try' if they know you and like you.

Testing the product

Once the e-learning object is working, try it out on colleagues or even family members (they may welcome the chance to find out what you have been up to all this time). People who have already attempted similar projects may be happy to assist, particularly if you contacted them when you were doing the initial reconnaissance. Systematic peer review of e-learning materials will become very useful once there is a consensus on how to do it (Ruiz *et al*, 2007).

The most important evaluation will be with volunteer students. You should seek feedback from them on the following:

- *Utility*. Each screen needs to be assessed in terms of how easy it was to follow the text and graphics. Students need to comment on how easily they could navigate through the various screens.
- *Accuracy*. Is the material presented consistent with/complementary to what they have learned elsewhere on the course? Be alert to discrepancies and eliminate them because students will not be able to raise their hands to clarify details when the module goes into general use.
- *Effectiveness of learning*. Could the students identify an improvement in their knowledge or skills after they had completed the module?
- *Enjoyment*. If they did not feel excited or intrigued or happy, the module was not as effective as it could have been.

Planning for future modification

You are not going to get the e-learning materials right first time, because nobody does. The project oversight group needs to agree at the outset that feedback will have to happen – and therefore modification will have to happen.

You will be making changes after the initial student evaluation, but it is just as important to build in a capacity to make changes arising from routine student use during your course. The key factors that will drive later changes are:

- *Usage data*. If some materials do not get used much, why is that? If some elements of the module give students consistently low or high scores, why is that? The system that hosts your learning materials should be able to capture usage data every time a student logs on.

- *Student feedback*. Each element of the module must give clear instructions on how to submit a comment. 'Would you recommend this module to another student?' is a useful question to pose.

Research into e-learning in medical teaching

Collecting information about how students use e-learning materials is relatively easy, since it is possible to embed systems to collect data on who uses what and for how long, and to measure the difference between pre- and post-test scores. This information can also provide helpful feedback to students (Benjamin *et al*, 2006). Finding out how much *behaviour* has changed is a bit more relevant and harder to quantify.

How best to evaluate the impact of your e-learning depends on the audience. Those more scientifically inclined will expect quantitative data, while those from a purely educational background are perhaps more likely to understand that qualitative methods may be more relevant to measuring changes in skills and attitudes. A rapidly evolving discipline such as e-learning does not readily lend itself to double-blind randomised controlled trials, since there are so many confounding variables. For example, students may additionally use other material from the web (Trinder *et al*, 2008).

Another limiting factor is the difficulty of identifying meaningful outcomes. Students may report satisfaction and improved knowledge, but does that actually lead to changes in performance? Research into e-learning is still in its infancy. There is as yet no single model that can usefully compare the efficacy of different learning materials, or the comparative costing of electronic as opposed to traditional teaching methods (Krain *et al*, 2007). Research should perhaps first concentrate on evaluating the discrete component parts of learning materials, such as the optimal length of a video-clip. Continuous refinement may need to be a pragmatic compromise.

While currently the research base is weak, aspects of good design can be identified. So, decide what you want to teach, to whom and when. Keep the text concise and use images, audio-clips and interactions only to convey difficult material or to reinforce important elements. Ensure that students find the technology easy to use, and that they can see how they are progressing through the materials. The content should be interesting, relevant and progressively challenging. Reward the students for their efforts and give timely opportunities to put the lesson into practice.

Issenberg *et al* (2005) conducted a meta-analysis of studies that had evaluated the impact of medical simulations on learning outcomes. This revealed those key features of simulated cases that are likely to enhance success. In summary, simulated cases should (in order of importance):

- provide feedback
- allow repetitive practice of skills
- be integrated into the curriculum

- allow practice with increasing levels of difficulty
- be usable in a variety of teaching settings, from large-group teaching to individual use
- feature clinical variation by offering a range of cases and treatment responses
- provide a controlled environment so that teachers can pick up on student difficulties
- promote individualised learning, so that students can learn skills at different rates
- have absolutely clear learning outcomes
- feature tasks as close to everyday clinical practice as possible.

On the horizon

With the majority of medical students now using the internet (Sandars *et al*, 2008), the need for medical schools to provide courses on computer literacy may recede but should remain an option. As e-learning becomes mainstream, standards are being adopted to ensure materials are easy to use, accessible by users with various kinds of disability, and can be shared between systems.

The dichotomy of providing set courses or modules remains in tension with constructivist educational methods, where the students embrace the so-called 'web 2.0 phenomenon' of creating content, rather than just being passive recipients. These include discussion boards or blogs (web-logs, where students can comment on the course and pose problems which can be answered by students as well as staff), and wikis (collaborative websites which can be extended and edited by anyone who has access). Discussion boards need to be moderated to maintain quality and this activity is another skill the students can gain experience in. However, since not all students are keen to collaborate, recognition should be given that some can learn through viewing the discussion as 'lurkers' (Anagnostopoulou *et al*, 2008).

Lakhan & Jhunjhunwala (2008) have produced a review of the 'open source' movement in higher education, including useful information as to what resources are available. The so-called SCORM (Sharable Content Object Reference Model) standards have been developed by the US government to ensure the software systems and specifications used to create learning materials permit them to be exported and shared on the web (see http://www.adlnet.gov/Technologies/scorm/default.aspx). However, it seems likely that a mixed economy will prevail, with some institutions favouring open-access approaches, while others will look to the sale or licensing of access in order to recoup production costs and fund further developments.

Further developments might include the creation of 'serious games', where students can explore a virtual world in the role of a personalised avatar. Currently, such applications are resource greedy, in terms of both time taken for staff and students to learn the system and the high

Table 6.3 Risks and safeguards in the development of e-learning materials

Risk	Safeguard
Project runs out of time and people to do it	Get in touch with people who have developed similar learning materials to discuss the reality of what is required
Project is difficult for the institution's IT team to implement	Meet the technical team as early as possible with a clear plan of what the final product will have to look like
Learning materials duplicate what has been done elsewhere	Carry out a web search for publicly accessible sites that might hold the e-learning materials you need
Learning materials are dull	Make a conscious effort to engage students' emotions, for example by telling a great story, introducing surprise elements or encouraging reflection
Students see no reason to use the materials	Run your initial plans past a student focus group, and ensure that the learning modules are fully part of the timetable and included in assessment

specification of computers and bandwidth of connection required. In medical education such immersive simulations have been used to teach triage and teamwork in a simulated disaster zone (de Freitas, 2008). While working in a multidisciplinary team is an important aspect of psychiatry, patience and perseverance are arguably more necessary skills than making decisions against the clock. However, virtual worlds may prove useful in developing empathic interview skills through role-play, where the student can experience the effect that changing age, sex, race or acquiring a disability can have on their interactions.

Summary

This chapter has aimed to give the reader a sense of the ways in which e-learning can enrich the teaching of psychiatry, as well as to provide guidance on how to get such a project going. It is hoped that the possibilities offered by e-learning will inspire readers to 'have a go' themselves. However, the realistic reader will know that there must be traps and snares. Table 6.3 addresses some of the commonest risks, and suggests how the prudent teacher can safeguard against them. The e of e-learning should begin with education, include engagement, enthusiasm, enterprise, ever-present, evaluation, economic, experiential, equality and only lastly electronic.

References

Agrawal, V. (2007) Podcasts for psychiatrists: a new way of learning. *Psychiatric Bulletin*, **32**, 270–271.

Anagnostopoulou, K., Parmar, D. & Priego-Hernandez, J. (2008) *Managing Connections: Using e-Learning Tracking Information to Improve Retention Rates in Higher Education.* Available at http://mancons2.middlesex.wikispaces.net/file/view/Final+Report+(Anagnostopoulou,+Parmar+&+Priego-Hernandez,+2008).pdf

Benjamin, S., Robbins, L. I. & Kung, S. (2006) Online resources for assessment and evaluation. *Academic Psychiatry*, **30**, 498–504.

Brookfield, S. D. (1986) *Understanding and Facilitating Adult Learning.* Open University Press.

Chan, C. H. & Robbins, L. (2006) E-Learning systems: promises and pitfalls. *Academic Psychiatry*, **30**, 491–497.

D'Alessandro, D. M., Lewis, T. E. & D'Alessandro, M. P. (2004) A pediatric digital storytelling system for third year medical students: the virtual pediatric patient. *Biomedical Central Medical Education*, **4**, 10.

de Freitas, S. (2008) *Serious Virtual Worlds. A Scoping Document.* Joint Information Systems Committee (JISC). Available at http://www.jisc.ac.uk/media/documents/publications/seriousvirtualworldsv1.pdf

EDINA (2011) Film & Sound Online. JISC National Data Centre, Edinburgh University (http://www.filmandsound.ac.uk/?purl_key=isan&purl_id=0012-0000-1279-0000-0-0000-0000-0&message=continue_purl).

Evans, P., Suzuki, Y., Begg, M., *et al* (2008) Can medical students from two cultures learn effectively from a shared web-based learning environment? *Medical Education*, **42**, 27–33.

Fitzmaurice, B., Armstrong, K., Carroll, V., *et al* (2007) Virtual Interviews for Students Interacting Online for Psychiatry (VISIOn): a novel resource for learning clinical interview skills. *Psychiatric Bulletin*, **31**, 218–220.

Gaines, K. (2004) *701 e-Learning Tips* (ed E. Masie). The Masie Center. Available at (http://www.scribd.com/doc/3222398/701-eLearning-Tips).

General Medical Council (2003) *Tomorrow's Doctors* (2nd edn). GMC.

Guerandel, A., Felle, P. & Malone, K. (2003) Computer-assisted learning in undergraduate psychiatry (CAL-PSYCH): evaluation of a pilot programme. *Irish Journal of Psychological Medicine*, **20**, 84–87.

Hare, E. H., Evans, P., McIntosh, C. E., *et al* (2007) Case-based online e-learning for medical undergraduates. *Psychiatric Bulletin*, **31**, 73–75.

Issenberg, S. B., McGaghie, W. C., Petrusa, E. R., *et al* (2005) Features and uses of high-fidelity medical simulations that lead to effective e-learning: a BEME systematic review. Medical Teaching, **27**, 10–28.

Kirkpatrick, D. L. (1998) *Evaluating Training Programmes: The 4 Levels* (2nd edn). Berrett-Koehler.

Krain, L. P., Bostwick, M. & Sampson, S. (2007) 'It's high tech but is it better?' Applications of technology in psychiatry education. *Academic Psychiatry*, **31**, 40–49.

Lakhan, S. E. & Jhunjhunwala, K. (2008) Open source software. *EDUCAUSE Quarterly*, **31**(2). Available at http://www.educause.edu/EDUCAUSE+Quarterly/EDUCAUSEQuarterlyMagazineVolum/OpenSourceSoftwareinEducation/162873

Martin, V. L. & Bennet, D. S. (2004) Creation of a web-based lecture series for psychiatry clerkship: students' initial findings. *Academic Psychiatry*, **28**, 209–214.

Ruiz, J. G., Candler, C. & Teasdale, T. A. (2007) Peer-reviewing e-learning: opportunities, challenges and solutions. *Academic Medicine*, **82**, 502–507.

Sandars, J., Homer, M., Pell, G., *et al* (2008) Web 2.0 and social software: the medical student way of e-learning. *Medical Teaching*, **14**, 1–5.

Trinder, K., Guiller, J., Margaryan, A., *et al* (2008) *Learning from Digital Natives: Bridging Formal and Informal Learning. Research Project Report. Final Report.* The Higher Education Academy (http://www.academy.gcal.ac.uk/ldn/LDNFinalReport.pdf).

Williams, C. & Harkin, P. (1999) Multimedia computer-based learning: a developing role in teaching, CPD and patient care. *Advances in Psychiatric Treatment*, **5**, 390–394.

Wilson, P., Petticrew, M. & Booth, A. (2009) After the gold rush? A systematic and critical review of general medical podcasts. *Journal of the Royal Society Medicine*, **102**, 69–74.

CHAPTER 7

How to give a lecture

Nisha Dogra

Introduction

There can be a tendency to assume that formal lectures have little function in education today. However, they remain an effective teaching tool, if used in the right context. Lectures are a teaching strategy that we can easily learn to do well, but it is also easy to deliver them badly. In the past, it often seemed that doctors were all expected to be able to lecture, in one context or another. The professionalisation of medical education has changed this, but the lecture remains a key teaching method.

In this chapter, I will take a very practical approach, in large part informed by Reece & Walker (2000), Minton (1997) and Sullivan & McIntosh (1996), three sources that have helped me to develop my own lecturing style. The chapter begins with a brief consideration of why lectures continue to be used. It then moves on to consider how a lecturer can best prepare and deliver a lecture. Because a degree of interactivity can enhance a lecture, suggestions are made for how lecturers can make their own teaching more interactive. The chapter also discusses some common problems and possible solutions before it outlines some techniques for continuing professional development.

First, spend a little time on the exercise presented in Box 7.1.

Box 7.1 A reflective exercise on lecturing

Think of good and bad lectures you have attended. Now reflect on what, from your perspective, made them that way. Then:

- Make a list of the characteristics of a good lecturer.
- Make a list of features of a good lecture.

Lectures as an effective teaching technique

For the purposes of this chapter, a lecture is considered to be a formal presentation to an audience of 50 students or more. If the student number is less than 50, it is much easier to incorporate features of small-group teaching (see Chapter 8) and to minimise the disadvantages of the lecture methods. The audience number will usually dictate the venue. A traditional lecture theatre is not conducive to interaction between students and the focus is largely on the lecturer.

The lecture is still the method most commonly used to impart key basic knowledge to students in medical education. It may now be considered unfashionable but that does not reduce its value. Box 7.2 lists the principal benefits of the lecture. Price & Mitchell (1993) discussed improving lectures through the use of interactive techniques (discussed below) such as questioning, demonstrating and reviewing. Case reports and problem-solving exercises are also effective ways of engaging learners.

There is considerable debate about the optimal length of a lecture. However, often those delivering lectures do not have the power to set the time, and lengths can vary from a few minutes to over 90 minutes. In my experience lectures over 1 hour without a break rarely engage the audience. Attention spans of even the most enthusiastic do not last that long. Group size will also limit the interaction with the lecturer, but that does not mean interaction has to be limited. Box 7.3 lists the principal limitations to the use of lectures and Box 7.4 specific difficulties that can be encountered.

Costa *et al* (2007) found that while lectures were rated equally with interactive discussion groups for content, students preferred the latter and also performed better at the end-of-placement examination. However, the differences were small and, as the authors point out, they did not examine cost-effectiveness. Increasing technological advances now enable many universities to post video lectures. Cardall *et al* (2008) in the USA

Box 7.2 The benefits of lectures

- Lectures remain the most effective method for delivering low-level learning of the 'cognitive skills' type, that is, giving basic information rather than synthesis or evaluation.
- They enable dissemination of information quickly to large audiences.
- They provide an overview and/or the context or framework for other activities (for example, using a lecture to lay the foundation for a topic before having small-group work to build on this learning).
- They can encourage students to want to learn more by arousing their curiosity.
- The teacher has control over the direction of the teaching.

> **Box 7.3** When lectures are not the right approach
>
> Lectures are not the right method to deliver information to students when:
>
> - learning outcomes relate to students' attitudes or feelings
> - teaching psychomotor skills (students need to be able to practise these)
> - the aim is to impart high-level cognitive skills such as evaluation
> - a large quantity of detailed information is to be given (if given in a lecture, much of the information is unlikely to be retained).

> **Box 7.4** Difficulties with lectures
>
> - Communication is largely in one direction, from teacher to student.
> - There is little or no feedback regarding the effectiveness of the learning.
> - Students may adopt very passive roles and be disengaged.

found that students felt they were more likely to increase their speed of knowledge acquisition, look up additional information, stay focused and learn more when using accelerated video-recorded lectures compared with live lectures. An accelerated lecture is one that students watch at their own pace, from normal speed to two-and-a-half times the normal speed. While students cited the benefits of a live lecture as talking with the lecturer, asking questions and learning from others asking questions, these perceived benefits were not frequently applied. Whether the perceived increased learning from recorded lectures actually occurred was not verified.

First considerations

Effective teaching depends on effective preparation. When you are invited to give a lecture, there are important issues to clarify, such as the time you have, the audience and the context. Are the learning outcomes for you to set or are there predefined outcomes?

It is important to familiarise yourself with students' previous learning associated with the subject on which you are teaching. If it is some time since they previously covered important issues and you plan to revisit them, let students know the purpose of your including them.

Use the lecture as a means of hooking students and encouraging them to learn more, rather than seeing it as a way of covering everything about the subject in an hour or so.

Structuring your lecture

A single lecture or a series of lectures?

Preparation will need to take account of whether you are delivering a series of lectures or a single lecture (if the latter, it may still be one of a series, given by a variety of lecturers). One-off lectures as learning experiences have limited efficacy but can stimulate interest.

Pacing and pausing

The attention span of most people is 15–20 minutes, so incorporate appropriately spaced summaries, in case they drift off at a crucial point. Pausing is an effective way of allowing the students to catch up and refocus. Pausing and summarising are also strategies to ensure that the lecture has a clear structure.

Introduction

Give students a guide as to what to expect, and signpost as you move from one topic to another. Provide a clear context and be explicit about the relevance of the teaching to their needs; highlight the learning expected.

Main body

'Less is more', so avoid giving students too much information that they can get from any textbook. Use the contact time to highlight key issues and focus on the principles rather than the detail.

Summary

Recap the main points. Do not introduce new material at the summary stage.

Questions

Leave time for questions, even if only a few minutes (see below).

Preparing your materials

Preparation is key to a good lecture. It is easy for the audience to tell whether the lecturer has spent enough time preparing. The less experienced you are, the more time preparation takes, but experience does not render preparation unnecessary.

> **Box 7.5** The use of slides in lectures: guidelines and pitfalls
>
> - Keep your slides simple.
> - Just because you can spin words on to the slide does not mean you should.
> - Use animation sparingly.
> - Use a font that is easily read (such as Arial, which does not have serifs). If you have to use a small text size, you have too much material on one slide.
> - Use a colour scheme that offers good contrast.

Slides

Some people suggest that you are better off not using slides in lectures, as they allow you to fall into too many traps. I would argue that awareness of the potential pitfalls allows you to deal with them (Box 7.5). Few of us will be such charismatic speakers that we can hold an audience for 45–60 minutes without the use of some audiovisual aids. The purpose of slides is to provide a guide to the audience and an aide memoir to the lecturer. Slides do not require full sentences.

It is important to ensure the number of slides and their contents fit the time allocated. Do not have one long presentation and hope that you can adapt it to fit the time 'on the hoof'. This rarely works and often just ends up losing the audience. Skipping though irrelevant slides indicates poor preparation and disrespect for the audience. However, if you have mistimed your talk and are running out of time, it is preferable to skip over non-essential slides than to run over time. Handouts can provide further details if necessary.

If during the lecture you need to refer back to an earlier slide, copy the slide rather than flick back and forth, as the chances are that, under pressure, you will find it difficult to locate the right slide and you are likely to waste time and to risk losing the audience.

Handouts

It can be disadvantageous to distribute handouts before the presentation, as students may not attend the actual lecture. I personally do not mind this, as I see them as adults who need to be able to make decisions about their own learning. It can be useful for students to have the handouts so they can follow the lectures, but many may read it and then 'rest easy'. However, other learners will be more engaged in the learning, knowing they do not have to take notes and that they can really listen.

Handouts can be a very effective way of engaging students and making the learning more interactive. Activities such as students having to complete lists where a stem is provided or where they have to annotate a diagram or fill in missing words may enliven the lecture process.

Charlton (2006) argues against the use of handouts, as he feels note taking by the students themselves ensures they process the information actively. However, if handouts are used in the ways suggested above, they can help students learn. It is likely that students who learn by writing their own notes will do so irrespective of whether a handout is provided or not.

Using CDs/DVDs

If you wish to use excerpts from a longer film or presentation, it is usually advisable to copy them onto a separate CD/DVD. Waiting for lecturers to find the right point at which to play a DVD is frustrating and can ruin the momentum. It is probably not the best idea to try some fancy complex visual presentation for the first time in front of a large audience. It is worth considering a fallback position in case the technology lets you down.

Questions

Before the lecture, spend a little time thinking about the questions you might ask the audience and also questions they might ask you. If they have had to undertake some preparation for the session, it may be worth checking out what they made of the work they had to do.

Rehearsing the lecture

Early on in your career, and later perhaps for just the more important ones, rehearse your lectures. This helps to build confidence and provides an opportunity to get feedback from supportive colleagues. If I am lecturing on something that might be difficult, I will usually get a colleague to cast an eye over my presentation. This can also be useful when you are presenting a subject on which you are passionate, as a first draft may be more about you than about the needs of the learner.

Delivering the lecture

It sounds obvious, but do go to the bathroom and have a drink of water before the lecture. If you are uncomfortable it will show and may minimise your impact. Arrive on time at the very least but early if you are not familiar with the venue. Appear confident and, as some would say, 'fake it if you have to'. A nervous or anxious speaker does not inspire confidence. Make sure you know how the audiovisuals work or have enough time to find out. Survey the room and remove any distractions such as materials from a previous teaching session.

Box 7.6 Delivering the lecture: some 'do's and 'don't's

Do:

- speak with conviction and commitment
- speak clearly
- make good eye contact across the room
- relate the contents of the lecture to student needs
- keep to time.

Don't:

- read from notes or read out the slides verbatim.
- try to cover too much.

The old adage of 'tell them what you are going to tell them, tell them and then tell them what you have just told them' is still an effective strategy. Box 7.6 outlines some basic points relating to the delivery of the lecture.

First impressions count for a lot, so the introduction to the lecture– the first few minutes – warrants a special mention here. Some lecturers use quotes, anecdotes or jokes to engage with the audience (discussed more under 'Use of the self' below), but be careful with using strategies that are at odds with your personality. The first few minutes can be a very useful time to obtain clarity about where the students are with their learning and then to indicate how the lecture builds on that.

Making a lecture interactive and engaging

Evidence on the effectiveness of interactive lectures

There is limited evidence in this area about lectures specifically. However, we do know that most adults learn better when they can interact with the teaching. Nonetheless, Huxham (2005) cites some concerns about using interactive techniques in lectures:

- reduction in content (in practice this may be positive, as most lectures cover too much)
- student resistance to the style
- the teacher may lose control if peer discussions take over
- loss of teaching time as shifts are made between different teaching styles.

Huxham then argues that these can be overcome and actually most students can be persuaded that engaging in the learning is in their interest.

Use of the self

Verbal communication is clearly the basis of almost any lecture, but it can be reinforced with effective and positive non-verbal communication. Simple things such as looking interested in the audience can make a difference, as can looking as though you actually want to be there. Using eye contact to gauge responses is a very useful way of obtaining feedback on whether you are pitching your talk at the right level. Avoid gazing at one member of the audience, though, and cover all areas of the room.

Humour can be effective but risqué jokes may be deemed inappropriate. It is worth developing your own style by watching many others and using the techniques that fit with your personality. Clinical examples and anecdotes can bring theory and facts to life, and as you have a wealth of clinical experience that is usually a great way of engaging students as future doctors.

If you are giving a personal perspective, particularly one that challenges certain contexts, be explicit about that. This can be an excellent way of modelling good practice but it is poor practice to pass off personal perspectives as evidence.

The use of questions

Questions are an excellent way of engaging others. In lectures, the time constraints, audience size and the context can make it difficult to engage for any length of time with students, but it can happen. Asking students to write down their answer to a question tends to improve their level of attention and can engage them; it is also less time consuming than having a discussion.

Questions are a useful means of checking whether students have understood what you have told them. Getting them to raise their hands to indicate learning can provide quick and effective feedback.

It is worth repeating students' questions as the audience may not have heard them and questions are sometimes imprecise. Keep your answers brief and to the point. Depending on time constraints, rather than answer the question yourself, you might want to throw it open to the audience. Again, if it is about something you have covered, it is an excellent way of getting relatively quick feedback about how you have communicated a concept or idea.

Enhancing interaction

A simple and effective technique is to ask a question, get students to call out the answers, and ask one of them to write up. This makes the teaching a more shared experience and also recognises that students are able to contribute to their own learning.

Making it relevant

Be explicit about the links between the taught material and students' future clinical practice.

Audiovisual aids

Ensure that the audiovisual aids help to deliver the material you want to get across rather than distract from it. If you feel you need more than one slide at the same time, consider having other aids, such as flip charts or white boards.

Handling difficult situations

Difficult students

Some students can at times be surprisingly rude and disrespectful. It is not uncommon to find some trying to talk throughout your lecture or passing notes to each other. When an examination is looming, some may be sitting in your lecture with textbooks relating to other subjects open beside them. It is tempting to be sarcastic and/or rude to deal with your frustrations but this should be avoided.

It is not unreasonable to expect students to turn off their mobile phones but it is also reasonable then that yours does not ring during the lecture (unless of course you are on call, in which case let students know – is there any better example of the reality of being a doctor?).

Some students may not grasp what you are teaching and persist in asking questions. You should try to address their concerns but remember that they are not the only ones in the audience; if they continue to struggle, ask them to see you after the lecture. It is, though, worth checking whether other students are struggling, because this may be an indication that you need to modify the level of your lecture for the audience as a whole.

Hostile questions may come from defensive students, especially in psychiatry. You should try to avoid getting defensive yourself, as that only weakens your position.

Even after over 20 years in practice, if I do not know the answer to a question I will happily admit I do not know. If I think I should know, I will add that I should. This is unlikely to happen when teaching medical students but it is worth being prepared for it should it happen. If you do not understand the question, ask for it to be repeated.

Audiovisual aids fail to work

After the initial panic, remember you do know what you are talking about and the aids are just that – aids. They are not the lecture.

Being asked to lecture on a subject of little interest to you

There is no doubt that this is a challenge and one that you may not be able to avoid. However, it can be useful to consider this as an opportunity to really think about what the audience needs to know. Sometimes not being an expert is useful, as you may prepare more effectively.

The timing of the lecture

It may be that the lecture slot you get is at the end of the day, when students have sat through too much other teaching. It can be useful to acknowledge that they might be tired (as you might be, too). Some lecturers use physical exercises such as star jumps and the like to awaken the students. I personally have always cringed at such techniques, but if you are comfortable using them and can make them work, use them. It can be frustrating if there are few students left but it is unfair to give them a hard time – after all, they are the ones who stayed to attend!

Being unable to deliver the lecture

It is absolutely unacceptable for a lecturer simply to fail to turn up. It is unprofessional and a poor example to set students. If for any reason you cannot honour your commitment, make sure the students are informed. Sickness may prevent you from being in a position to say how you will remedy the situation, but, as soon as you can, get in touch with the students and let them know how they can access the teaching you would have delivered. If you are going to be late, let students know – most of them will understand that clinical responsibilities can get in the way.

Having a bad day

We all have bad days. Sometimes you can deliver a lecture and, despite your best efforts, the audience and you just do not connect. It is important not to let that put you off future lecturing. After the initial disappointment has worn off, reflect on what might have happened. If there are learning points, then take those on board, but do not beat yourself up over it. Effective preparation usually reduces the likelihood of a lecture going badly but it will happen to most of us. Without becoming unduly negative, it may focus your attention on ways in which your lecturing could be improved, as mentioned below.

Developing and improving your lectures

Giving lectures can be improved with practice, but then you can hit a plateau. I try to avoid giving the same lecture more than three times. It is easy to get lazy, especially when there are other demands on your time.

Student feedback

It can be useful to ask for student feedback. Formal evaluations may not always be available, as students can be overwhelmed with the number of evaluations now requested from them. However, teachers often do not receive the feedback for their teaching. I have always been fairly open with students and, as well as any formal evaluations, I try to get informal feedback after the teaching. If I am trying a new technique, I am honest with students and say that I really need to know their experience of it, because if it does not work I would stop using it. I have found that students in these situations often give constructive and honest feedback, as they value your commitment to their education.

Peer or senior colleague feedback

This can be a very useful way of developing your lecturing skills. General feedback can be uninformative and your colleague should be specific about good and bad points, so that weaknesses can be constructively addressed.

Filming teaching

Video feedback can augment peer observation. The first time you watch yourself giving a lecture can be painful. It is worth remembering that you probably had a similar experience with clinical interviewing, but practice made you better and that happens with teaching too. Watching yourself is a powerful way of picking up on mannerisms that can be annoying from an audience's perspective. Directly visualising your strengths and limitations allows you to use the former and to work on the latter.

Summary

- The lecture enables the delivery of key principles or the opportunity to provide an overview to a large audience.
- Ensure that the *context* of the lecture is declared at the beginning.
- Large numbers may make it difficult to engage with the audience and to be clear about their needs.
- When agreeing to a lecture, establish whom it is for and what the context is. Ensure you make adequate connections to existing knowledge.
- Have a clear and logical structure, which you share with the audience.
- Do not try to cover too much – 'less is more'. Use a variety of presentational techniques, such as overheads, slides, video.
- Use a variety of techniques to increase audience participation (e.g. questions, buzz groups, interactive handouts, questionnaires, multiple-choice questions).

- Keep the audience thinking and if possible ask challenging questions, even if they are rhetorical.
- Have a beginning (tell them what you are going to tell them), a middle (tell them what you want to tell them) and an end (tell them what you have told them).
- Always leave adequate time for questions and then a summary.

References

Cardall, S., Krupat. E. & Ulrich, M. (2008) Live lectures versus video-recorded lectures: are students voting with their feet? *Academic Medicine*, **83**, 1174–1178.

Charlton, B. G. (2006) Lectures are an effective teaching method because they exploit human evolved 'human nature' to improve learning. *Medical Hypotheses*, **67**, 1261–1265.

Costa, M. L., van Rensburg, L. & Rushton, N. (2007) Does teaching style matter? A randomised trial of group discussion versus lectures in orthopaedic undergraduate teaching. *Medical Education*, **41**, 214–217.

Huxham, M. (2005) Learning in lectures: do interactive windows help? *Active Learning in Higher Education*, **6**, 17–31.

Minton, D. (1997) *Teaching Skills in Further and Adult Education* (revised 2nd edn). Macmillan.

Price, D. A. & Mitchell, C. A. (1993) A model for clinical teaching and learning. *Medical Education*, **27**, 62–68.

Reece, I. & Walker, S. (2000) *A Practical Guide to Teaching, Training and Learning* (4th edn). Business Education Publishers.

Sullivan, R. & McIntosh, N. (1996) *Delivering Effective Lectures*. JHPIEGO Strategy. Available at http://www.reproline.jhu.edu/english/6read/6training/lecture/delivering_lecture.htm

CHAPTER 8

How to do small-group teaching

Nisha Dogra & Khalid Karim

Introduction

In this chapter we begin by defining small-group teaching. We review the strengths and limitations of various types of small-group teaching before considering when it is an appropriate teaching strategy. Practical tips follow on how to prepare for such teaching. As small-group teaching can be quite difficult, we discuss issues and challenges that might arise and how these might be addressed.

First, though, spend a little time on the exercise presented in Box 8.1.

Box 8.1 A reflective exercise on small-group teaching

Consider the last learning event that you attended that had small-group learning as a strategy.

- How effectively was this managed by the facilitator?
- What were the strengths of the facilitator?
- What would have helped the session to run better?

What is small-group teaching?

Small-group teaching is a generic term that can be used to mean tutorials, seminars, discussion and problem-based learning (PBL) groups, or workshops. For the purposes of this chapter, small-group teaching is defined as teaching that aims to promote student learning through working with peers and a facilitator. The most common types of small-group teaching format are outlined on the following page.

Tutorials

Students are set a task or assignment and the tutorial is a mechanism for providing them with support to meet that task. In teaching undergraduate medical students, for example, this might be a format used for helping them prepare their clinical portfolios.

Seminars

Students research a topic and present their findings to their peers, with more learning from the ensuing group discussion. Seminars therefore tend to be led by the learners, but the context and preparation need to be clearly identified. A suitable topic for an undergraduate seminar might be the use of antidepressants.

Participation is to be encouraged. Once one student has presented the topic, the others might want to ask questions or share their experiences. The facilitator can clarify and add to the students' learning. If students are not experienced, their presentations can be lengthy and/or poorly prepared, so the facilitator needs to monitor this carefully. At the end of the seminar, the facilitator or a student assigned the role should summarise the learning.

Discussion groups

The students discuss a specific issue with specific learning tasks, for example how to manage a particular disorder or situation. This format is very useful when you want students to explore their own attitudes, but requires careful and sensitive facilitation. Discussion groups can readily lose focus and it can be a lengthy process to hear the perspectives of all students.

Problem-based learning (PBL) groups

In PBL curricula, these are a pivotal method of learning. There are usually some supplementary lectures but most of the learning is through group work. PBL is discussed in Chapter 9.

Workshops

Students have an opportunity to develop skills in a simulated situation and to link theory with practice.

When is small-group teaching appropriate?

The primary purpose of small-group teaching is not to impart facts, key concepts or principles but to help students analyse, evaluate and critique their learning and understanding. Small-group teaching can also be an excellent opportunity for students to explore their attitudes in a safe environment and to practise the application of their learning.

Entwistle *et al* (1992) suggested that the goal of small-group teaching should be to develop the following in students:

- higher cognitive understanding, by building on key principles
- key competencies
- effective communication skills
- particular personal qualities
- independence
- group management skills.

Size of the small group

The numbers in a 'small' group can vary from 4 to 60! Realistically, the most effective group size is 8–12 students, as this prevents quiet students from 'hiding' but enables the tutor to manage the group and direct the learning. Small-group teaching for more students needs very careful planning. In such circumstances it helps to consider all that needs to be covered and to divide the tasks between subgroups. This ensures that students actively listen to each other, as they are aware they are not covering all of the material. It also prevents feedback from becoming too repetitive. Jaques (2003) and Reece & Walker (2000) provide an overview of other techniques that can be used.

Strategies for small-group teaching

Brainstorming

This is a problem-solving technique used to generate a number of ideas or solutions very quickly – usually in just a few minutes. It is often used to generate as many ideas as possible, only some of which are thereafter given more detailed attention. It can be a useful warm-up exercise and allows freedom to 'think outside the box', thereby encouraging creativity.

Group round (round robin)

Each person has a short period of time to say something in turn to the whole group. The direction round the group can be decided by the first speaker or the facilitator. Jaques (2003) argues that more interest is usually generated if the first person chooses who should go second, the second who goes third and so on. This is less likely to be successful where members of the group are not familiar with each other.

Buzz groups

Students are asked to turn to their neighbour and discuss an issue or problem. This is good at ensuring everyone has an opportunity to express an opinion and also enables sharing of perspectives that may be difficult with a larger audience. This can be an effective method for developing listening and communication skills, as students can be asked to relay back what their partner said.

Snowballing

Snowball groups (also sometimes called pyramid groups) are an extension of buzz groups. The discussion work begins in pairs, and two pairs then become a four, four become eight and the eight share to the group as a whole. In this way the group's learning from each other increases in a staged way. However, it is important to keep the group task focused and to prevent too much repetition, for example by building in layers of complexity as the group size increases.

Fishbowls

The usual configuration has an inner group discussing an issue or topic while the outer group listens with a specific task in mind, for example to identify key themes raised, or issues not raised. If the inner group was role-playing, the outer group may provide structured feedback on specific topics, such as communication skills.

Crossover groups

Students are divided into an initial set of subgroups, and then are shuffled around into different subgroups; learning from the previous subgroup is then shared with the new subgroup. Keeping tabs on this kind of activity can be difficult if there are many students and the facilities are limited. It can be useful to give students a number or colour and to ask the 1s or reds to move, to ensure smoother movement between group formations.

Role-plays

Role-play is often done in triads, for example one student playing the patient, another the doctor and a third acting as an observer. The observer usually provides specific feedback. This is very useful way of helping students to gain different perspectives but it does require the facilitator to move between groups to ensure effective learning. There needs to be clarity about the observer role to maximise the learning.

Specific tasks for subgroups

Subgroups work on specific tasks which they then feed back to the larger group. For example, one group might consider the biological aetiological factors in a particular case, a second group the psychological factors and a third group the social factors. In this way more material can be covered. It also encourages student engagement and attentiveness to each other.

It can be helpful to focus discussion by asking students to write key points on a flip chart to present their outcomes to their peers or for the flip charts to be displayed and students to view them. A discussion of what they have seen can then take place as a way of giving the learning context and relevance.

The role of the facilitator

The London Deanery (2009) outlined the three main tasks that the small-group facilitator has to manage simultaneously:

- the group and the dynamics within it
- the activities
- the learning that takes place.

Exley & Dennick (2004) summarised the specific roles of the facilitator as:

- ensuring the objectives are achieved
- finding meaning in the experience and actions of the group
- confronting resistance and task avoidance
- acknowledging feelings within the group
- providing structure through discussion and activities
- valuing autonomy and individual needs but also understanding the group dynamics.

To coordinate the students' learning, the facilitator during any session may need to act as one or more of the following (London Deanery, 2009):

- an *instructor*, who provides information that students can build on or information about the tasks to be undertaken
- *chair* of the session, who ensures different perspectives are given space (it is important to retain neutrality in a discussion and for students to lead the debate)
- an *expert adviser*, who clarifies student understanding as issues are raised through discussion
- *leader* of the discussion, especially for difficult or sensitive subjects
- *devil's advocate*, who challenges the students (which may be especially important if the students are comfortable with each other and have accepted positions that are no longer challenged)

101

- a *commentator*, who summarises the learning or comments on the process
- a *supporter* of the discussion, who moves between subgroups (especially important if the group is large)
- a *role-model* to the students
- the *timekeeper*.

Preparing for small-group teaching

For many teachers, the outcomes and contents of small-group sessions will be predefined. However, even if this is the case it is still worth reviewing them with the students to ensure there is a shared understanding and that, as a teacher, you do not make assumptions about their knowledge base.

It is more difficult to predict exactly what will happen in a small-group session than in a lecture, for example, and so can be more anxiety provoking. However, avoid the temptation to make your small group a lecture to a smaller audience. It is crucial that small-group teaching is interactive.

When small-group teaching is conducted over a period with the same groups of students, the relationship between the facilitators and students has time to develop. This can allow more flexible learning than in one-off sessions, as there can be a better sense of shared goals.

It is worth reviewing the goals and allocating specific amounts of time for the various tasks and activities. A session plan for a workshop on diversity at a child psychiatry conference serves as a working example in Box 8.2.

If small-group learning builds on a lecture, ensure that you are familiar with the lecture material, as you may need to clarify student misunderstanding or elaborate on aspects of it.

Ensure that instructions for the various exercises are clear and students have access to them. During small-group discussions students can become side-tracked and lose focus. Having the exercise visible helps them to keep to task.

It can be helpful to have students prepare ahead of the teaching session, but you can anticipate that at least half will not have prepared; you can plan how you are going to manage this and ensure that those who have prepared are not bored while the others catch up.

If group work is to be assessed, be clear about how this is to be done, as it can cause a great deal of inter-student friction. If you are not setting the assessment it can still be important to understand the process, as you may be asked about it as the facilitator.

Room layout

The various ways in which rooms may be set up to ensure maximum student participation are shown in Fig. 8.1 (based on Jaques, 2000). The

---

Box 8.2 The objectives and session plan for a diversity workshop

Objectives

By the end of the session participants should be able to:
- evaluate the use of the word 'culture' and related concepts
- identify how practitioner culture may influence clinical practice
- describe the impact of culture on children's mental health
- identify strategies to ensure that services are culturally appropriate for diverse families.

Session plan

- From your perspective, how does culture affect family life? (15 minutes)
- How does this influence presentation of problems to services (child and adolescent mental health services and others)? (30 minutes)
- What is your experience of working with diversity? (10 minutes)
- Exercise to consider participants' own cultural identity as a means of understanding the diversity of culture (diversity shuffle and multicultural self). (30 minutes)
- Presentation to pull the learning together. (20 minutes)
- Discussion of the morning session and the difficulties faced in delivering culturally appropriate services, with a view to developing strategies that individuals can take back to the workplace. (30 minutes)

Note that although a total of 150 minutes was allowed for the workshop, only 135 minutes were allocated, to build in some flexibility for participants to organise themselves.

---

common factor in all the layouts is that members of the group can see each other or turn easily to see other members, as face-to-face interactions are a common feature of small-group sessions. The room is often not within the tutor's control but it should be possible to secure one of these layouts. In options 1 and 2 in Fig. 8.1, everyone can see each other but there is potential for the focus to be on the teacher. In the other options the teacher is an integral part of the group. Tables can be helpful if students need to write or refer to texts, although some can see them as a physical obstacle and a possible barrier. Option 3 may be less useful, as the teacher has a better view of some students than others and this can lead to some students being accidentally excluded. Often the person next to us in such a formation is the one we can interact with least well because we don't tend to see those immediately to our side as we have to turn to look at them.

Running the group

If members of the group are familiar with each other, only minimal introductions may be required. In other contexts (for example at conferences)

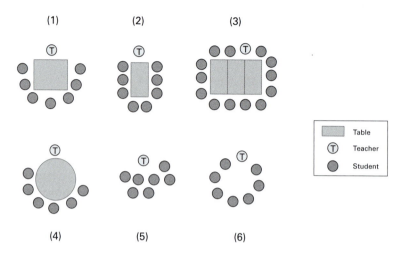

Fig. 8.1 Ways in which rooms may be set up to ensure maximum student participation in a small-group session (based on Jaques, 2000).

introductions can be helpful to the facilitator in better understanding the learners' needs; nonetheless, it is important not to spend a disproportionate amount of time on introductions. At the start, state the learning outcomes and outline how you expect the session to pan out.

When the students are engaged in tasks it is useful for the facilitator to move between groups to help move the discussion and also to help students to stay focused.

If the student group is used to working together, they are already likely to be familiar with the 'ground rules', but it can be useful to reiterate them. The usual ground rules for group work comprise:

- safe learning environment
- respect for different perspectives
- listen to others respectfully (no put-downs)
- views to be challenged respectfully
- everyone needs to do their share and prepare appropriately
- keep to time
- leave any personal agendas outside the session
- group members should only share information about themselves that they feel comfortable sharing
- if discussing particularly personal or sensitive issues, confidentiality may need to be emphasised

It is important that the group is allowed to challenge different perspectives, otherwise learning is unlikely to be effective; it is the facilitator's role to ensure that this is done respectfully and in a professional manner. However, it is likely that some issues may evoke strong emotional responses. It is appropriate to allow expression of these as long as any conflict is resolved; this is an important part of group functioning and learning, so should not be avoided if the situation arises.

At the beginning of each exercise or task the facilitator should check that the students have understood the instructions – students may start talking about other things if they have not understood.

If students are asked to make presentations, the facilitator's role in keeping time is crucial. It is frustrating for students who have prepared if they do not have the opportunity to present because of poor time keeping.

To ensure the participation of all students, it can be useful to ask them to take turns in giving feedback to the larger group or in acting as note takers. In established groups, roles are often assumed and sometimes these need to be challenged. Using the phrase 'I would like to hear from someone who hasn't yet spoken' is a gentle way of encouraging quieter members to speak up.

Potential problems and how to address them

Although small-group teaching is a rewarding process, it can pose particular difficulties. The many potential problems can be broadly grouped as relating to goals, to group interactions, to students or to tutors (Tiberius, 1999). These areas will be discussed in turn.

Goal-related problems

Tiberius (1999) identified three possible problems with group goals, in that they may be unclear, unattainable or unacceptable.

It is important that students understand clearly the goals of the course from the beginning. Indeed, if possible they should be involved in deciding them; Parkin *et al* (2001) provide an example of this with general practice trainees. It is advisable that tutors remain flexible enough to negotiate any difficulties that may arise at this point and modify the goals if appropriate.

Difficulties arise in attaining goals for a variety of reasons. Some group structures are better for providing information, while others encourage participative listening to develop the learner's own perspectives and understanding. The structure should be aligned with the group's goals. Poor time management can lead to problems and it is important that tutors lead the group and provide appropriate direction.

Some students can find the group's goals unacceptable. They may not see the relevance of what they are learning or they may find the materials unduly personal. These situations need to be managed by the tutors in a clear and sensitive manner, perhaps with support and feedback from colleagues. Reiterating the group's ground rules (see above) can help in these situations.

Group interaction problems

These can be summarised as: lack of interaction; the teacher dominates the interaction; students participate unequally.

Lack of interaction between tutor and students is the commonest of these problems. This could arise either because the students or the tutor have little experience of what is required in a group, or because the students feel intimidated by the tutor, who is seen as both expert and assessor. In this situation it is important for tutors to keep their input to a minimum and be supportive of the students' contributions. Students do better when they feel their input is a positive experience and it is essential to avoid sarcasm or harsh comments. Sometimes students feel they lack the knowledge to make a contribution and in this situation it is important that teaching material is available before the session.

The group dynamic is especially important for good interaction. If the members of the group are new to each other, they may need to build a level of trust before they feel able to express opinions openly. The tutor should facilitate this process and develop a non-threatening atmosphere in which students feel safe. This dynamic can be influenced by factors such as group size and physical surroundings, including the seating arrangement. Interaction is often stifled in groups that are too large.

In any group there is a tendency for individuals to participate unequally. A common problem is for a dominant speaker to monopolise the discussion. This can antagonise the tutor and others in the group but needs to be handled sensitively. It may be necessary to speak to the student privately, or can be helped by assigning that person a specific task. Getting members of the group to take turns can be used but may affect the natural flow of ideas.

Another common problem is the silent student. Students can be silent for a number of reasons. Personality type, cultural factors and group dynamic are influential. It is important that these students feel comfortable and the tutor facilitates their inclusion.

Cliques may develop and can be either silent or domineering. In extreme cases it may be necessary to split the group up to manage this situation.

Student-related problems

Many of these have been incorporated into the previous discussion. Specific problems in this area include:

- inadequate preparation by the student
- students who do not participate or do so grudgingly
- students who dominate the session
- students who want certainty and 'answers' rather than to work through the issues
- students who are hostile.

A multitude of factors can affect students' performance in a group and it is essential that the tutor is aware of the environment in which the group is held. For example, upcoming examinations can have a significant effect on students' attitudes, particularly if the work being done in the small-group session is seen as irrelevant. Other factors that the tutor could explore include the personal motivation of an individual to do the course and the necessary skills for small-group learning. Often students like certainty and answers, particularly when stressed, but it is essential that the tutor resists this approach and instead encourages more mature learning.

Hostility from students is rare but can be difficult. Students may have preconceived assumptions that are challenged by the group or may feel it is necessary to challenge the tutor's authority. This can sometimes be used to help facilitate debate but the student should not be allowed to dominate the discussion or to take it in an inappropriate direction. Students who are actively competing or who are insensitive to the feelings of others may need to be spoken to privately or given tasks in the session to direct their actions.

Tutor-related problems

The tutor is an essential part of the group process and it is important to recognise the difficulties that can affect the tutor's function. It should not be assumed that everyone can do this effectively from the beginning: the skills required do need development.

Tutor-related problems include:

- inadequate preparation
- failure to use the small-group environment effectively
- not engaging the students
- excessive criticism
- failure to recognise or acknowledge student responses, especially if difficult issues are raised
- over- or under-controlling the session.

Tutors do not teach in a vacuum. The institution can have a profound effect on performance and there can be external stresses on the tutor which affect teaching, such as pressure to produce research. Personal factors can often have a profound impact, and produce 'off days', but if feedback is consistently poor then the tutor will need to re-examine his or her teaching style. Inadequate preparation may be secondary to poor time management or an excessive workload.

Many of the problems a tutor may encounter can be helped significantly by feedback from both students and colleagues. The latter may be essential if one encounters a particularly difficult group. Feedback is useful only if it is acted upon. The tutor needs to ensure that comments are treated in a constructive manner. As with lectures, tutors can learn a lot from experienced colleagues, either through observation or through acting as a co-facilitator.

Summary

In this chapter we have focused on the purpose of small-group teaching, the different types of small-group teaching and the strategies that are most commonly used. We have also reviewed the facilitator role and the factors teachers need to consider in preparing for and running small groups. We have then considered potential problems and how these might be resolved.

- Small-group teaching is used to get learners to talk, debate, discuss and engage in problem solving. It is an opportunity to maximise learner participation.
- Get students to question, criticise, analyse, evaluate, speculate, think and understand.
- Set a context and ensure that the discussions are directed towards the achievement of the learning objectives.
- Make sure the learners know what is expected of them; if they need to prepare anything in advance, ensure that they have plenty of notice.
- Be prepared with questions that cover a wide range of cognitive skills, from recall through application to problem solving.
- Be prepared to elaborate and rephrase questions if necessary.
- Ensure an adequate wait time after asking a question and be prepared to listen actively to the answer.
- Respond to answers by providing explanations, sensitive feedback on misunderstandings and praise for understanding.
- Encourage learners to talk with each other; break the group up into smaller groups if necessary.
- Ensure that there is time to summarise the results of the discussion at the end.
- Refer to the context of the learning objectives to provide a sense of cohesion, completeness and achievement.

References

Entwistle, N. J., Thompson, S. & Tait, H. (1992) *Guidelines for Promoting Effective Learning in Higher Education*. Centre for Research and Learning and Information, University of Edinburgh.

Exley, K. & Dennick, R. (2004) *Small Group Teaching: Tutorials, Seminars and Beyond*. Routledge Falmer.

Jaques, D. (2000) *Learning in Groups: A Handbook for Improving Group Learning* (3rd edn). Kogan Page.

Jaques, D. (2003) ABC of learning and teaching in medicine: teaching small groups. *BMJ*, **326**, 492–494.

London Deanery (2009) *Small Group Teaching*. London Deanery. Available at http://www.faculty.londondeanery.ac.uk/e-learning/small-group-teaching/Small%20group%20teaching.pdf

Parkin, A., Dogra, N. & Platts, P. (2001) Negotiated learning and teaching in child psychiatry for general practice registrars. *Education for General Practice*, **12**, 80–86.

Reece, I. & Walker, S. (2000) *A Practical Guide to Teaching, Training and Learning* (4th edn). Business Education Publishers.

Tiberius, R. (1999) *Small Group Teaching: A Problem Shooting Guide*. Kogan Page.

CHAPTER 9

Problem-based learning

Angela Cogan & Craig Melville

Introduction

Education: that which reveals to the wise, and conceals from the stupid, the vast limits of their knowledge. (Mark Twain)

Problem-based learning (PBL) was introduced as a teaching method in undergraduate medical education at McMaster University Medical School, Ontario, in 1969. Since then it has been integrated into medical curricula worldwide and has been endorsed by bodies such as the World Health Organization (Spencer & Jordan, 1999); it was first adopted in Europe by the University of Maastricht Medical School in 1974. In response to the recommendations made by the General Medical Council (1993) in *Tomorrow's Doctors*, in 1996 the University of Glasgow was the first UK medical school to adopt PBL as the core educational method in the medical undergraduate curriculum. Around 30% of medical schools in the UK have since moved to a PBL curriculum.

Considerable research has examined the effectiveness and outcomes of PBL curricula. Although it seems early to suggest that the approach encourages recruitment into psychiatry, there is evidence that PBL has specific advantages in the acquisition of skills relevant to the specialty and that it may improve performance in psychiatric examinations.

What is problem-based learning?

Strategies for PBL were developed as part of an exploration of educational theories of adult learning. There is an emphasis on active learning, facilitated by a constructive, self-directed, collaborative and contextual learning process (Dolmans *et al*, 2002). Key concepts within PBL are that its use with small groups should enable students to explore their existing knowledge, identify gaps, carry out independent learning and return to the group to discuss and share this new knowledge. This allows students to establish links more readily between different learning experiences and the process equips the student with skills that can be applied to self-directed, lifelong learning.

Despite the strong theoretical basis behind PBL, its use in medical schools has been shown to be heterogeneous, in terms of both the format used and the amount of PBL within various curricula (Maudsley, 1999; Kelson & Distlehorst, 2000). Regardless of these differences, three common features of PBL occur across medical undergraduate curricula:

- students work in small groups
- learning is activated by clinical problems
- a facilitator has a key role.

To illustrate one PBL model, an outline of the system used in Glasgow is provided. The PBL groups run through years 1–3, with years 4 and 5 of the curriculum comprising clinical attachments. Other aspects of the curriculum that complement the small-group PBL in years 1–3 are fixed-resource sessions (similar to a workshop) and plenary sessions (similar to a lecture or seminar). Vocational studies, providing structured experience in clinical techniques and patient contact, are integrated with the PBL. The students are allocated to a PBL group of up to eight students for blocks organised around a coherent theme, such as 'Homeostasis' or 'Conception, growth and development'. At the end of each 10-week term, the student is moved to a new group. Facilitators work with a group for one or two 5-week blocks.

An example of a PBL scenario, designed to facilitate the learning process of the small group, is shown in Box 9.1. Students are not given the clinical problem in advance and see it for the first time when they meet with the group's facilitator. At the start of each session, the group selects a student chair and student scribe. The chair actively leads the group to apply the seven-stage process set out in Box 9.2, activating learning around the clinical problem contained in the PBL scenario in Box 9.1.

Thus, students learn material in the context of a clinical scenario rather by specialty or in a curriculum-based sequence. Advocates of PBL suggest

---

Box 9.1 An example of a problem-based learning scenario

You are working in an inner-city general practice.

George Mackay, a 22-year-old man, comes to see you about problems he is having at his work as a telesales operative. He tells you he is worried about his boss and other colleagues. George is obviously scared and tells you that he has heard them talking about ways to get rid of him. Last week George noticed his computer screen was flickering and thinks his boss might have done something to it.

George's mother came with him and is unsure of what is happening to her son.

Consider the relevant assessment and management issues for this case.

Box 9.2 A seven-stage approach to problem-based learning: the Glasgow steps

1 Grasp the meaning of the scenario. (Are there any words you need to define?)
2 List the main issues in the scenario.
3 Activate your mind. (Brainstorm to generate explanations of the main issues based on your existing knowledge.)
4 Specify the exact questions on which you need to work.
5 Got what you need? (Plan your use of resources.)

The enquiry

6 Offer your answers to the group. (Pool and test the new knowledge and apply it to the scenario. Reflect on the adequacy of your answers and the appropriateness of your questions.)
7 What's our role in this? (Reflect on the group process.)

that the process – students discussing the scenario, exploring the definitions involved and identifying learning objectives related to the case – emphasises relevance to students and improves retention. The main learning objectives identified are explored using any *a priori* knowledge the students have, for example from previous studies or learning within the medical curriculum. Discussion with the group leads to a list of questions and relevant methods and materials to be used in answering these questions. The students then research the subject matter with a view to sharing their findings with the group in the next session. The emphasis is thus on actively seeking answers to clinically relevant questions from a range of sources, such as textbooks, journals and internet resources, rather than passively receiving information from lectures, lecture handouts and a prescribed book list. Within this context the role of the facilitator is to promote discussion, and not to teach the subject matter.

Towards the end of each scenario, the student chair invites the PBL group to consider how well they worked together. This allows the group to develop an awareness of issues that arise while working as part of a team and group members are encouraged to find solutions to problems within the group process, such as one person dominating the group or someone who is not participating in the work of the group. In addition, the facilitator meets with students individually towards the end of the 5-week block to discuss their approaches to the work done.

The experience in Glasgow has been that although coming to terms with this new style of learning in year 1 can provoke anxiety, by the end of the first term the vast majority of students are comfortable with the process and are able to use it effectively.

What does the PBL group facilitator do?

In the original conception of PBL in medical education proposed by Barrows & Tamblyn (1980), facilitators were encouraged to guide the learning of students via approaching the problem-based scenario at a 'metacognitive level'. For example, a PBL group with no prior direct learning or experience of psychiatry may struggle to work together on a PBL scenario describing someone presenting to a general practitioner with low mood. Understandably, the PBL group may view the facilitator (expert) as a source of the solution and ask a direct question. In this instance, a metacognitive response from the facilitator would be one that encourages the students to look beyond the scenario and ask themselves broader questions, such as 'What circumstances can affect someone's mood?', which might activate prior knowledge of relevance. A key role of the facilitator is to enable students within the group to develop both the skills to probe and question around a scenario and an awareness of what questions they should ask themselves. However, a recent review (Taylor & Miflin, 2008) recognises several different models for the role of the PBL facilitator and notes there is considerable variation between medical schools.

Despite considerable debate over these differing models, the exact role of the facilitator in PBL groups remains uncertain – there is a lack of clarity about how active the facilitator should be in group sessions, what makes a good facilitator and the best way to train and support facilitators for this demanding role (Maudsley, 1999). On the one hand, there is a clear consensus that facilitators should resist the temptation to act as experts, imparting their own knowledge to the students. However, research has suggested that PBL groups with expert facilitators from a clinical background report higher levels of satisfaction, achieve better scores on relevant examinations and more readily identify learning objectives in keeping with the PBL scenario (Davis *et al*, 1992; Schmidt & Moust, 1995; Hendry *et al*, 2002).

McLean & Van Wyk (2006) suggest there is value in recruiting facilitators from a wide variety of healthcare backgrounds, such as general practitioners, pharmacists, physiotherapists and nursing practitioners, as it heightens awareness among students of the team approach to patient care. Indeed, the pure PBL facilitator role as envisaged by Barrows & Tamblyn (1980) actually allows people from different backgrounds to be trained and work as facilitators, which is important in terms of keeping costs down and creating sufficient numbers of staff.

To allow recruitment of facilitators from diverse backgrounds, different models of training for facilitators have been developed. Wetzel (1996) gives the Harvard Medical School tutor training programme as an example. This involves:

- one 2-hour session for a new tutor, with a short presentation of the principles of PBL followed by practice tutorial groups led by experienced tutors

- a course orientation meeting for all tutors 1 week before the course begins
- weekly tutorial meetings for all tutors to explore issues arising from the groups and to preview cases for the coming week
- observation of and feedback to all new tutors by an educator.

It should be noted that PBL is one of a number of small-group methods employed in medical student education (see Chapter 8 of the present volume, and Walton & Matthews, 1989). Walton & Matthews (1989) emphasise that 'small group work enables participants to gain a great deal from their fellows, in a type of communication that cannot take place in a lecture hall'. They define a group as 'a number of people interacting in a face-to-face situation'. Examples include a seminar, defined as a leader-centred rather than participant-centred group with a specific aim presented by the leader, who also ensures that it is adequately explored. A free-discussion group is participant-centred, generating its own issues, which are clarified on the initiatives of the participants themselves.

Is problem-based learning effective?

Although it has been widely implemented and well received by medical educators, the evidence for PBL is equivocal. Two prominent reviews have suggested that the outcomes for students in a PBL curriculum are less favourable than the outcomes for students in traditional curricula (Colliver, 2000; Newman, 2003). Albanese & Mitchell (1993) point to its relative inefficiency and suggest that PBL curricula cover about 80% of what might be covered in a traditional curriculum in the same period. Costs are great in terms of staff training, time and production of PBL materials. It has been argued that, given the considerable resources required for PBL curricula, greater benefits would be expected than have been demonstrated to date (Colliver, 2000). Other weaknesses cited include student frustration at the apparent lack of structure, groups becoming preoccupied by trivial topics and interpersonal conflicts undermining a group's effectiveness (Gillespie, 1995). In spite of the best efforts of a facilitator, some students may do a disproportionate amount of the group's work and other students may either dominate group discussion or be reluctant to contribute at all in the group context. A fuller list of identified strengths and weaknesses of PBL is given in Table 9.1.

Advocates of PBL suggest that the approach promotes a deep rather than surface learning style. Deep learning involves understanding underlying theories and concepts as well as their practical application. This is postulated to improve retention as well as application of this knowledge in different areas (El-Sayeh *et al*, 2006). However, McParland *et al* (2004) compared two cohorts of year 2 clinical students, one taught using a traditional psychiatry curriculum and the other taught using a PBL curriculum, and found that

Table 9.1 Advantages and disadvantages of problem-based learning

Advantages	Disadvantages
Students develop generalisable skills (e.g. self-directed learning)	Student anxiety and uncertainty during initial phase of skills acquisition
Experience of small groups highly relevant to working within teams	Increased resources required (facilitators, space for groups, etc.)
Increased motivation for learning	Clinicians' concerns that students lack knowledge
Development of extensive, flexible knowledge base	More costly for universities
Improved communication and psycho-social skills (e.g. negotiation)	May be more suited to mature students
Can be used flexibly across the curriculum	Unfamiliar to teachers and other staff

although the PBL groups were more successful in their examination, there were no significant differences in learning styles between the two groups.

Other positive findings suggest that students from PBL curricula perform better in examinations (Blake *et al*, 2000) and feel better prepared to work independently (Schmidt & Molen, 2001). A longer-term follow-up of Harvard Medical School graduates has suggested they have better psychosocial skills and relational skills than students from the original curriculum (Clark, 2006).

The reviews discussed above have largely focused on randomised that delivered at the same medical school. It has been argued that these types of study are inappropriate when evaluating educational interventions (Norman & Schmidt, 2000; Dolmans, 2003; Farrow & Norman, 2003) as it is impossible to conduct a truly blind study and the complexity of interventions militates against the use of these study designs. Instead, in order to develop a clear picture of the effectiveness of the various components, there is a need to focus more on the theoretical concepts underlying PBL. For example, some studies have examined the impact of the role of the PBL facilitator on student outcomes (Dolmans *et al*, 2002), while others have examined the effects of different levels of cooperation between PBL group members on achievement scores (Bahar-Ozvaris *et al*, 2006).

Despite the lack of consistent findings, PBL is popular among students and educators (Antepohl *et al*, 2003; Prince *et al*, 2005). Importantly for psychiatry, PBL curricula have been shown to have a positive impact on outcomes relating to communicating with service users, working within multidisciplinary teams and developing the psychosocial competence of students (Block, 1996; Antepohl *et al*, 2003; Prince *et al*, 2005). Koh *et al* (2008) carried out a systematic review of the evidence of the effects of PBL on physician competency after graduation and concluded that it has had positive effects in the following areas – coping with uncertainty, appreciation of the legal and ethical aspects of healthcare, communication skills, and self-directed continuing learning.

Problem-based learning and psychiatry

There is interest in whether PBL curricula for medical undergraduates may have different benefits in relation to different specialties. For example, does it prepare students preferentially for some specialties but not others, and will it have a longer-term impact on recruitment and retention into particular specialties? From the evidence outlined above, it would appear that PBL curricula are likely to have a positive outcome for psychiatry. However, results to date have been mixed. McParland *et al* (2004) compared the learning styles, attitudes to psychiatry and performance of two groups of students – one taught using a traditional psychiatry curriculum, the other using a PBL curriculum. The students on the PBL curriculum had significantly better outcomes as measured by examination performance, but there were no differences between the groups on learning styles or attitudes to psychiatry.

A second study has demonstrated that performance outcomes in psychiatry were better in a PBL curriculum compared with a standard curriculum (Distlehorst *et al*, 2005). Interestingly, in the same study there was no significant difference in outcomes for the other branches of medicine studied, including surgery, paediatrics, obstetrics, medicine and family medicine. Alongside the finding that PBL also has a positive impact on communication skills, working with others and psychosocial competence (Block, 1996; Antepohl *et al*, 2003; Prince *et al*, 2005), the suggestion is that psychiatry as a specialty may do well from the introduction of PBL into medical undergraduate curricula. It may also produce graduates in other specialties who have skills relevant to psychiatry.

Perhaps there is value in considering incorporating elements of PBL into postgraduate psychiatry training and continuing professional development (McCarthy *et al*, 2000; Smits *et al*, 2005; Bhugra, 2008). This has already happened in some centres worldwide. In Birmingham and Solihull Mental Health Trust, PBL and other small-group teaching techniques have been incorporated into the foundation year (FY1 and FY2) programme in psychiatry and there are plans to roll out a similar format for the teaching of the MRCPsych curriculum (Vassilas *et al*, 2008). PBL as a part of psychiatry residency education was incorporated into the Harvard Longwood Residency Training Program (McCarthy *et al*, 2000) and the New South Wales NSW Institute of Psychiatry postgraduate course (Burke, 2001). The authors concluded that, with some modification, PBL could be one of a number of educational methods introduced into postgraduate psychiatry training.

Summary

Both in the UK and internationally, PBL is an established part of the undergraduate curriculum in a growing number of medical schools. As the learning style has a theoretical basis and clearly delineated structures and processes, its effectiveness is amenable to research and evaluation. Following earlier claims that PBL is ineffective, there is growing evidence that it does not diminish the academic achievements of students and has a positive impact on attitudes and skills relevant to working as a doctor.

It should become clear within the next 5–10 years whether experience of PBL as undergraduates promotes recruitment and retention into psychiatry. Initial findings suggest that graduates from medical schools that have adopted a PBL curriculum may be better equipped for a career in psychiatry. Communication skills, working within multidisciplinary teams and psychosocial competence are central to all branches of psychiatry and all seem to be positively targeted by undergraduate medical PBL curricula.

References

Albanese, M. A. & Mitchell, S. (1993) Problem-based learning: a review of literature on its outcomes and implementation issues. *Academic Medicine*, **68**, 52–81.

Antepohl, W., Domeij, E., Forsberg, P., *et al* (2003) A follow-up of medical graduates of a problem-based learning curriculum. *Medical Education*, **37**, 155–162.

Bahar-Ozvaris, S., Cetin, F. C., Turan, S., *et al* (2006) Cooperative learning: a new application of problem-based learning in mental health training. *Medical Teacher*, **28**, 553–557.

Barrows, H. S. & Tamblyn, R. M. (1980) *Problem Based-Learning: An Approach to Medical Education*. Springer.

Bhugra, D. (2008) Psychiatric training in the UK: the next steps. *World Psychiatry*, **7**, 117–118.

Blake, R. L., Hosokawa, M. C. & Riley, S. L. (2000) Student performances on step 1 and step 2 of the United States Medical Licensing Examination following implementation of a problem-based learning curriculum. *Academic Medicine*, **75**, 66–70.

Block, S. D. (1996) Using problem-based learning to enhance the psychosocial competence of medical students. *Academic Psychiatry*, **20**, 65–75.

Burke, D. (2001) A new model for postgraduate and continuing education in psychiatry. *Australasian Psychiatry*, **9**, 215–218.

Clark, C. E. (2006) Problem-based learning: how do the outcomes compare with traditional teaching? *British Journal of General Practice*, **56**, 722–723.

Colliver, J. A. (2000) Effectiveness of problem-based learning curricula: research and theory. *Academic Medicine*, **75**, 259–266.

Davis, W. K., Nairn, R., Paine, M. E., *et al* (1992) Effects of expert and non-expert facilitators on the small-group process and on student performance. *Academic Medicine*, **67**, 470–474.

Distlehorst, L. H., Dawson, E., Robbs, R. S., *et al* (2005) Problem-based learning outcomes: the glass half-full. *Academic Medicine*, **80**, 294–299.

Dolmans, D. (2003) The effectiveness of PBL: the debate continues. Some concerns about the BEME movement. *Medical Education*, **37**, 1129–1130.

Dolmans, D. H., Gijselaers, W. H., Moust, J. H., *et al* (2002) Trends in research on the tutor in problem-based learning: conclusions and implications for educational practice and research. *Medical Teacher*, **24**, 173–180.

El-Sayeh, H. G., Budd, S., Waller, R., *et al* (2006) How to win the hearts and minds of students in psychiatry. *Advances in Psychiatric Treatment*, **12**, 182–192.

Farrow, R. & Norman, G. (2003) The effectiveness of PBL: the debate continues. Is meta-analysis helpful? *Medical Education*, **37**, 1131–1132.

General Medical Council (1993) *Tomorrow's Doctors* (1st edn). GMC.

Gillespie, R. S. (1995) Problem-based learning redefines medical education. *Impact*, 1(4), 1–6.

Hendry, G. D., Phan, H., Lyon, P. M., *et al* (2002) Student evaluation of expert and non-expert problem-based learning tutors. *Medical Teacher*, 24, 544–549.

Kelson, A. C. M. & Distlehorst, L. H. (2000) *Groups in Problem-Based Learning: Essential Elements in Theory and Practice*. Lawrence Erlbaum Associates.

Koh, G. C., Khoo, H. E., Wong, M. L., *et al* (2008) The effects of problem-based learning during medical school on physician competency: a systematic review. *Canadian Medical Association Journal*, 178, 34–41.

Maudsley, G. (1999) Do we all mean the same thing by 'problem-based learning'? A review of the concepts and a formulation of the ground rules. *Academic Medicine*, 74, 178–185.

McCarthy, M. K., Birnbaum, R. J. & Bures, J. (2000) Problem-based learning and psychiatry residency education. *Harvard Review of Psychiatry*, 7, 305–308.

McLean, M. & Van Wyk, J. (2006) Twelve tips for recruiting and retaining facilitators in a problem-based learning programme. *Medical Teacher*, 28, 675–679.

McParland, M., Noble, L. M. & Livingston, G. (2004) The effectiveness of problem-based learning compared to traditional teaching in undergraduate psychiatry. *Medical Education*, 38, 859–867.

Newman, M. (2003) *A Pilot Systematic Review and Meta-analysis on the Effectiveness of Problem-Based Learning*. Newcastle University Learning and Teaching Support Network.

Norman, G. R. & Schmidt, H. G. (2000) Effectiveness of problem-based learning curricula: theory, practice and paper darts. *Medical Education*, 34, 721–728.

Prince, K. J., van Eijs, P. W., Boshuizen, H. P., *et al* (2005) General competencies of problem-based learning (PBL) and non-PBL graduates. *Medical Education*, 39, 394–401.

Schmidt, H. G. & Molen, H. T. (2001) Self-reported competency ratings of graduates of a problem-based medical curriculum. *Academic Medicine*, 76, 466–468.

Schmidt, H. G. & Moust, J. H. (1995) What makes a tutor effective? A structural-equations modeling approach to learning in problem-based curricula. *Academic Medicine*, 70, 708–714.

Smits, P. B. A., Verbeek, J. H. A. M. & de Buisonje, C. D. (2005) Problem based learning in continuing medical education: a review of controlled evaluation studies. *BMJ*, 324, 153–156.

Spencer, J. A. & Jordan, R. K. (1999) Learner centred approaches in medical education. *BMJ*, 318, 1280–1283.

Taylor, D. & Miflin, B. (2008) Problem-based learning: where are we now? *Medical Teacher*, 30, 742–63.

Vassilas, C., Haeney, O. & Brown, N. (2008) What is the role of the MRCPsych course for the new specialist training grade in psychiatry? *Psychiatric Bulletin*, 32, 108–110.

Walton, H. J. & Matthews, M. B. (1989) Essentials of problem-based learning. *Medical Education*, 23, 542–558.

Wetzel, M. S. (1996) Developing the role of the tutor/facilitator. *Postgraduate Medical Journal*, 72, 474–477.

CHAPTER 10

Teaching trainee psychiatrists how to teach medical students: the Southampton model

David Dayson & Faith Hill

Introduction

This chapter offers an example of education development in practice – a case study of how many of the ideas in this book can come together in the context of a particular medical school. The chapter focuses on ways that junior staff can be trained for education roles and illustrates how the recommendations of the General Medical Council (GMC) and the core competencies of the Royal College of Psychiatrists (RCPsych) can be delivered through a bespoke training programme. The chapter raises a number of issues that all practitioners embarking on the development of a training programme need to consider and also presents evaluation data that confirms the success of the approach adopted at the Southampton School of Medicine.

Background

The School of Medicine

The School of Medicine at the University of Southampton is widely recognised as one of the leading institutions in the UK for undergraduate medical education. Following a successful bid to the Department of Health, student numbers at the School have expanded rapidly over the past few years, with a 47% rise to an intake of 250. The School has also developed two innovative and ambitious new programmes: a 4-year graduate entry programme for graduates of all disciplines; and a 6-year widening access programme. These two programmes are closely integrated with the traditional 5-year, school-leaver programme. The three programmes vary in detail but all the students experience early patient contact, an integrated basic science curriculum, student-selected modules and a curriculum designed to offer 'spiral' learning from one year to the next. All students experience extensive training on clinical rotations throughout the South

Central Region of the National Health Service (NHS) and neighbouring areas – involving staff from a total of 21 NHS trusts, including nine mental health trusts.

The expansion at Southampton has increased the need for staff development, for new staff and for staff at newly established medical student teaching centres around the region. The School has a Medical Education Division, which runs a highly successful staff development programme, recently commended by the General Medical Council (Hill & Stephens, 2004; General Medical Council, 2008). The Division has worked closely with the undergraduate leads for the mental health attachments to ensure timely and effective training for psychiatrists involved in teaching. Initially, this training was aimed at senior staff and mostly involved consultant psychiatrists attending our 4-day educators' training course. This course was effective for training senior staff but we recognised that much of the teaching is delivered by trainees. We therefore developed a bespoke programme to meet the specific needs of trainees – Teaching Skills Part I and Part II.

Psychiatry programme

The psychiatry programme for our students has constantly evolved over the past 10 years in response to the large increase in student numbers and the newly developed programmes. We have dispersed teaching and no longer place medical students solely within in-patient settings, but include community mental health teams (CMHTs) and specialist services. Medical students are now attached to CMHTs in Southampton, Winchester and the New Forest, as well as with teams providing services in older persons' mental health and child and adolescent psychiatry. Within these settings, medical students receive their teaching and clinical experience from lead tutor teams. Each lead tutor team consists of: a consultant psychiatrist; an additional educator, who is typically from a nursing or psychology background; and local administrative support staff.

There are many innovations in the Southampton programme. Possibly the foremost of these has been to embed education money within posts. The budget for teaching sessions is therefore readily identifiable and in due course will be held centrally, within the undergraduate department. Other innovations have included: a portfolio that links the student learning outcomes to the needs of the early postgraduate years; a student fellowship scheme that identifies students who are keen on psychiatry as a career and fosters their development; establishment and support of a student-led society to encourage interest in psychiatry; and special study modules in psychiatry. Also, we are the only UK undergraduate programme to include adult mental health, older persons' mental health and child and adolescent mental health services in our core teaching.

An important annual event, the third- and final-year teachers' training day, brings all of the key teachers across the region together for a lively and inspiring day-long seminar on a current topic of interest. In the past 3 years, we have addressed the following areas: how we can tailor a programme to fit better with the needs of the postgraduate years; how we can motivate medical students and encourage recruitment into mental health; and how we can incorporate the teaching of professionalism within our programme. Our forthcoming training day will cover the use of the arts and humanities in undergraduate teaching.

Needs assessment

The drivers for our Teaching Skills Part I and Part II course have evolved since its inception in 2004. Initially, we surveyed the cohort of trainees about their perceived lack of training in areas necessary for undergraduate teaching. The results of this initial survey are presented in Table 10.1. Although learning outcomes and ethics were at the top of the list, we decided that these were best addressed by dedicated teaching sessions, rather than a workshop. We noted that assessment and feedback were third in the list, followed later by creating interest and communication skills. Thus, we reasoned that a workshop devoted to feedback would be the best place to start, complemented by some teaching theory about how people learn by incorporating new information into what has already been learnt.

In addition, we noted the central drivers from the GMC in two of its key documents. *Tomorrow's Doctors* stated the following: 'you must understand the principles of education as they are applied to medicine; you will be familiar with a range of teaching and learning techniques; and you must recognise your obligation to teach' (General Medical Council, 2003). These themes were elaborated on in the document *Good Medical Practice*, which stated that 'teaching, training, appraising and assessing ...

Table 10.1 Psychiatric trainees' perceptions of their requirements for further training in areas necessary for undergraduate teaching

Area	No. of trainees indicating training requirement ($n = 23$)	%
Learning outcomes	19	83
Ethics	18	78
Assessment and feedback	15	65
Diversity	12	52
Multidisciplinary working	7	30
Creating interest	6	26
Communication skills	4	17
Enabling access to patients	2	9

Responses were returned by 23 senior house officers, who ranked the training requirements.

students are important for the care of patients now and in the future. You should be willing to contribute to these activities; you must develop the skills, attitudes and practices of a competent teacher; you must be honest and objective when appraising or assessing the performance of students' (General Medical Council, 2006). More recently the competency-based curriculum for specialist training in psychiatry has developed this further by stating that major competencies include being able to 'plan, deliver, and evaluate teaching and learning in a variety of environments; to assess, appraise and evaluate learning and learners; and to supervise and mentor learners' (Royal College of Psychiatrists, 2007). Furthermore, these major competencies have then been elaborated into what should be achieved under supervision and what would be a measure of competency and mastery.

These GMC and core competency drivers are cited at the beginning of the Teaching Skills Part I day to impress upon the attendees the importance of them gaining appropriate teaching skills. Furthermore, aside from the statutory and curriculum requirements, the attendees are encouraged to realise that acquiring teaching skills has immense personal benefit. Principally, it is argued that there are the following advantages:

- being able to teach consolidates skills you will need throughout your career
- teaching produces an improved fund of knowledge and forces the organisation and review of existing knowledge, while students' questions will readily identify your own learning gaps
- teaching develops a deep approach to learning which leads you to make your own thought processes explicit and enables you to remain in touch with basic information while integrating this with more advanced learning
- teaching in psychiatry offers a unique opportunity to develop reflective practice for the learner, which will be of great value in clinical work
- the role of teacher gives you influence on students' career paths and an investment in the future of your specialty.

It is argued that teaching skills can transfer to patient–doctor interactions. In particular, the skills that apply to teachers can be a key component of the negotiation and persuasion skills used in the following: compliance with therapy, motivational interviewing and challenging abnormal reasoning in a patient with delusions. We further suggest to trainees that the development of a deep learning style, through teaching on the subject, develops resilience in the workplace. This is one of the main findings of a paper entitled 'Stress, burnout and doctors' attitudes to work', which we introduce to the trainees (MacManus *et al*, 2004). MacManus *et al* demonstrate that a deep learning style leads to an approach at work that integrates new and previously learned information, produces a sense of control and autonomy in the workplace and consequently protects against the symptoms of burnout when staff are faced with perpetual organisational and career change within the NHS.

Teaching Skills Part I

The Part I course was developed with a number of processes in mind. Most of the day is spent with the attendees actively participating as opposed to listening to didactic talks (which account for only about a sixth of the day). Throughout the day, the attendees cycle through a process of engagement, short didactic teaching, small-group learning, large-group learning and activities to consolidate what has been learned. Thus, the attendees are exposed to a variety of teaching methods within a variety of group settings. The duration of activities is kept relatively short: the didactic teaching lasts no more than 20 minutes, whereas group activities may last 30 or 40 minutes.

Attendees are asked to reflect on how the giving out and timing of handouts can influence the teaching process. On the course, handouts are given out at the beginning of the day, but they are described and signposted for future learning at the end of the day. Most importantly, we make it explicit that we are modelling paired delivery of teaching (i.e. the simultaneous use of two teachers), in the hope that the trainees will take forward this way of delivering educational sessions in the future. Throughout the day there is interplay between the two presenters, with alternating periods of activity, observation and reflection. This in turn produces an ongoing conversation throughout the day; the collaborators can reflect back on each other's performance and review how the day is proceeding. Furthermore, this collaboration extends before and after the teaching day itself. Each teaching day is preceded by at least 2 hours of reflection and discussion on previous feedback, with subsequent modification of the next workshop. At the end of the day, time is taken to review the participants' feedback sheets, with some personal thoughts on what was successful and what needs further improvement.

The content of the Part I course is intentionally kept simple in order that we have time to model and reflect on the processes described above. We open with an ice-breaker and then encourage the trainees to articulate their learning outcomes for the day. We then introduce a number of key learning and teaching principles, including topics such as:

- student learning needs (e.g. meaningfulness; connection with past learning; challenging tasks and milestones; some control over learning)
- the learning pyramid (retention rates for different methods)
- balancing task, group and individual needs
- the learning environment, including the social and emotional needs of learners
- student-centred learning (e.g. active learning, teachers as facilitators, critical thinking, reasoning and reflection)
- the learning cycle and different learning styles associated with the cycle
- giving and receiving feedback.

The trainees work in groups to develop teaching methods appropriate to different learning situations. We do not advocate any particular style of teaching but encourage the trainees to assess the advantages and disadvantages of different methods and to try out new approaches and to vary their styles. We facilitate discussion of the opportunities for encouraging learners to increase control over their learning and also the relative advantages of active learning versus didactic teaching. The trainees work in groups to identify examples of each of the following approaches, and consider when it might be best to use each approach:

- active learning, with the teacher in control
- active learning, with the learner in control
- didactic teaching, with the teacher in control
- didactic teaching, with the learner in control.

We also give particular attention to the importance of constructive feedback and spend time on a role-play in which the trainees give each other feedback on their teaching skills. Usually the trainees identify from the role-play the main elements of good feedback, but we also have a checklist and make sure they cover key points from the interactive feedback model (Hill, 2007). This model includes asking the person for his or her personal self-assessment: what went well and what could be improved? Areas of reinforcement are clearly pointed out, along with areas needing improvement. A realistic improvement plan is negotiated. Importantly, following this model, time is spent reviewing understanding and checking the feelings of the learner.

A key feature of the Part I course is the involvement of medical students. We invite three or four of them to take part in all the activities. They are always impressed that so much attention is being given to their training needs. They are able to offer a student 'voice' during the day and to validate our conclusions. For example, trainees are often cynical and disbelieving when we, as staff, explain the importance of introducing students to each other at the start of attachments. Trainees assume that by the third year students will all know each other really well. They are amazed when the students confirm that they have often not met before and emphasise the importance of our advice. We have also noticed that trainees are inclined to take the day more seriously when students are present!

Teaching Skills Part II

We developed Part II of the course as a direct consequence of the written feedback from Part I. Trainees requested more detailed feedback on their actual teaching skills, as opposed to their feedback skills. We therefore developed the further workshop, with a main focus on 'micro-teaching', where the participants work in pairs to design and deliver a piece of teaching lasting 15 minutes. Each micro-teaching presentation then receives focused feedback on its process and content.

We consider it important that the trainees have participated in the earlier workshop so that they can give appropriate feedback in a positive manner, which will inspire change for the better as opposed to demoralising the aspiring teachers. Moreover, the short piece of micro-teaching cannot be seen in isolation. Before the workshop, the trainees team up in pairs to plan their teaching. This is a further piece of modelling, which attempts to recreate the planning relationship of the co-presenters. The attendees are encouraged to continue with this collaborative approach after the workshop, with further teaching in pairs. They are particularly encouraged to engage in the following behaviours, which are associated with successful teaching: talking with one another about teaching; observing each other teaching; and planning, organising, monitoring and evaluating teaching together. In effect, the trainees are then continually teaching each other to teach (Little, 1982).

In addition to the micro-teaching and its feedback, there is a session on different learning styles and how teaching might be adapted to these. We focus on the four main learning styles identified by David Kolb: innovative learners; analytic learners; common-sense learners; and dynamic learners (adapted from Kolb, 1984). Trainees work in groups to establish how they might modify their teaching to accommodate each of these styles. The trainees also complete an inventory assessing their own learning styles and are invited to consider how their learning style might influence their teaching style. We stress that there is no right or wrong learning style and that, indeed, the most effective learners are those who can function in different ways according to the specific content and context of the learning.

Finally, part of the day is used flexibly and adapted to incorporate topics of interest. For instance, in the first workshop we were given a presentation by a trainee and a medical student on their study of what makes for inspirational teaching from the perspectives of trainees and medical students. In our second workshop we used this slot instead to explore how cultural differences between the teacher and learner can affect the teaching process.

Evaluation

Each training day consistently receives overwhelmingly positive scores from the attendees. The success of the training days is measured against each of their learning objectives. Examples of two such sets of feedback are presented in Tables 10.2 and 10.3.

In addition to the quantitative evaluation, we routinely invite the participants to offer free-text comments. They are usually very generous in the praise they offer us. Examples have included:

Really made me think; not what I expected.

Thanks to the entire team ... the day has given me the motivation to be more mindful when I teach medical students ... might consider pursuing an MSc in medical education.

Table 10.2 Participants' evaluation of the Part I course

	Average score (poor = 1; excellent = 6)
Overall rating	5
Learning objective 1 (attitudes): to explore attitudes to the teaching of medical students	5
Learning objective 2 (skills): to gain an understanding of how to provide constructive feedback and formative assessment to undergraduate medical students	5
Learning objective 3 (knowledge): to examine some key theories of student learning and approaches to teaching	6

Ratings provided by all 24 senior house officers attending the February 2008 course, except for the overall rating, made by 22.

Table 10.3 Participants' evaluation of the Part II course

	Average score (poor = 1; excellent = 6)
Overall rating	6
Learning objective 1 (attitudes): to increase confidence and motivation towards the teaching of medical students	6
Learning objective 2 (skills): to develop small-group teaching skills	6
Learning objective 3 (knowledge): to increase understanding of effective teaching methods, student motivation and learning styles	6

Ratings provided by all 13 senior house officers attending the June 2008 course.

Micro-teaching particularly useful, highlighting how important it is to prepare and have a structure, but adapt your teaching style according to your students – cultures and learning styles.

A number of themes for improvement have also emerged from the comments and we respond to these wherever possible. For example, participants have suggested:

- the need for specific training on teaching large groups
- a desire to have students present on both days (rather than one day, as at present)
- the importance of prior reading.

Over and above the immediate evaluations from the trainees, we also look at the data we have from the medical students. The undergraduates are asked to give an overall rating for each of their clinical rotations (see Fig. 10.1). As described above, there have been many positive changes in

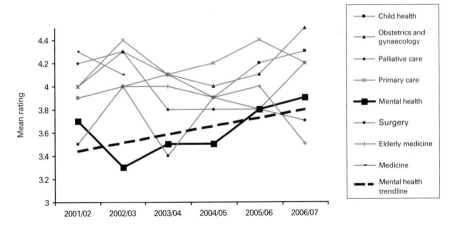

Fig. 10.1 Medical students' evaluation (poor = 1; excellent = 6) of the specialty components of their undergraduate teaching (final-year feedback).

the delivery of our undergraduate programme. Nevertheless, the consistent rise in satisfaction with the programme does coincide with the introduction of the teaching skills workshops since 2004.

Lessons learned

The programme of teaching skills development has grown as a close collaboration between the Director for Undergraduate Medical Education within the trust and the Director of the Division of Medical Education within the university. Neither person in these positions would have been able to collaborate in such a way without the generous support of their respective organisations. In particular, the Hampshire Partnership Foundation NHS Trust has fostered and encouraged undergraduate teaching from the outset by establishing posts – such as the Director for Undergraduate Education – with allocated funding. Likewise, the School of Medicine has fostered and encouraged such collaborative work through recognising the importance of teacher development across the undergraduate programme. We are also fortunate to have excellent logistical support to underpin the whole process – a factor that we consider essential to our success.

In retrospect, it seems entirely sensible to have based the first workshop around feedback skills, because in the second workshop those very feedback skills are employed in the micro-teaching sessions to enhance the teachers' skills.

In the micro-teaching a number of themes continue to re-emerge that require further development. These revolve around packaging the teaching content with the appropriate behavioural, speech and language skills to enable its communication and retention. The behavioural skills that need to be consistently improved are: developing teachers' expressive body language; and using as fully as possible the theatrical space available in front of learners. In terms of voice skills, trainees consistently need support with varying the pace and rhythm of their speech, alongside developing the capacity for gaps and changes in tone and volume for emphasis and dramatic effect. Finally, in terms of their use of language they frequently need supporting with the following: to place the information they are communicating within a narrative context; to use analogy and appropriate visual metaphor; and finally to allow themselves to use repetition and rhetorical skills to emphasise the information being communicated.

Our focus on these behavioural skills links to our observation that trainees typically pay far more attention to the content of their teaching than the needs of their learners. Perhaps understandably, trainees are anxious that they may not have the necessary knowledge to impart to students. They are also concerned that they may be asked questions that they are unable to answer. These fears tend to lead to an over-preparation of content and an over-reliance on a didactic teaching approach. One of the main challenges for us, in teaching trainees how to teach, is to instil a level of confidence where 'not knowing' is seen as acceptable and trainees can confidently engage in shared learning and enquiry with the students.

A teaching skills project such as ours always needs to be regarded as a work in progress. At least 6 months before each workshop, the co-facilitators need to spend time together discussing the forthcoming workshop and considering the changes needed to keep it fresh for both the presenters and the attendees. We suggest that co-facilitation is vital, with a regular cycle of feedback, reflection and subsequent change. Involving undergraduate students at some stage in the process is also an important ingredient. Ultimately, though, the workshops depend on the enthusiasm and engagement of the participants. In conclusion, therefore, we would like to express our appreciation and thanks to all the highly committed trainee psychiatrists who have attended the teaching skills courses in Southampton.

References

General Medical Council (2003) *Tomorrow's Doctors* (2nd edn). GMC.

General Medical Council (2006) *Good Medical Practice*. GMC.

General Medical Council (2008) *Quality Assurance of Basic Medical Education*. Report on School of Medicine, University of Southampton. Available at http://www.gmc-uk.org/static/documents/content/Southampton.pdf

Hill, F. (2007) Feedback to enhance student learning: facilitating interactive feedback on clinical skills. *International Journal of Clinical Skills*, 1, 21–24.

Hill, F. & Stephens, C. (2004) Negotiating strategic direction for education staff development. The Southampton experience. *Medical Teacher*, 26, 645–649.

Kolb, D. A. (1984) *Experiential Learning: Experience as the Source of Learning and Development*. Prentice Hall.

Little, J. W. (1982) Norms of collegiality and experimentation: workplace conditions for schools success. *American Educational Research Journal*, **19**, 325–340.

MacManus, I. C., Keeling, A. & Paice, E. (2004) Stress, burnout and doctors' attitudes to work are determined by personality and learning styles: a twelve year longitudinal study of UK medical graduates. *BMC Medicine*, **2**, 29.

Royal College of Psychiatrists (2007) *A Competency Based Curriculum for Specialised Training in Psychiatry*. RCPsych.

CHAPTER 11

Involving trainees in teaching

Neil Masson & Clare Oakley

Introduction

Teaching is an important role for all practising psychiatrists. However, many studies have shown that psychiatric trainees are in fact the primary educators of medical students (Kaufman, 1970; Callen & Roberts, 1980; Bing-You & Sproul, 1992). Medical students often work more closely with trainees than consultants during their psychiatry attachment and this allows trainees a unique opportunity to enhance the knowledge and skills of medical students, as well as to influence their values and behaviour through role-modelling and professional socialisation. For psychiatric trainees in particular, working with medical students provides a critical forum for addressing misconceptions and stigma about mental illness (Foreman *et al*, 2007). This chapter highlights the important role trainees have in teaching undergraduates, the potential benefits for students and trainees, and the unique ways in which trainees can contribute to the teaching of undergraduates.

The role of psychiatric trainees in undergraduate education

The transition from undergraduate medical student to postgraduate psychiatric trainee brings with it a multitude of new responsibilities, including that of teaching. Trainees regularly gain experience of teaching, for example through formal case presentations and journal clubs, departmental inductions and conference presentations. They teach a variety of learners such as peers, other professionals, patients and of course medical students. Trainees must rapidly develop teaching skills when they progress from student to teacher, often without any formal training in how to teach (Bramble, 1991).

Many studies have shown that trainees in all specialties are the main educators of medical students and can spend 20–25% of their time in this role (Kates & Lesser, 1985). Medical students in turn claim that up to a third of their education is derived from trainees alone (Busari *et al*, 2000). A study by Callen & Roberts (1980) found that the average psychiatric trainee will spend 3.67 hours per week teaching undergraduates and they feel they should spend more time doing so. A survey by Bramble (1991) found that psychiatric trainees spent 13.8% of their time teaching and that they viewed teaching as an important skill. While senior psychiatrists will have overall responsibility for the education of medical students on their placements, the job of teaching, appraising and assessing medical students is often given to trainees (Curran & Bowie, 1998; Vassilas *et al*, 2003). With the increase in medical student numbers over recent years, trainees may play a greater role in teaching, and while this is often to free up clinical time for senior psychiatrists and is seen as good experience for the trainee, there are also distinct advantages that trainees bring to undergraduate teaching, for both the student and the trainee (American Psychiatric Association, 2002; Bloor *et al*, 2006).

How undergraduates benefit from trainee teaching

There is evidence from other medical specialties that the quality of trainee teaching correlates with better academic performance by students (Morrison & Hafler, 2000). There are several potential reasons why trainee teaching can be particularly useful for medical students. Trainees are in an intermediate position of having knowledge, authority and experience that is greater than a medical student but less than a senior psychiatrist; students are therefore less intimidated by trainees and more likely to express concerns, ask questions and seek more teaching (Stewart & Feltovich, 1988). Medical students are also following behind trainees on a continuum of professional development, where they gradually acquire knowledge, skills, attitudes and professional values (Stritter *et al*, 1988). As their stages of professional development are similar, it is easier for trainees to adapt their teaching to concentrate on 'early skills' such as basic psychopathology or asking sensitive questions. As they are more closely related on the career ladder, when students are on a placement with trainees they are seeing the job they could soon be doing, which can also generate enthusiasm for the specialty and potentially influence career choice.

As trainees have themselves been undergraduates relatively recently, they may be more familiar with the needs and concerns of students and the level of competence expected of students during medical school. They are also likely to have first-hand experience of the undergraduate course and the nature of upcoming examinations. Psychiatric trainees may also be more familiar with the problem-based learning style that is common in undergraduate curricula (see below and Chapter 9), as trainees may have experienced this style of learning themselves. There are also similarities in examinations and assessments, with both psychiatric trainees and medical students tending to have mutual exposure to objective structured clinical examinations, multiple-choice questions, observed clinical encounter assessments, observed procedure assessments and portfolio assessments. Such similarities mean that trainees are in an ideal position to teach students.

An important by-product of trainee teaching is vicarious learning, where students learn through role-modelling and professional socialisation. Role-modelling, or teaching by example, is itself is a powerful way of transmitting attitudes, beliefs and behaviour to students (Bandura, 1986). This type of learning is particularly important for trainees, as students may spend more clinical time with them than with senior psychiatrists, owing to their availability during working hours and when on call. Furthermore, studies have found that psychiatric trainees are considered by students to be the most influential role-models, ahead of consultants, and that students select recent graduates as important role-models, as they have 'survived the system' (Kaufman, 1970; McLean, 2004; Joubert *et al*, 2006). This has important implications for influencing career choices, as both clinical experiences during attachments and influential role-models have been the factors most often cited as affecting specialty choice by medical students (Wright *et al*, 1997; Althouse *et al*, 1999; Elzubeir & Rizk, 2001). When student-identified role-models themselves have been asked about what characteristics they rated as most descriptive of themselves, they chose their enthusiasm for their specialty and their enthusiasm for teaching (Ambrozy *et al*, 1997). This emphasises why devotion to teaching, among trainees in particular, can foster role-modelling and the resultant benefits of learning by example.

How trainees benefit from teaching undergraduates

While teaching should of course benefit the intended recipient, the act of teaching undergraduates also benefits trainees in many ways. Undergraduate teaching allows trainees to improve their knowledge base, communication skills, appraisal skills, examination skills and motivation for learning, all of which help maintain lifelong professional development. The process of planning, organising, delivering and evaluating teaching can be extremely rewarding and research has shown that trainees' job satisfaction is augmented by teaching duties (Moffic, 1982; Morrison *et al*, 2005). The skills learned from teaching students will also be used by trainees for the rest of their career and when teaching other groups, such as other psychiatrists, trainees and patients.

Teaching itself can be a powerful motivator for self-directed learning. As the trainee will have less knowledge than a senior psychiatrist, the topics they choose to include in teaching may be more limited. This can highlight gaps in current knowledge, often emphasised by searching questions from medical students, which will galvanise trainee learning (Painter *et al*, 1987).

Previous research has shown that teaching leads to better knowledge acquisition in trainees compared with self-study or lecture attendance (Weiss & Needlman, 1998). Given that both trainees and medical students are often preparing for upcoming examinations, which are often in a similar format, any preparatory teaching given by trainees can be of benefit for their own examination. Both medical students and trainees are also subject to appraisal and the experience of giving feedback to students can be of benefit to how they handle their own evaluations. Also, learning to provide effective feedback on performance is an essential skill which will be needed by higher trainees when they supervise and assess more junior colleagues in the workplace (Brown & Cooke, 2009).

Teaching is a core component of practising as a medical professional and teaching and training have been listed as one of the 12 key attributes of a good psychiatrist (Royal College of Psychiatrists, 2009a). As some form of teaching is considered to be an essential element of working as a consultant psychiatrist, this is reflected in the expectations for psychiatric trainees. The new curriculum for psychiatric trainees, developed by the Royal College of Psychiatrists and approved by the Postgraduate Medical Education and Training Board, has as one of its 18 intended learning outcomes 'develop and utilise the ability to teach, assess and appraise' (Royal College of Psychiatrists, 2009b). Core trainees are expected to demonstrate an understanding of the principles of adult learning, identify learning outcomes, have a professional attitude towards teaching and ensure that feedback from teaching activities is used to develop their teaching style. The competencies expected of advanced trainees include identifying learning styles, using a variety of teaching methods, organising educational events and facilitating the learning process, and assessing performance. Therefore, it is necessary for psychiatric trainees to develop skills in teaching and to be involved in delivering teaching to a variety of groups. Trainees are required to provide evidence to show that they have been involved in teaching and have achieved the required competencies. This portfolio of evidence can include a logbook of teaching activity, feedback forms from recipients of teaching sessions and Assessments of Teaching. The Assessment of Teaching is the workplace-based assessment specifically developed to assess teaching skills and can be used when delivering small-group teaching sessions or lectures. This evidence is presented at the trainees' Annual Review of Competence Progression, which will determine whether they have achieved the necessary competencies to progress to the next stage of postgraduate training.

Trainees' concerns

Despite the amount of undergraduate teaching that trainees are expected to do, and the potential benefits of trainee teaching, the vast majority of trainees do not receive formal training in education (Dewey et al, 2008). A survey in the UK revealed that as few as 30% of psychiatric trainees had received specific training in teaching (Bramble, 1991). A similar national survey of trainee psychiatrists in the USA showed that only 13% of them had received any formal training to improve their teaching (Painter *et al*, 1987). Owing to the limited amount of formal training in teaching, it is important that trainees discuss their teaching with their consultant during educational supervision to ensure they are receiving appropriate support.

Other common concerns raised by trainees about teaching include feelings of inadequacy, its stressful and time-consuming nature and doubts about what to teach, particularly when trainees are learning themselves (Stritter *et al*, 1988). Kates & Lesser (1985) consider the common problems encountered by psychiatric trainees when teaching medical students as being lack of role clarity, insufficient knowledge of the students' learning objectives and inadequate teaching support for the trainee. Given these findings it is therefore important to highlight the practical areas of medical student education that psychiatry trainees can most influence.

Clinical teaching

Induction

Medical students often feel unsure of themselves when they start a placement in psychiatry, as it can seem very different from the other placements they have experienced. In order for them to gain the most out of the placement, it is important that they quickly become orientated to psychiatry and what is expected of them and what they should aim to achieve in the placement. This is a task that the trainee of the consultant with whom they are working is well placed to undertake. The junior trainee will have been in the same situation as the medical student a few years previously and will remember the uncertainties and misunderstandings. At the beginning of an attachment, students can be assisted by the trainee in developing learning objectives for their time in psychiatry and planning what learning opportunities and experiences will be available to them in order to meet those objectives. Although the primary goal will be for the student to pass the examination in psychiatry, different students will have different areas of interest, and these should be identified and cultivated. While trainees may feel particularly enthusiastic about teaching students who are keen to pursue a career in psychiatry, teaching should be tailored, where possible, to suit other career interests as well. For example, students may wish to gain experience in liaison psychiatry, where there is more cross-over with medical specialties. The trainee can facilitate interesting experiences for students, for example arranging for them to accompany the community psychiatric nurse on home visits or accompanying them to a tribunal.

The introduction to a placement in psychiatry should include familiarising medical students with what may be unfamiliar terminology, the differences in history taking and the unique skill demanded by the mental state examination. There are important 'on the ground' issues that trainees may be best placed to teach, such as interview safety and how best to interact with and interview patients. The basic skills of assessing patients presenting with mental health problems should be outlined initially and students should be encouraged to attempt formulations for the patients they see. Trainees will remember the things that they found difficult to understand when they first encountered psychiatry and should highlight the key points of assessing, formulating, diagnosing and treating the common mental disorders. It will be helpful for students to have a practical sense of this to relate to when they are gaining knowledge from what they have read and been taught in lectures. There is a complexity in teaching psychiatry because there are essential components of being a good psychiatrist that are not related to factual knowledge but to personal qualities, such as empathy and skills such as active listening. Obtaining these skills requires repeated patient interactions with direct observation, supervision and opportunistic discussion. The psychiatric trainee as a teacher can facilitate the medical student's fledgling efforts at diagnostic and therapeutic interviewing by serving as a role-model and a constructive critic (Foreman *et al*, 2007).

In-patient-based teaching

Once induction is complete, students may want initially to see patients in pairs but should be encouraged to see patients alone eventually. Students should be supported to follow up the care of patients from admission to discharge, although this may be difficult owing to the brief nature of student placements. Ward rounds can be the ideal place for focused teaching; however, there must be appropriate modifications to the ward round to ensure that the student is not just a passive observer but is considered to be a valued member of the multidisciplinary team. Medical students should document their findings in case notes and should be encouraged to present patients they have seen in a similar way that a trainee may do. It is important to allow time in the ward round to discuss and explain specific management issues and ethical dilemmas (El-Sayeh *et al*, 2006). The trainee and student can be allocated joint tasks to complete between ward rounds, such as obtaining the views of carers or arranging physical tests. Under supervision from the trainee, students can also directly contribute to the care of in-patients by completing tasks that are more familiar to them, such as taking medical histories, doing physical examinations and performing practical procedures such as taking blood.

On call

Medical students can gain valuable experience by shadowing trainees when they are on call. This may take the form of daytime on call or, if the student is keen and available, evenings and weekends on call. Such students are more likely to obtain experience of psychiatric disorders that commonly present out of hours, such as acute psychosis, mania, substance misuse, self-harm and acute anxiety (Dunn & Fernando, 1989). As students are often encouraged to follow patients on their journey through hospital care, this provides an ideal opportunity for them to see patients when they are most unwell, before admission. They are able to learn by observing the on-call doctor prioritise cases, manage time, assess and manage acute presentations, formulate risk assessments and use the mental health legislation where appropriate. Students can also reciprocate by assisting the trainee with appropriately delegated tasks such as documenting the interview, performing a physical examination and obtaining blood samples. As out-of-hours work often involves liaison with other specialties, it is useful for medical students to see this interface from the point of view of psychiatry and appreciate the skills that psychiatrists can offer other specialties. As the work intensity when on call can be variable, quieter periods can be the ideal time to discuss any acute cases seen or to give an informal tutorial on a related topic.

In clinic (see also Chapter 13)

Although students are more likely to sit in with consultants in clinic, the increasing numbers of students at medical school mean that trainees are now more likely to be involved in clinic teaching also. It can again be potentially useful to have a student in clinic to take on tasks such as obtaining a collateral history from a carer or relative or summarising a set of case notes. Medical students will tend to prefer to observe clinic assessments early on in their attachment, until they gain enough experience to see patients, either alone or under supervision. If they are observing, it is important that they are given a particular task to keep them focused, such as describing an aspect of the patient's mental state or considering what the diagnosis is. A more active approach is 'hot-seating', where the student leads part of the consultation; this has the advantage that the student's interaction with the patient is observed, which gives an opportunity for feedback to be given later (Spencer, 2003). When students are interviewing patients alone, they should have sufficient details about the case and be given a specific task with a time frame in which to complete it. The student can then present findings to the trainee and the patient can be seen jointly to agree a management plan. The trainee should ensure that time is set aside to provide feedback to students on how they have performed; feedback should be fair, specific and collaborative (Brown & Cooke, 2009). Attempts should be made for students to follow up any patients who have been discharged from hospital, so they can appreciate recovery from mental illness. Many students are also required to keep a logbook of cases they have seen and if a student is interested in a particular case he or she may want to see the patient alone after the clinic appointment to complete a full assessment. The consent of patients should always be obtained first when students are in clinic and if patients do not consent then a contingency plan should be in place to avoid students being left with nothing to do. This could include asking them to review the notes of the next patient or to read up on a particular topic of interest.

Formal teaching

While the more informal clinical teaching described above can often be undertaken by core trainees, in many training centres it is only higher or advanced trainees who are permitted to undertake formal teaching of medical students. This is because the award of the MRCPsych is viewed as a demonstration of a broad knowledge base sufficient to teach undergraduates. While improving the quality of teaching is important for all trainees, those who do regular formal teaching should pay particular attention to improving these skills by reflection, seeking feedback and attending relevant teaching courses. Some of the types of formal teaching mentioned below are discussed in more detail in other chapters of the present book, but we focus here on the perspective of the trainee as the teacher.

Lectures (see Chapter 7)

Higher trainees will commonly be asked to lecture medical students either in place of their supervising consultant or as part of a regular teaching timetable. Common weaknesses are that an inexperienced trainee may be particularly prone to include lacking confidence, saying too much too quickly, poor timing, not stressing key points and not providing a summary (Curran & Bowie, 1998). Practical tips that are of relevance to trainees who may be new to lecturing include researching the audience and their needs, developing key aims to base the lecture on, preparing thoughtful support materials such as handouts and reading lists, and structuring the lecture so that there are activities and exercises that break up the presentation. Lectures can be particularly stressful for trainees and arriving early to be more familiar with the physical environment and speaking informally to early attendees can help. As trainees are likely to give standalone lectures, it will be more important to establish the ground rules, such as asking students to turn off mobile phones and encouraging interaction and questions. It is important to explain the title, content, objectives and length of the presentation and to set the content in context. If the lecture is long and theoretical, then attention and recall can be improved by changing the format of the lecture to include 'brainstorming', 'buzz groups' or mini-assessments (Cantillon, 2003). The final part of the lecture should include a summary of the key points, further sources of information and enough time for questions. At the end of the lecture it is important to reflect on what went well, what went badly and what could be improved. Feedback from the audience and peer observers can be of particular benefit in improving the presentation skills of trainees (El-Sayeh *et al*, 2005).

Small-group teaching (see Chapter 8)

Some medical schools organise formal small-group seminars as part of the curriculum, but trainees are more likely to be involved in teaching groups of students on an informal basis during clinical placements. Although there is a tradition of teaching students in groups as part of so-called 'bedside teaching', there are particular topics that are best dealt with through group discussion. For example discussion of issues such as stigma in mental health, preparation for examinations and practical skills such as cognitive testing are ideal for group settings. Although trainees will be more comfortable with teaching predetermined topics using a leader-centred style, it is also important to use participant-centred 'free discussion groups', where students generate issues that are important to them and to which they can bring their own subjective experiences (Walton, 1997; El-Sayeh *et al*, 2005). As students may be less intimidated by trainees, they may be more likely to express worries or ask questions during small-group teaching (Stewart & Feltovich, 1988).

Problem-based learning (see Chapter 9)

Problem-based learning (PBL) has been increasingly used in undergraduate curricula over the past few decades as a means of enhancing 'deep' learning, motivation and retention of knowledge, as well as of developing skills in collaboration and teamwork (McParland *et al*, 2004). The use of this style of learning in educating psychiatric trainees has also been described and promoted and it is therefore important that trainees are familiar with this method of teaching (McCarthy *et al*, 2000). As undergraduate PBL curricula require more staff, this provides more opportunities for trainees to receive training in PBL and to act as facilitators or tutors in PBL groups. The learning methods used in PBL can also be adapted for clinical small-group teaching, as described above, if the discussion of clinical cases flags up areas of uncertainty. This can then form the basis of learning objectives, followed by self-directed learning and a subsequent group discussion on the knowledge acquired (Hughes & Williams, 1998).

Summary

Psychiatric trainees are key figures in undergraduate teaching and undertake a significant proportion of the teaching medical students receive in psychiatry. Benefits for medical students include trainees' familiarity with their learning needs and the fact that their relative lack of seniority may make them more approachable. Benefits of teaching for trainees include improving their own knowledge and the development of essential teaching skills. Trainees should involve themselves in both clinical and formal teaching of medical students and should receive appropriate training and consultant supervision for this important role.

References

Althouse, L. A., Stritter, F. T. & Steiner, B. D. (1999) Attitudes and approaches of influential role models in clinical education. *Advances in Health Sciences Education*, **4**, 111–122.

Ambrozy, D. M., Irby, D. M., Bowen, J. L., *et al* (1997) Role models' perceptions of themselves and their influence on students' specialty choices. *Academic Medicine*, **72**, 1119–1121.

American Psychiatric Association (2002) *Psychiatric Residents as Teachers: A Practical Guide*. APA.

Bandura, A. (1986) *Social Foundations of Thought and Action*. Prentice Hall.

Bing-You, R. G. & Sproul, M. S. (1992) Medical students' perceptions of themselves and residents as teachers. *Medical Teacher*, **14**, 133–138.

Bloor, K., Hendry, V. & Maynard, A. (2006) Do we need more doctors? *Journal of the Royal Society of Medicine*, **99**, 281–287.

Bramble, D. J. (1991) 'Teaching the teachers' – a survey of trainees' teaching experience. *Psychiatric Bulletin*, **15**, 751–752.

Brown, N. & Cooke, L. (2009) Giving effective feedback to psychiatric trainees. *Advances in Psychiatric Treatment*, **15**, 123–128.

Busari, J. O., Scherpbier, A. J. J. A., Van Der Vleuten, C. P. M., *et al* (2000) Residents' perception of their role in teaching under-graduate students in the clinical setting. *Medical Teacher*, **22**, 348–353.

Callen, K. E. & Roberts, J. M. (1980) Psychiatric residents' attitudes toward teaching. *American Journal of Psychiatry*, **137**, 1104–1106.

Cantillon, P. (2003) Teaching large groups. *BMJ*, **326**, 437–440.

Curran, S. & Bowie, P. C. W. (1998) Teaching psychiatry to medical undergraduates. *Advances in Psychiatric Treatment*, **4**, 167–171.

Dewey, C. M., Coverdale, J. H., Ismail, N. J., *et al* (2008) Residents-as-teachers programs in psychiatry: a systematic review. *Canadian Journal of Psychiatry*, **53**, 77–84.

Dunn, J. & Fernando, R. (1989) Psychiatric presentations to an accident and emergency department. *Psychiatric Bulletin*, **13**, 672–674.

El-Sayeh, H., Waller, R., Budd, S., *et al* (2005) The steep learning curve of medical education. *Psychiatric Bulletin*, **29**, 312–316.

El-Sayeh, H., Budd, S., Waller, R., *et al* (2006) How to win the hearts and minds of students in psychiatry. *Advances in Psychiatric Treatment*, **12**, 182–192.

Elzubeir, M. A. & Rizk, D. E. E. (2001) Identifying characteristics that students, interns and residents look for in their role models. *Medical Education*, **35**, 272–277.

Foreman, T., Dickstein, L. J. & Garakani, A. (eds) (2007) *A Resident's Guide to Surviving Psychiatric Training* (2nd edn). American Psychiatric Association.

Hughes, T. & Williams, C. (1998) Teaching general psychiatry to medical undergraduates. *Advances in Psychiatric Treatment*, **4**, 177–182.

Joubert, P. M., Kruger, C., Bergh, A. M., *et al* (2006) Medical students on the value of role models for developing 'soft skills' – 'that's the way you do it'. *South African Psychiatry Review*, **9**, 28–32.

Kates, N. S. & Lesser, A. L. (1985) The resident as a teacher: a neglected role. *Canadian Journal of Psychiatry*, **30**, 418–421.

Kaufman, P. (1970) Problems of undergraduate psychiatry teaching. *Seminars in Psychiatry*, **2**, 145–161.

McCarthy, M. K., Birnbaum, R. J. & Bures, J. (2000) Problem based learning and psychiatry residency education. *Harvard Review of Psychiatry*, **7**, 305–308.

McLean, M. (2004) The choice of role models by students at a culturally diverse South African medical school. *Medical Teacher*, **26**, 133–141.

McParland, M., Noble, L. M. & Livingston, G. (2004) The effectiveness of problem-based learning compared to traditional teaching in undergraduate psychiatry. *Medical Education*, **38**, 859–867.

Moffic, S. H. (1982) Educating psychiatry residents to become psychiatric educators. *Journal of Psychiatric Education*, **6**, 107–111.

Morrison, E. H. & Hafler, J. P. (2000) Yesterday a learner, today a teacher too: residents as teachers in 2000. *Pediatrics*, **105**, 238–241.

Morrison, E. H., Shapiro, J. F. & Harthill, M. (2005) Resident doctors' understanding of their roles as clinical teachers. *Medical Education*, **39**, 137–144.

Painter, A. F., Rodenhauser, P. R. & Rudisill, J. R. (1987) Psychiatric residents as teachers: a national survey. *Journal of Psychiatric Education*, **11**, 21–26.

Royal College of Psychiatrists. (2009a) *Good Psychiatric Practice* (3rd edn). College Report 154. RCPsych.

Royal College of Psychiatrists (2009b) *A Competency Based Curriculum for Specialist Training in Psychiatry*. RCPsych.

Spencer, J. (2003) Learning and teaching in the clinical environment. *BMJ*, **326**, 591–594.

Stewart, D. E. & Feltovich, P. J. (1988) Why residents should teach: the parallel process of teaching and learning. In *Clinical Teaching for Medical Residents* (eds J. C. Edwards & R. L. Marier), pp. 3–14. Springer.

Stritter, F. T., Shahady, E. J. & Mattern, W. D. (1988) The resident as professional and teacher: a developmental perspective. In *Clinical Teaching for Medical Residents* (eds J. C. Edwards & R. L. Marier), pp. 15–31. Springer.

Vassilas, C. A., Brown, N., Wall, D., *et al* (2003) 'Teaching the teachers' in psychiatry. *Advances in Psychiatric Treatment*, **9**, 308–315.

Walton, H. (1997) Small group methods in medical teaching. *Medical Education*, **31**, 457–464.

Weiss, V. & Needlman, R. (1998) To teach is to learn twice: resident teachers learn more. *Archives of Pediatrics and Adolescent Medicine*, **152**, 190–192.

Wright, S., Wong, A. & Newill, C. (1997) The impact of role models on medical students. *Journal of General Internal Medicine*, **12**, 53–56.

CHAPTER 12

Involvement of service users in psychiatric education

Nisha Dogra & Tracey Holley

Introduction

The literature on the involvement of service users or patients in medical education almost suggests that this is something that has happened only over the past decade or so. Anyone involved in clinical medical education will be aware that service users have always been a central component of teaching – you cannot teach clinical medicine without them. However, over the past couple of decades the roles played by service users have changed and diversified and service users have become more active partners. As an example, many service users/survivors and carers have emphasised the need for training in 'emotional care' and the need for clinical competence to be coupled with humanity. Within this model, human relationships are deemed to be at the core of mental health and practitioners demonstrating a shared humanness (Carson *et al*, 2008) with their clients increase the likelihood of successful outcomes.

In this chapter we begin with a brief discussion of terminology and the political drivers that have influenced the process. Where possible, we have referred to the literature as it relates to the teaching of psychiatry; otherwise we have used evidence from other medical disciplines. We consider the different levels of service user involvement in medical education. There is then a review of different stakeholder perspectives with respect to service user involvement – the key stakeholders being service users, medical students and teachers. There is then a discussion of the nature of service user involvement. Finally, the challenges are considered. We do not address the advantages and disadvantages of using real versus simulated patients, since Chapter 19 focuses on this. As the literature relating to service user involvement in medical education has grown, this chapter focuses on that literature but acknowledges that other disciplines, such as nursing, have developed practice in these areas (e.g. Langton *et al*, 2003; Felton & Stickley, 2004).

Terminology

The Royal College of Psychiatrists has argued that the preferred use by those to whom the term refers is 'service users and carers'. However, although we shall use this term as it is now widely used in psychiatry and mental health, we note that this does not necessarily reflect the views of the majority (Swift *et al*, 2000; McGuire-Snieckus *et al*, 2003). For the sake of ease we use the term 'service users' to include carers, although we appreciate that carers may not use services directly. Rees *et al* (2007) also highlight the lively debates that exist about appropriate terminology. The term 'experts by experience' recognises the value of experiential expertise (on a par with professional expertise) and encompasses those involved in training who have never used services as well as service users. When citing the literature we shall use the terms used by the authors.

Policy frameworks

The literature suggests that until the political drivers came into play, the involvement of service users in teaching was not on the medical education agenda. In fact, as far back as 1993, the General Medical Council (GMC) in its first edition of *Tomorrow's Doctors* stated that medical students should have early patient contact and community placements to promote a better understanding of patients' experience of ill health, of the social determinants of health and disease, and of the needs of the community. It is of note, however, that many schools were doing this well before 1993. The National Service Framework for Mental Health (Department of Health, 1999a), which reflected the recommendations of *Pulling Together* (Sainsbury Centre for Mental Health, 1997), stated that 'service users and carers' should be involved in planning, providing and evaluating training for all healthcare professionals (Department of Health, 1999a,b). With the establishment in 2002 of the Commission for Patient and Public Involvement in Health (Department of Health, 2005) there was further expectation that educators would consider service user and carer involvement more than they might previously have done. The patients' forum INVOLVE also seeks to ensure that there is a framework for active patient involvement in all aspects of healthcare, including training. In 2005 the Royal College of Psychiatrists deemed it to be mandatory for psychiatric trainees to receive training directly from people who experience mental health problems and their carers (Fadden *et al*, 2005).

Shifts in the policy framework reflect the changing role of patients and also the changing relationships between the public and doctors. The previously 'done to' and 'spoken to' service user was becoming the 'doer of' and the 'speaker of' their condition. Along with the rise of the 'expert patient' came the emergence of the importance of narratives of distress

– a non-medicalised language. This should be coupled with a more 'level playing field' in the future in the context of recovery-oriented interventions, where discerning psychiatrists will see their role as being 'on tap' rather than 'on top'.

Levels of involvement

The involvement can be direct with students at the clinical level but can also include broader involvement in other aspects of education, such as curriculum development, student recruitment and the development of policy. Dogra *et al* (2008) asked mental health service users how they thought mental health service users might contribute to medical student education with respect to psychiatry. The following key themes were identified:

- Service users can provide a contextualisation of individuals who have mental health problems, for example combining humanity with professionalism. This includes seeing the individual person (not just the illness) and looking beyond the case study towards a more holistic, psychosocial model of care.
- Service user involvement can emphasise positive aspects of mental health, counterbalancing negative media constructions and helping to dispel myths, fears and fantasies about mental ill-health.
- The engagement of service users as active partners in the learning process can be a means to illustrate the importance of hope and recovery. This may also act as a reminder that recovery begins with the assessment process.
- Involving service users in teaching can help students to recognise diversity, including the range of ways in which people experience mental ill-health, and the diversity that can exist within a single diagnostic category.
- Service user involvement can reinforce students' sense of the expertise they bring through their own experience. This should encourage the establishment of some common ground between students and service users and encourage a shared humanness.

Others have suggested that service users can provide support for interviewing skills and giving feedback, although the latter can be difficult if the care process is still active, so teachers should give close attention to service users' well-being.

Livingston & Cooper (2004) describe methods of delivery that might be deployed by service users. These include formal presentations, demonstrations to small groups and acting as personal tutors, as well as being observers in assessing a student's interpersonal skills. Service users can also become involved in course planning and development.

Box 12.1 The skills and attitudes that service users expected of a medical student

In the study by Dogra *et al* (2009) service users identified the following attitudes and skills that students require in psychiatry.

Attitudes

- Interpersonal qualities such as caring, listening, spending time, being non-judgemental
- Valuing and respecting patients, seeing the patient as a whole person, demonstration of non-stigmatising behaviour and non-stereotypical views of patients with mental illness
- Empathy and sympathy
- Conveying hope and a positive outcome
- Respect for diverse perspectives such as spirituality and homeopathy
- Accepting their own limitations and valuing teamwork

Skills

- Effective at engaging patients and developing a partnership with them
- Good and effective communication skills
- Basic counselling skills:
- Making an assessment and being able to diagnose and manage the problem in a way that is collaborative.

When asked about the knowledge, skills and attitudes that might be expected of a medical student, service users were more likely to identify the attitudes and skills that students require in psychiatry (Box 12.1) than the knowledge base (Dogra *et al*, 2009). This may be partly because many service users, while they are often the 'experts of their own experience' and even their condition, will be less familiar with other conditions. In this study there was little discussion about specific content within the 'knowledge' themes. When content was raised, it reflected personal experience of having received poor care in that area (e.g. side-effects of medication).

Service users also feel that they can contribute to the organisation of teaching (Dogra *et al*, 2008) and suggested that:

- teaching on mental health should be integrated and happen early in the course (with a view to addressing negative attitudes)
- teaching of mental health should be recurring
- more time should be given to this area than is currently devoted to it.

Similarly, they might influence policy and guidelines, as identified by Livingston & Cooper (2004). Users also have also suggested they might be involved in student selection, and this may merit further consideration.

The ladder of involvement

Tew *et al* (2004) presented a model named 'the ladder of involvement', with five levels at which service users can be included in the organisation and delivery of teaching.

- *Level 1: No involvement*. The course is delivered and managed with no consultation with or involvement of service users (except perhaps in more traditional passive roles).
- *Level 2: Limited involvement*. Service users have some involvement, when they are invited, but this is dependent on course leaders choosing this option. There is no opportunity for service users to shape the course as a whole.
- *Level 3: Growing involvement*. Service users contribute to at least two of several functions, such as course planning, delivery, student selection, assessment or management. Involvement is financially remunerated but service users are not part of decision-making forums.
- *Level 4: Collaboration*. Service users are involved in at least three formal functions but also are part of the decision-making forums concerned with, for example, curriculum content, style of delivery, learning outcomes, assessment criteria and methods, student selection and evaluation criteria. Service users contributing to the programme have the opportunity to meet for training, supervision and support. Steps are taken to enable service users to access programmes as students.
- *Level 5: Partnership*. Service users and teaching staff work together systematically and strategically across all areas and key decisions are jointly made. One of the authors (TH) has worked at this level and can attest to its efficacy.

However, some of the issues that this type of model raises are not discussed by Tew *et al* (2004). If service users actually become students on programmes through their involvement, how does this comply with equal opportunity legislation? Additionally, some users see their value as being heightened when they are *not* part of the 'delivery' system. This was an issue also identified by Livingston & Cooper (2004) and Rees *et al* (2007).

Curriculum design and planning

Curriculum design and planning require significant skill and most service users do not have a relevant educational background. Livingston & Cooper (2004) argued that quality assurance needs to address appropriate training to enable effective partnerships to be establsihed with service users in this area. Rees *et al* (2007) discussed some of the practical difficulties in implementation of service user involvement because of training needs and other aspects of service users' lives.

Stakeholders' perspectives

Service users' perspectives

Most of the research into service users' perspectives is about their involvement in clinics or on wards rather than in other roles. Much of the work has taken place in the USA, but where it has been undertaken in the UK, Australia and even Saudi Arabia, the overwhelming evidence indicates that service users are generally happy to participate in medical student education. Spencer *et al* (2000) argued that much of the work with respect to patient perspectives looks at their satisfaction with teaching encounters as opposed to what patients can contribute beyond just 'being there'.

Doshi *et al* (2006) found that in-patients with mental illness were generally happy to be seen by medical students and most felt they benefited from seeing students. It is of note that patients are not passive teachers or learning tools but part of a human interaction that can affect both those involved. Indeed, the student is also 'being seen' by the patient!

Patients' enablement and satisfaction were not impaired by student participation in general practice (Benson *et al*, 2005). The impact in psychiatry has not yet been explored, although it is often noted that the vulnerability of patients and the dynamic nature of this needs recognition. Informing patients that their participation is beneficial to the student's learning only if patients are seen and respected as part of the teaching team is crucial if patient involvement is to be non-exploitative and fully informed.

Qualitative analysis by Benson *et al* (2005) showed that patients generally supported the teaching of medical students but wanted to know when their doctor was absent because of teaching commitments (which they felt was a reasonable reason for absence), the characteristics of students (patients worried about undressing alone with students of the opposite sex) and the nature of the teaching planned. They wanted to have greater choice and felt it was better if they were asked about teaching in advance, when they booked their appointment, rather than at the time of the appointment, when it was harder to decline. It is also of note that they felt they could exert greater choice in the community context than in hospitals.

Coleman & Murray (2002) presented the reasons given by patients in primary care for the benefits of their involvement in education (in this case of general practitioners). They categorised these as either altruistic or reflecting some form of personal gain. The reasons are summarised below (where a finding has also been reported by others, the reference is added in parentheses). The altruistic reasons were:

- providing a service to the community by helping to train doctors (also Spencer *et al*, 2000)
- repaying a system that had helped them
- providing a service for no financial reward.

Reasons given for patient involvement that involved personal gain included:

- improved knowledge of their own condition (Stacy & Spencer, 1999; Spencer *et al*, 2000)
- enhanced self-esteem
- relief from social isolation and the opportunity for company (Stacy & Spencer, 1999)
- reassurance of well-being (as received several examinations and checks)
- a better perceived service (through general practitioners' improved understanding of their condition and because when general practitioners teach they have to keep up to date).

Coleman & Murray (2002) also reported the difficulties of patient involvement in the education of medical students, from the service users' perspective:

- embarrassment and anxiety (Benson *et al*, 2005; Doshi *et al*, 2006)
- reinforcement of feelings of ill-health and continuation of a focus on the illness
- extra time expended
- consent and confidentiality (Spencer *et al*, 2000).

In more general terms, involvement can be a negative experience if the power differentials of the traditional patient–doctor relationship are upheld. If there is shared humanness and a sense of a level playing field, the experience can become a self-affirming one that is beneficial to the journey of recovery and self-discovery.

Service users' experience of adverse effects

Benson *et al* (2005) and Spencer *et al* (2000) found no evidence of any adverse effects of participation. However, this appears not to have been well explored and it may also be difficult to separate out distress caused by participation (e.g. from inexpert or insensitive students) as opposed to distress from the disorder itself. Livingston & Cooper (2004) indicate that it would be useful to identify the distinguishing characteristics of those who benefit from involvement in medical education and those who might be distressed by it. However, distress is a transient state and it may be that those looking after patients in a vulnerable state would advise them against participation in student teaching. Briefing and debriefing of service users by teachers should help to minimise adverse effects.

Students' perspectives

Unsurprisingly, students value contact with patients and carers – it is this experience that gives them a real sense of 'doing the job' (Butterworth & Livingston, 1999). However, many medical students bring with them some negative attitudes towards patients with mental health problems (Dixon *et al*, 2008).

147

Psychiatric trainees are generally enthusiastic about patients contributing to their education and assessments, although fears were expressed about the latter (Vijayakrishnan *et al*, 2006)

Teachers' perspectives

Very little work has been undertaken to explore teachers' perspectives on the involvement of service users in their teaching of medical undergraduates. Tang & Skye (2008) looked at teacher characteristics when patients declined participation in medical education. Patients were more likely to decline participation when the teacher was uncomfortable discussing student involvement and when he or she was a member of faculty as opposed to a resident. The latter is a little surprising. In psychiatry, senior staff often develop long-term relationships with their patients and it may be more difficult for such patients to decline participation.

The nature of service users' involvement

Who?

Jackson *et al* (2003) argue for the need to ensure that service user involvement embraces all types of service users. They discuss how to ensure the involvement of less affluent service users. Their study found that patients living in areas of deprivation were positive about involvement in medical education and considered their personal experience and knowledge of illness to be an important aspect of student learning. However, there is also a need to ensure the involvement of those service users who are not vocal or politically powerful.

Spencer *et al* (2000) argued for the need to ensure diversity of student exposure, for example to the narrative experiences of service users (Holley, 2008). It is important that students do not use the experience of diverse groups in a stereotypical way; for example, the experience of one Indian patient with depression is not representative of other Indians with depression. Dogra & Karim (2005) argued for a more patient-centred approach, to fundamentally change the way we think about patients and their uniqueness. We need to ensure that when students meet patients they recognise that the perceptions of that individual are part of a particular narrative, with meanings that might be interpreted very differently by another person.

Where?

The move away from hospitalised care has often led to a lack of access to patients, as most are no longer 'captive' on wards, where participation was often welcomed if only to relieve boredom. People with illness in the community may be less inclined to participate, as they may have other priorities.

When?

There is no reason why service user involvement cannot begin early on in medical student careers and continue throughout. Early contact may help them to understand that illness should not be seen as a defining feature of an individual.

Why?

Beyond the political drivers, it is worth considering why service users should be more actively involved in medical education. As yet the research in this area has not shown differences between traditional service user involvement and more collaborative involvement.

The question of payment

In Coleman & Murray's (2002) study, discussed above, the patients felt that choosing to be involved for money alone would be to do it for the wrong reason (although refund of expenses was seen as acceptable). In contrast, Livingston & Cooper (2004) argued that the ability to earn money is an advantage and also that payment indicates that the service user's involvement is properly valued, a point also identified by Rees *et al* (2007). Some service users express the concern that payments for their contribution will affect their state benefits (see Scott, 2003). However, it is important to note that not all service user trainers are on benefits and some may find a new career and meaningful work as a professional service user, that is, someone with both professional training and experiential expertise.

Concerns over the involvement of service users

Psychiatrists operate with clear boundaries between them and their patients, and work to establish trusting, professional relationships. Having their patients as colleagues may blur some of these boundaries and present difficulties for both parties.

There are concerns that service user involvement can be token, lack clarity of purpose and result in a poor experience all round (Felton & Stickley, 2004; Ahuja & Williams, 2005; O'Keefe & Britten, 2005). Therefore it is imperative that educators and service users and carers consider the rationale for involvement at any specific point and have clarity about its purpose.

Over a decade ago, Spencer *et al* (2000) argued that further work with respect to patient involvement needed to address the following areas:

- whether there was 'added value' by engaging real patients rather than simulated patients
- whether there were benefits for the patients, beyond their personal satisfaction

149

- whether and how patients should have a role in student assessment
- the strengths and limitations of different models of patient involvement.

Much of this work remains to be done. Nevertheless, we hope in this chapter we have identified the enormous value service users can bring to the educational experience.

References

Ahuja, A. S. & Williams, R. (2005) Involving patients and their carers in educating and training practitioners. *Current Opinion Psychiatry*, **18**, 374–380.

Benson, J., Quince, T., Hibble, A., *et al* (2005) Impact on patients of expanded, general practice based, student teaching: observational and qualitative study. *BMJ*, **331**, 89.

Butterworth, M. & Livingston, G. (1999) Medical student education: the role of caregivers and families. *Psychiatric Bulletin*, **23**, 549–550.

Carson, A. M., Fairbairn, G., Lloyd, M., et al (eds) (2008) *The Narrative Practitioner Developing Excellence in Research, Education and Practice: 2007 Conference Proceedings*. North East Wales Institute, Glyndwr University.

Coleman, K. & Murray, E. (2002) Patients' views and feelings on the community-based teaching of undergraduate medical students: a qualitative study. *Family Practice*, **19**, 183–188.

Department of Health (1999a) *Patient and Public Involvement in the New NHS*. TSO.

Department of Health (1999b) *The National Service Framework for Mental Health*. Department of Health.

Department of Health (2005) *New Era in Patient and Public Involvement in the NHS*. Department of Health.

Dixon, R. P., Roberts, L. M., Lawrie, S., *et al* (2008) Medical students' attitudes to psychiatric illness in primary care. *Medical Education*, **42**, 1080–1087.

Dogra, N. & Karim, K. (2005) Training in diversity for psychiatrists. *Advances in Psychiatric Treatment*, **11**, 159–167.

Dogra, N., Anderson, J., Edwards, R., *et al* (2008) Service user perspectives about their roles in undergraduate medical training about mental health. *Medical Teacher*, **30**, e152–156.

Dogra, N., Cavendish, S., Anderson, J., *et al* (2009) Service user perspectives on the content of the undergraduate curriculum in psychiatry. *Psychiatric Bulletin*, **33**, 260–264.

Doshi, M., Acharya, S. & Wall, D. (2006) Mentally ill inpatients' experiences and opinions on seeing medical students: a questionnaire study. *Medical Teacher*, **28**, 568–570.

Fadden, G., Shooter, M. & Holsgrove, G. (2005) Involving carers and service users in the training of psychiatrists. *Psychiatric Bulletin*, **29**, 270–274.

Felton, A. & Stickley, T. (2004) Pedagogy, power and service user involvement. *Journal of Psychiatric and Mental Health Nursing*, **11**, 89–98.

General Medical Council (1993) *Tomorrow's Doctors*. GMC.

Jackson, A., Blaxter, L. & Lewande-Hundt, G. (2003) Participating in medical education: views of patients and carers in deprived communities. *Medical Education*, **37**, 532–538.

Langton, H., Barnes, M., Haslehurst, S., *et al* (2003) Collaboration, user involvement and education: a systematic review of the literature and report of an educational initiative. *European Journal of Oncology Nursing*, **7**, 242–252.

Livingston, G. & Cooper, C. (2004) User and carer involvement in mental health training. *Advances in Psychiatric Treatment*, **10**, 85–92.

McGuire-Snieckus, R., McCabe, R. & Priebe, S. (2003) Patient, client or service user? A survey of patient preferences of dress and address of six mental health professions. *Psychiatric Bulletin*, **27**, 305–308.

O'Keefe, M. & Britten, N. (2005) Lay participation in medical school curriculum development: whose problem is it? *Medical Education*, **39**, 651–652.

Rees, C., Knight, L. V. & Wilkinson, C. E. (2007) 'User involvement is a sine qua non, almost in medical education': learning with rather than just about health and social care service users. *Advances in Health Sciences Education*, **12**, 359–390.

Sainsbury Centre for Mental Health (1997) *Pulling Together: The Future Roles and Training of Mental Health Staff*. Sainsbury Centre for Mental Health.

Scott, J. (2003) *A Fair Day's Pay: A Guide to Benefits, Service User Involvement and Payments*. Mental Health Foundation.

Spencer, J., Blackman, D., Heard, S., *et al* (2000) Patient-oriented learning: a review of the role of the patient in the education of medical students. *Medical Education*, **34**, 851–857.

Stacy, R. & Spencer, J. (1999) Patients as teachers: a qualitative study of patients' views on their role in a community-based undergraduate project. *Medical Education*, **33**, 688–694.

Swift, G., Zacharia, M. & Casey, P. R. (2000) A rose by any other name: psychiatric outpatients' views on dress and address. *Irish Journal of Psychological Medicine*, **17**, 132–134.

Tang, T. S. & Skye, E. P. (2008) When patients decline medical student participation: the preceptors' perspective. *Advances in Health Sciences Education: Theory and Practice*, **14**, 645–653.

Tew, J., Gell, C. & Foster, S. (2004) Learning from experience: involving service users and carers in mental health education and training. National Institute for Mental Health in England (West Midlands), Trent Workforce Development Confederation.

Vijayakrishnan, A., Rutherford, J., Miller, S., *et al* (2006) Service user involvement in training: the trainees' view. *Psychiatric Bulletin*, **30**, 303–305.

CHAPTER 13

Time-efficient clinical teaching

Greg Lydall

Introduction

As service pressures increase, so do demands on clinician teachers. Yet opportunities for effective clinical teaching abound, even in a busy service. Nearly every aspect of a psychiatrist's work offers educational value and may be imparted through different teaching methods. This chapter provides illustrations of evidence-based approaches to the time-efficient clinical teaching of one or two medical students on attachment, and should apply to any psychiatric specialty.

Teaching may be integrated into ward rounds, out-patient clinics, home visits and other clinical encounters. The challenge is to provide simultaneous high-quality teaching and clinical care without compromising either (Cantillon, 2003; Doshi & Brown, 2005). With adequate planning and team involvement, integrated teaching can achieve more than the educational objectives expected by students. It may also enhance positive role-modelling, reflective practice and both trainee and trainer satisfaction. Ultimately, it is hoped that a positive clinical experience will encourage more students to choose a career in the exciting field that is psychiatry.

Educational background (see also Chapter 1)

Patient-based teaching offers improved relevance and recall, lifelike preparation and transferable skills (Dent, 2001; Hartley et al, 2003; Spencer, 2003). Integrating time-efficient, patient-based teaching into ambulatory and ward settings is challenging not least because of the competing demands on the clinician's time. Student participation may decrease productivity and lengthen the working day, hence the need for time-efficient integrated teaching strategies (Usatine et al, 1997).

One intention of clinical teaching is to foster deep learning, a process which, through seeking connection and thinking about the whole picture, results in improved understanding. Deep learning is the opposite style to surface learning, which is largely about memorising (Marton & Saljo, 1976). Students who adopt a surface learning approach are more likely to fail and to gain poorer, lower-marked degrees (Butcher, 1995). Fostering a deep approach to learning involves enhancing student motivation and involvement, interaction with others and a well-structured knowledge base (Butcher, 1995).

The experiential learning model states that learning is most effective when based on direct experience (Kolb, 1984). The model describes a cycle that involves engagement in a new experience, feedback and reflection, formulation of sound theories, and application of these theories in new situations.

The process of learning from patients was described by Cox (1993). It involves a figure of 8, where the experience cycle (preparation, briefing, clinical interaction and debriefing) leads into an explanation cycle (reflection, explication, working knowledge). This leads back into preparation for the future and the experience cycle.

Role-modelling is another important process that occurs during clinical teaching (Paice *et al*, 2002). Role-models can display positive and negative behaviours, which are imparted to learners through conscious and unconscious processes. Their positive characteristics comprise: clinical competence, teaching skills and personal qualities (Cruess *et al*, 2008). Observed behaviours and attitudes are incorporated into the belief patterns and behaviours of the student. Clinicians can improve upon this important aspect of their teaching through awareness of their own behaviours and reflection on their actions and unconscious processes; role-modelling is also enhanced by the provision of protected teaching time (Schon, 1987).

Along with gaining skills, an important aspect of learning to become a professional is joining the 'community of practice', by being given tasks that contribute to the enterprise (Lave & Wenger, 1991). In psychiatric practice, students may partake of this through detailed history taking (which demands active listening), discussing treatment options and psycho-education (for example regarding the illness or proposed therapeutic strategies). Feeling useful during the psychiatric attachment, seeing positive role-models, witnessing effective treatment and enjoying the time are all predictors of the choice of psychiatry as a specialty (McParland *et al*, 2003; Pidd, 2003; Thomas, 2008). All of these can be addressed in time-efficient clinical teaching.

Arrangements

Preparation

Preparation is crucial. For optimal time-efficient teaching, the teacher will need to balance the demands of the curriculum and students' learning objectives with the available resources: time, clinical space, staff and patients.

The teacher should read through the relevant medical school curriculum to find out which themes occur commonly in clinical examinations or objective structured clinical examinations (OSCEs). If possible, the teacher should examine the weekly timetables of the clinicians on the team and map these to the medical students' timetable. Medical student attachments are increasingly split between lectures and visits to general practices and other sites, which leaves less continuous time in one specialty, and thus more need for time efficiency. Delegating some teaching to enthusiastic and educationally interested junior doctors and other team members (e.g. mental health nurses, psychologists) increases the variety of clinical exposure and time efficiency.

Before students arrive, the learning environment should be prepared. This includes alerting the team members and administrative staff, and ensuring that rooms, desks and equipment are available. It is helpful to ask staff in advance to identify suitable cases, which can then be added to your list of resources and matched to the students' learning objectives.

Teaching on ward rounds
(adapted from Murdoch & Cottrell, 1998)

Allocating an appropriate patient for whom the student is 'responsible' for the duration of the attachment has many advantages. The student gets to know the person and problems in detail, can participate in treatment (supervised by qualified doctors) and can witness the patient's recovery. Selection of a relatively low-risk patient likely to engage with a student and improve rapidly is helpful. Ideally, patients should be seen from community or emergency presentation until discharge, so allocating sessions for these is recommended. Allocating tasks before the ward round for feedback during the round can save time; such tasks might be taking a history, gathering collateral information, discussing medication side-effects or psycho-education about diagnosis. At each ward round, the student can focus on a particular learning goal in relation to the patient, and present using one of the models described below.

Safety on the ward is paramount. Students should be inducted into safety policy, including alarms and breakaway techniques.

Teaching in out-patient clinics
(adapted from Spencer, 2003)

Initially, it is recommended to book a lighter clinic than usual, to allow time for feedback and teaching. As your skills and the student's familiarity with the models improve, time may be regained as efficiency increases. Nevertheless, teaching students does generally impact on service. Some time can be saved by asking students to read patients' case records before the clinic commences. You can ask students to complete specific tasks (from their agreed goals), such as writing down the mental state or differential diagnosis. With the student's and the patient's agreement, try placing the student in the 'hot-seat' by asking him or her to lead part or all of the consultation (it will be important to provide feedback to the student afterwards). Students should see patients on their own once they are familiar with the clinic, and then can present using one of the models below.

'Wave scheduling' allows for efficient use of clinician/teacher time, with minimal impact on the number of patients seen (Ferenchick *et al*, 1997). The student assesses about half the cases on his or her own, and then presents to the teacher in a combined session. In a typical 9.00–12.00 morning clinic, the trainee sees patients 1, 3 and 5 for half an hour each and presents them to the trainer for 30 minutes on the half hour. The trainer sees patients 2, 4 and 6 on the hour and without the student. Planned allocation of interesting cases to the odd numbers requires significant foresight but can be done (patient choice of times notwithstanding).

Teaching in community settings

When planning a home visit with a student, safety again becomes paramount. In addition, it will be necessary to select a patient appropriate for the student's level of experience. Students may initially shadow or actively observe (see below) the teacher at work, but can later take on specific areas of history or mental state to assess. The journeys to and from the assessment may represent further teaching time.

Time-efficient clinical teaching: four approaches

For all four models described below, it is important to explain what is required from the learner and to allow for flexibility between models. The four are summarised in Table 13.1, which includes the traditional approach, for comparison.

Activated demonstration

This model is useful early on in the attachment or where the student's knowledge level is low. It demonstrates clinical expertise and role-modelling, while actively engaging the learner.

The teacher scans the case notes and learner's goals, and anticipates which areas will be important to the patient (although the latter is of course unpredictable). The learner is given a specific set of assignments to complete while observing the teacher (Wilkerson & Irby, 1998). Examples are: 'Watch how I ask questions about suicide and self-harm with Mr Smith' and 'Please write down the questions and answers to the mini-mental state

Table 13.1 Summary of teaching models

Model	Student level of experience/ confidence	Suitable setting	Process in brief
Classical case presentation	Any	Any	Student does full psychiatric history/ examination and presents to teacher, followed by discussion and feedback
Activated demonstration	Low	Any	Learner has specific assignments to complete while observing
One-minute preceptor	Medium–high	Ambulatory settings and ward rounds	Get a commitment Probe for underlying reasoning Teach general rules/principles Provide positive feedback Correct errors
Aunt Minnie	Medium– high	Ambulatory settings	Focused history/examination on main complaint Present main complaint and presumptive diagnosis Teacher then sees patient, makes diagnosis, and creates a management plan Learner writes up notes/observes Feedback and discussion Checking and signing medical record
SNAPPS	Medium –high	Ambulatory settings	Summarise the findings Narrow down the differential diagnosis Analyse pros/cons of each diagnosis Probe the teacher Plan management Select a case-related problem for self-directed learning

examination as we go through it with Mrs Jones'. After the demonstration the learner is 'activated' by reporting the findings; this is followed by a brief discussion. The learner should be encouraged to ask questions about the clinician's rationale. Lastly, independent study linked to the student's educational goals is agreed and assigned.

The one-minute preceptor

This widely known and researched model is also known as the one-minute teaching model. It is applicable to ambulatory settings and psychiatric ward rounds and focuses on diagnostic reasoning skills. In a pilot study within general medicine, learners reported strong satisfaction with this model, and teachers rated learners' skills and knowledge higher than with the traditional approach (Aagaard *et al*, 2004). The learner sees the patient beforehand and the process can be integrated with clinics using 'wave scheduling' (described earlier). This model is based on five 'micro-skills' on the part of the teacher (Neher *et al*, 1992):

- get a commitment from the learner about the likely issues
- probe for underlying reasoning or alternative explanations
- teach general rules (map the case to agreed learning goals)
- provide positive feedback about what the learner did right
- correct errors by making suggestions for improvement.

The application of these micro-skills is illustrated in Box 13.1.

Box 13.1 Illustration of the application of the five micro-skills of the one-minute preceptor model

A patient with treatment-refractory schizophrenia is attending a consultant psychiatrist, the teacher, who is accompanied by a medical student, the learner.

Micro-skill 1: Get a commitment
Teacher: 'What do you think is going on?'
Learner: 'I think Mr X has treatment-resistant schizophrenia.'

Micro-skill 2: Probe for underlying reasoning or alternative explanations
Teacher: 'What led you to that conclusion?'
Learner: 'Mr X is a 21-year-old man with a 3-year history of first-rank psychotic symptoms suggestive of paranoid schizophrenia, specifically thought broadcasting and second-person auditory hallucinations. He has been treated with two different types of antipsychotics without sufficient response.'
Teacher: 'How would you manage his condition?'
Learner: 'I would consider initiating clozapine after discussion with the patient and ruling out any contraindications. I would discuss the pros and cons, including the risk of agranulocytosis.'

Micro-skill 3: Teach general rules (map the case to agreed learning goals)
Teacher: 'That sounds correct. He describes first-rank symptoms for at least 1 month with social withdrawal, which is sufficient to diagnose schizophrenia. Clozapine is the next pharmacological step and this choice is supported by the NICE and Maudsley guidelines. Bear in mind that prescribing clozapine is a commitment to regular blood tests. The NICE guidelines also recommend annual physical health monitoring and the use of cognitive–behavioural and/or family therapy.'

Micro-skill 4: Provide positive feedback about what the learner did right
Teacher: 'You did a good job of engaging with this patient and gaining diagnostic detail.'

Micro-skill 5: Correct errors by making suggestions for improvement
Teacher: 'You might want to explore substance misuse history in more detail because this co-occurs commonly in schizophrenia, and has been a problem for this patient in the past.'

Aunt Minnie

This model is designed to promote rapid diagnostic pattern recognition among students in an ambulatory setting (Cunningham *et al*, 1999) – in psychiatry typically in the out-patient follow-up clinic. It also allows for the development of note-taking skills, observation and role-modelling. The learner and patient need to understand the process, the teacher must also see the patient, and the teacher must be willing to admit to diagnostic uncertainty.

The learner sees the patient, takes a focused history and, if required, performs a physical examination on the basis of the main complaint. The student presents the main complaint and the presumptive diagnosis. Then the teacher independently sees the patient, makes a diagnosis and creates a management plan. The learner may write up the clinical notes or observe. Once the patient has left, feedback and discussion are followed by checking and signing the medical record.

SNAPPS

This learner-centred, out-patient case-presentation model encourages learners to engage in the teaching by challenging them to justify their thinking and explore what they do not understand (Wolpaw *et al*, 2003). Six steps take place after the learner has seen the patient and because it involves detailed differential diagnoses, which may be distressing, often does not occur in the presence of the patient. The six steps (summarise, narrow, analyse, probe, plan, select) give the acronym SNAPPS:

- *Summarise the findings* (maximum 3 minutes or 50% of allocated teaching time). Information should be condensed and relevant (the teacher can elicit further details if necessary). Use of semantic qualifiers (e.g. 'acute', 'recurrent') and psychiatric language is encouraged because successful diagnosticians use these qualifiers early in their presentations (Nendaz & Bordage, 2002).
- *Narrow down the differential diagnosis to the two or three most likely possibilities.* This step requires commitment by the learner, similar to the one-minute preceptor model (above).
- *Analyse the differential diagnoses by comparing and contrasting diagnostic options.* This allows learners to verbalise their thinking process and for interactive discussion.
- *Probe the teacher by asking questions for clarity, or to understand uncertainties or alternatives.* Here the learner is encouraged to reveal areas of knowledge weakness, by freely asking questions and using the teacher as an expert.
- *Plan management.* Again, this step requires commitment from the learner, and allows for questioning of the teacher.
- *Select a case-related problem for self-directed learning.* Here the learner may select further case-related reading, which may be suggested by the

teacher. It should occur soon after the teaching session and answer a specific question or set of questions for later feedback.

Feedback

To learners

Feedback is considered central to promoting learning, correcting misunderstandings, and improving self-confidence of learners, yet is often avoided (Ende, 1983). Nine recommended techniques have been described (Hewson & Little, 1998):

- creating a respectful, friendly, open-minded, unthreatening climate
- eliciting thoughts and feelings before giving feedback
- being non-judgemental
- focusing on behaviours
- basing feedback on observed facts
- basing feedback on specifics
- giving right amount of feedback
- suggesting ideas for improvement
- basing feedback on well-defined, negotiated goals.

The same authors also recommended a six-phase model for feedback, based on feedback from clinician educators (Table 13.2). A shorter version is the feedback sandwich: give a slice of negative feedback between two slices of positive feedback (Milan *et al*, 2006).

To teachers

It is often difficult receiving feedback even if it does serve to improve practice. This is one excellent reason to invite feedback from learners. Using the same model set out for learners (Hewson & Little, 1998), and after students have been graded (which makes it clear that their feedback does not affect their grade), the teacher should discuss what they enjoyed and what could be improved. Some schemes use standardised feedback forms, which will often be completed anonymously. These are useful for generating scores and for raising issues which are difficult to raise face to face. Another advantage of feedback to teachers is that the learners will gain confidence in giving it, which will be useful for when they are teachers.

Summary

This chapter has described how time-efficient clinical teaching can occur in different settings using four evidence-based teaching models. With

Table 13.2 Recommended six-phase feedback model (adapted from Hewson & Little, 1998)

Phase	Technique	Example
1. Prepare person for session	Inform ahead of time Select appropriate time and location Provide relaxed, respectful atmosphere Negotiate agenda	Let's make an appointment to review your performance What are your goals for this attachment? Remember your objective to carry out an accurate mini-mental state examination?
2. Ask person for self-assessment	What was done well How they felt Open-ended questions	How do you think it went? What was done well? What could be improved?
3. Diagnosis and feedback	Decide where person needs to improve; give reinforcing and positive feedback Feed back on observations of a specific behaviour/style/approach Give reasons in the context of well-defined shared goals	When you did/said … I was pleased/relieved/concerned/annoyed because…
4. Develop specific improvement plan	Invite suggestions Give your suggestions Suggest articles, consultations Teach (discuss, demonstrate, role-model, coach)	What could you do differently? This is my suggestion… Where will you get help? Let's reframe this problem … Let's talk about this…
5. Apply strategies to real situation	Agree to apply improvement plan to current or future problems	What will you do next time? Can you show me?
6. Review	Confirm person understands and agrees with feedback themes Person reviews behaviours benefitting from change Discuss consequences of lack of change	What did you do well? What changes will you make? By when? What if you don't?

adequate planning and team involvement, integrated teaching can cover students' learning objectives, enhance positive role-modelling and increase student and teacher enjoyment. Ultimately, it is hoped that a positive clinical experience will encourage more students to choose a career in the exciting field that is psychiatry.

References

Aagaard, E., Teherani, A. & Irby, D. M. (2004) Effectiveness of the one-minute preceptor model for diagnosing the patient and the learner: proof of concept. *Academic Medicine*, **79**, 42–49.

Butcher, C. (1995) *Active Learning and Teaching: Researching Learning and Teaching*. Staff and Departmental Development Unit, University of Leeds.

Cantillon, P. (2003) *ABC of Learning and Teaching in Medicine*. BMJ Books.

Cox, K. (1993) Planning bedside teaching – 1. Overview. *Medical Journal of Australia*, **158**, 280–282.

Cruess, S. R., Cruess, R. L. & Steinert, Y. (2008) Role modelling – making the most of a powerful teaching strategy. *BMJ*, **336**, 718–721.

Cunningham, A. S., Blatt, S. D., Fuller, P. G., *et al* (1999) The art of precepting: Socrates or Aunt Minnie? *Archives of Pediatric and Adolescent Medicine*, **153**, 114–116.

Dent, J. A. (2001) *Hospital Wards*. Churchill Livingstone.

Doshi, M. & Brown, N. (2005) Whys and hows of patient-based teaching. *Advances in Psychiatric Treatment*, **11**, 223–231.

Ende, J. (1983) Feedback in clinical medical education. *JAMA*, **250**, 777–781.

Ferenchick, G., Simpson, D., Blackman, J., *et al* (1997) Strategies for efficient and effective teaching in the ambulatory care setting. *Academic Medicine*, **72**, 277–280.

Hartley, S., Gill, D., Walters, K., *et al* (2003) *Teaching Medical Students in Primary and Secondary Care*. Oxford University Press.

Hewson, M. G. & Little, M. L. (1998) Giving feedback in medical education: verification of recommended techniques. *Journal of General and Internal Medicine*, **13**, 111–116.

Kolb, D. A. (1984) *Experiential Learning*. Prentice Hall.

Lave, J. & Wenger, E. (1991) *Situated Learning: Legitimate Peripheral Participation*. Cambridge University Press.

Marton, F. & Saljo, R. (1976) On qualitative differences in learning I – outcome and process. *British Journal of Educational Psychology*, **46**, 4–11.

McParland, M., Noble, L. M., Livingston, G., *et al* (2003) The effect of a psychiatric attachment on students' attitudes to and intention to pursue psychiatry as a career. *Medical Education*, **37**, 447–454.

Milan, F. B., Parish, S. J. & Reichgott, M. J. (2006) A model for educational feedback based on clinical communication skills strategies: beyond the 'feedback sandwich'. *Teaching and Learning in Medicine*, **18**, 42–47.

Murdoch, E. & Cottrell, D. (1998) Maximising the effectiveness of undergraduate teaching in the clinical setting. *Archives of Diseases in Childhood*, **79**, 365–367.

Neher, J. O., Gordon, K. C., Meyer, B., *et al* (1992) A five-step 'microskills' model of clinical teaching. *Journal of the American Board of Family Practitioners*, **5**, 419–424.

Nendaz, M. R. & Bordage, G. (2002) Promoting diagnostic problem representation. *Medical Education*, **36**, 760–766.

Paice, E., Heard, S. & Moss, F. (2002) How important are role models in making good doctors? *BMJ*, **325**, 707–710.

Pidd, S. A. (2003) Recruiting and retaining psychiatrists. *Advances in Psychiatric Treatment*, **9**, 405–411.

Schon, D. A. (1987) *Educating the Reflective Practitioner: Toward a New Design for Teaching and Learning in the Professions*. Jossey-Bass.

Spencer, J. (2003) Learning and teaching in the clinical environment. *BMJ*, **326**, 591–594.

Thomas, T. (2008) Factors affecting career choice in psychiatry: a survey of RANZCP trainees. *Australasian Psychiatry*, **16**, 179–182.

Usatine, R. P., Nguyen, K., Randall, J., *et al* (1997) Four exemplary preceptors' strategies for efficient teaching in managed care settings. *Academic Medicine*, **72**, 766–769.

Wilkerson, L. & Irby, D. M. (1998) Strategies for improving teaching practices: a comprehensive approach to faculty development. *Academic Medicine*, **73**, 387–396.

Wolpaw, T. M., Wolpaw, D. R. & Papp, K. K. (2003) SNAPPS: a learner-centered model for outpatient education. *Academic Medicine*, **78**, 893–898.

CHAPTER 14

Intercalated degrees

Rachel Upthegrove, Lisa Jones & Femi Oyebode

Introduction

The option of taking an extra year to complete an intercalated degree, either classed as a BSc or BMedSc, has long been a tradition for students in UK medical schools. Recently, more students have chosen this option, reflecting the increase in medical student numbers and the increasingly competitive market for foundation-year posts. Currently, just over a third of all British medical students obtain an intercalated degree. Likewise, the range of courses on offer has increased. The proportion of students taking an intercalated degree still varies widely from school to school, and it should be noted that in some (e.g. Oxford, Cambridge and Nottingham) a BSc degree is either obligatory or given to all students. In most schools, however, intercalating is an option only for students who have performed well in other parts of the course.

Traditionally, intercalating was taken in between the preclinical and clinical years, with basic science subjects of anatomy, biochemistry and pathology being the norm. The history of medicine was one of the few alternatives on offer. With the introduction of integrated teaching and the increase in student numbers, a wider range of subjects, including those in clinical areas, have been offered, from aerospace physiology to human genetics. Now in most medical schools students are able to intercalate at any point in their undergraduate course after their second year. Medical schools also increasingly compete to attract external students.

The General Medical Council (2003) identified two main purposes for the intercalated year: the development of research skills and an in-depth study in areas of particular interest over an extended period. This is reflected in the content of courses, where a strong research theme is a core feature. The second edition of *Tomorrow's Doctors*, published by the General Medical Council in 2003, and updated in 2009, also proposed that in the core medical degree (MB) course 'factual information must be kept to the essential minimum that students need at this [undergraduate] stage of their medical education'. Thus, students are not able to study subjects in any great depth; medical students' education must be spread thinly to cover all subjects needed to practise safely as doctors. Intercalated degrees offer an opportunity to dig beneath a superficial layer of knowledge in a self-directed manner, and to develop intellectual and practical tools that will allow students to become more effective medical practitioners. This is true not just for those with an academic future ahead; greater knowledge and practical experience of research methods will give tomorrow's doctors the analytical skills needed to appraise evidence critically.

In practice, the opportunity to study subjects closely related to psychiatry also offers those involved in undergraduate teaching a window of opportunity through which to encourage and nurture interest in this particular subject area. Students now are increasingly obliged to choose a future specialty at an early stage, to polish and improve portfolios and gain extra 'points' for shortlisting at the foundation-year stage. Psychiatry cannot afford to miss the opportunity intercalating offers to attract the interest of (and indeed recruitment of) the highest-calibre students.

Courses currently on offer in the UK

Medical schools throughout the UK now offer a wider range of intercalating options, with the aim of attracting the brightest and best students in an increasingly competitive market. Courses with themes relevant to psychiatry range from those in basic sciences (e.g. psychology or neuroscience) to those more clinically based (e.g. psychological medicine). Table 14.1 gives details of some of the courses relevant to psychiatry currently on offer at UK medical schools, by way of illustration (it is not an attempt to list all courses currently on offer). Common themes include a strong research content, with most courses including a research project as well as taught modules. For illustrative purposes, and since it is the course in which the authors have been involved, below we describe the recently established Birmingham intercalated degree course in some detail.

In contrast, the University of Cardiff Medical School has been running its BSc in psychology and medicine for a number of years. The course focuses on compulsory modules of critical analysis and behavioural science, with additional optional modules. The main objective of the degree course is to promote knowledge and understanding of psychology in medicine at both a conceptual and practical level. Students are encouraged to evaluate critically the theory and methodology of a variety of psychological subject areas. Specific topics include learning and memory, causal cognition, human cognitive neuroscience, social cognition and inter-group relations, abnormal child psychology, forensic psychology, attitudes and attitude change, animal learning and cognition, family psychology, developmental psychopathology and family. Hands-on research experience is obtained by conducting a project. A module on critical analysis aims to impart the basic skills of

163

Table 14.1 Some intercalated degrees on offer at UK medical schools relevant to psychiatry

Medical school	Course title	Overview of content
Birmingham	Psychological medicine	Research methodology together with original research project. Linked modules taught in themed weeks: neurobiology of psychological process, neurobiology of mental illness, psychiatry and psychopathology in the arts
Cardiff	Psychology and medicine	Compulsory modules of critical analysis and behavioural science with options including neuroscience of learning and memory, family process and child development, criminological psychology, attitudes and social cognition, stress and disease
Dundee	Medical psychology	Taught module psychology theory and treatment; students see two patients under supervision formally written up as case studies. Short research project
King's College London	Neuroscience	Research project together with taught modules of cognitive neuropsychology, systems neuroscience, experimental pharmacology of neurological and psychiatric disorders, pharmacology of neurological and psychiatric disease
Keele	Brain and behaviour	Laboratory-based research report in addition to lectures and tutorials with topics including behavioural neurobiology, neurobiological basis of brain disease
Leeds	Neuroscience	Taught modules include developmental neurobiology, neuronal signalling, brain behaviour and disorder, psychopharmacology of anxiety and depression
Leeds	Psychology	Both laboratory-based and clinical research projects offered, together with taught options including visual perception and language, developmental psychology and individual differences, biological and abnormal psychology, neuropsychology, learning and motivation
Manchester	Neuroscience psychology	Students choose modules from BSc programmes in bioscience and humanities subjects allied to medical programmes and are taught within that integrated course
Nottingham	Intercalated degree as an integral component of the course	All graduates receive a BMedSci degree as well as the MBBS required to graduate as a doctor. However, because the intercalated degree does not require an extra year of study beyond the normal length of the MBBS programme, it is considered inferior to the intercalated BSc degrees offered elsewhere
University College London	Neuroscience	Laboratory-based research project plus taught modules including: mechanisms of development, neural basis of learning and motivation, advanced neuroanatomy
University College London	Psychology	Research project and taught compulsory modules plus optional modules from third-year psychology programme. Options include concepts and methods in psychology and the psychology of individual differences.

data collection, collation, analysis and presentation that are common to all effective research, from the perspective of the historical development of the modern scientific method. Lectures are used to impart the theoretical aspects of the subjects covered but the emphasis is on the development of practical skills through participative seminars and practical work. The module is assessed by the critical analysis of an unseen paper and an oral presentation. A module behavioural sciences aims to provide students with an introduction to basic psychology and psychiatry. Psychological knowledge will have the opportunity to be further developed within advanced modules that focus on language, learning and memory, counselling and psychotherapy, and cognitive disorders. The course also seeks to provide an understanding of common psychiatric disorders. Teaching is science led and concentrates on aetiology, disease progression, and pharmacological and psychotherapeutic treatments. Assessment is via two examination papers in essay and multiple-choice format.

University College London (UCL) gives a good example of a psychology intercalated degree on offer. Core aims are stated as gaining an understanding of the biological, cognitive–behavioural and social approaches to psychology, methodological approaches and significant findings in scientific psychology. Again, research design and quantitative methods are both taught didactically and through the completion of a research project, which may be either laboratory or clinically based. A novel element to this course is a focus on weekly seminars across all modules. Students are expected to prepare and bring work to the seminar. Assessment includes evaluation of this preparation work and contribution during the seminar, together with multiple-choice questions and essays.

The Birmingham intercalated degree in psychological medicine

One example of the recently introduced courses relevant to psychiatry on offer to UK medical students is the Birmingham intercalated degree in psychological medicine. This was designed to offer students a unique opportunity to study in depth subjects with real relevance to clinical psychiatry, but in a way that enables students to explore areas of particular interest in a self-directed manner. Psychological medicine sits alongside other BMedSc degrees, in public health, history of medicine, ethics and law, and international health within the intercalation option strand of 'Medicine in society'. The course integrates the scientific disciplines of psychology and psychiatry and combines science and humanities through an exploration of how psychopathology is portrayed in the arts. These themes are the main focus of the taught programme in the first semester. As with the other intercalated BSc programmes, there is a strong focus on research and students spend the second semester completing a research project in an area of psychological medicine that interests them. Apart

165

from one January examination (for the research methods module), the assessments are all based on course work and students are given the freedom to determine their own areas for further study. The course began in 2005 and has proved extremely popular from the outset with both internal and external students.

Innovation in undergraduate teaching

Devised from the outset to stand alone within undergraduate medical teaching, the BMedSc course has used a number of innovative teaching formats and techniques:

- A thematic approach is taken to the taught component in semester 1, as detailed below, whereby weekly streams are designed to give the course a cohesive and integrated dimension.
- There is an explicit expectation, made clear from the outset to students, of active participation in all aspects of small-group teaching. This participation contributes in a small but significant way to their overall marks.
- The humanities are, as a result in part of the themed weeks, genuinely taught as an integrated component of the course and not 'tagged on' in a token fashion. This allows students to realise the full potential of striving for a wider understanding of the human experience within medicine.

Course objectives

On completion of the programme, students should have knowledge and understanding of:

- commonly used research methods and data analysis techniques within health and medicine
- legal and ethical frameworks of medical research
- the neurobiological basis of processes of the mind and behaviour
- the neurobiological basis of mental illnesses
- the portrayal of psychiatry and psychopathology in the arts
- the value of fictional narratives, poetry, biography, letters and journals in medical education.

In addition to enhancing knowledge and understanding we believe our teaching methods strongly support development of the following skills and attributes:

- the ability to critically read and appraise research evidence
- the ability to produce scientifically valid research
- the ability to manage a research project, from conception to completion, with enhanced project management skills, which will be transferable to other aspects of students' careers

- the ability to effectively communicate their ideas or scientific findings through a range of commonly used presentation mechanisms, including oral presentation, poster presentation, production of a journal article and essay writing
- enhanced independent learning skills
- greater awareness of team working and skills to support teamwork in clinical and academic settings
- improved ability to think logically and broadly about a range of problems, drawing on a variety of disciplines to support arguments.

Course details

Semester 1

The first semester lasts 9 weeks and largely comprises the following modules (in addition to which some research work is done and a plenary session presented):

- *Quantitative and qualitative research methods.* This module covers a range of research methods, for which the teaching draws on a range of disciplines, including epidemiology, psychology and the social sciences, to provide students with a 'toolbox' of methods. The module covers both theory and practice, so students should complete the module feeling confident about applying methods to their own research.
- *Neurobiology of psychological processes.* Building upon their core knowledge of psychology and the neurosciences, students explore topics such as perception, emotion, aggression, sex, sleep, learning, memory and language. Students identify an area of particular interest for independent in-depth study, which is assessed by a 2000-word essay. Examples of recent essay topics include the neurocognitive basis of love, attachment and creativity.
- *Neurobiology of mental illness.* This covers areas purposely distinct from syndromal diagnosis and treatment, as these will be covered by students in their clinical psychiatry placement. Topics include areas such as auditory hallucinations, language disorders, dementias and delusions. Weekly teaching is delivered in small groups over 2 hours with a mixture of didactic, group teaching and case examples. Students, again, are assessed by a 2000-word essay on a particular self-chosen area of interest. Recent essay titles have included 'The biological mechanisms behind obsessive–compulsive disorder', 'Functional magnetic resonance scanning in auditory hallucinations' and 'Molecular neurobiology of mood disorders'.
- *Psychiatry and psychopathology in the arts.* This module introduces students to the field of medical humanities. Students explore topics such as: the description of psychopathology in autobiographical narratives; the representation of madness in fictional narrative and feature films;

167

and the value of poetry, biography, letters and journals in medical education. Teaching is expert led and discussion based. Students identify an area of particular interest for independent in-depth study, which is assessed by a 2000-word essay. Recent essays have included 'The portrayal of madness in *Jayne Eyre*' and 'The portrayal of mental illness in film'.

The semester is designed and timetabled to include 'themed weeks'; thus, the teaching delivered in the last three modules (neurobiology of psychological processes, neurobiology of mental illness, and psychiatry and psychopathology in the arts) is presented as a cohesive whole, allowing the student to integrate understanding of the normal processes, how our knowledge of these processes underpins advances in the understanding of mental illness and the portrayal of illness in the arts and media.

As an example, week 2 involves:

- neurobiology of psychological processes: auditory perception
- neurobiology of mental illness: auditory hallucinations
- psychiatry and the arts: text from Daniel Schreber's *Memoirs of My Nervous Illness*.

See Table 14.2 for further details.

Plenary

Semester 1 concludes with a plenary session attended by two external speakers and all students, allowing students the chance to meet and question a humanities expert. There is an overt expectation of thoughtful contribution by all students to the discussion. We have been fortunate to attract a variety of excellent speakers from diverse backgrounds. These have included: Dr Allan Beveridge, speaking on 'The art of the mentally ill'; Dr Fiona Murray, on the life and works of Sylvia Plath; Elaine Rose, a poet and child and family social worker, talking about her writing; Dr Stephen Potts, screenplay writer and psychiatrist; and Fiona Shaw, author of *Out of Me*, speaking about her writing.

Semester 2

Semester 2 is devoted to a research module. That module actually spans the year, but with the bulk done in semester 2. It provides students with first-hand experience of undertaking research, from conception to presentation of findings. All students have a nominated supervisor and individually tailored support through all aspects of their research. Projects undertaken can be quantitative or qualitative in nature and conducted within the UK or abroad. Students design their research and obtain necessary approvals in semester 1 and conduct data collection and analysis in semester 2. Assessment of the research project includes an oral presentation of the research plan, written protocol, poster presentation of findings and a dissertation or journal-style submission.

Table 14.2 Birmingham psychological medicine BMedSc: weekly themed lectures semester 1

Week	Neurobiology of psychological processes	Neurobiology of mental illness	Psychiatry and psychopathology in the arts
1	Visual perception	Illusions and visual hallucinations	Seeing things: *The Black Monk*, by A. P. Chekhov; *The Doors of Perception*, by A. Huxley
2	Auditory perception	Musical and auditory hallucinations	Hearing voices: *Memoirs of My Nervous Illness*, by Daniel Schreber
3	Emotion and motivation	Pathological affect	Touched with fire: *An Unquiet Mind*, by Kay R. Jamison
4	Aggression and personality	Abnormal personality	Mad or bad? *Piano Teacher*, by Elfriede Jelinek
5	Human sexuality	Paraphillias	Aberrant love: *Enduring Love*, by Ian McEwan
6	Learning	Abnormal learnt responses	Abnormal learning: *Letter to His Father*, by Franz Kafka
7	Memory	Amnesias	Tell me who I am again: *Iris*, by John Bayley
8	Thinking and intelligence	Abnormalities of belief	Believe me, I'm right: *Dairy of a Madman*, by Nicolai Gogol; *Spider*, by Patrick McGrath
9	Language	Language disorders in psychiatric illnesses	Misuse of language: *The Curious Incident of the Dog in the Night-Time*, by Mark Haddon

Recent research projects have looked at:

- the influence of parental values and practices on the presence of coprolalia in Tourette syndrome
- the determinants and patterns of self-harm behaviours in individuals contributing to internet-based self-harm forums
- screening for attention-deficit hyperactivity disorder in children with intellectual disabilities using Conners' rating scales
- a review of pathological jealousy with specific reference to Othello
- the 'schizophrenia postdrome' – a study of low-level symptoms after full recovery from first-episode schizophrenia
- a systematic review of adverse birth outcomes in women taking selective serotonin reuptake inhibitors during the first trimester of pregnancy
- whether the severity of cognitive impairment in Alzheimer's disease is an accurate predictor of testamentary capacity.

Successes to date

Feedback

Positive feedback from students has been clear, with increased numbers applying for psychological medicine as an option in each successive year, often from outside Birmingham University. Written feedback includes:

Gave me time to think rather than just rote learn.

Now I have done the course I definitely want to be a psychiatrist.

I used to be scared of research but now I'm not.

I think I now understand better what it must be like to suffer from a mental illness.

This will be useful in whatever specialty I choose.

Thought provoking and challenging.

Feedback from external examiners has also been good. One comment read:

The programme content is appropriate for the degree level and also as an element intercalated into a medical degree programme. The structure appropriately balances taught content and self-directed/investigative learning. It is a positive element that there is an emphasis on the 'humanities' component of health care.

Publication and conference presentations

Numerous research projects have led to presentation at national and international conferences, poster presentations and publication in peer-reviewed journals (e.g. Deb & Burns, 2007; Gregory *et al*, 2007; Greeves *et al*, 2009; Patel & Upthegrove, 2009; Pearson & Oyebode, 2009). This high level of success has the potential to encourage those completing their psychological medicine degree to consider not only an academic career but also academic psychiatry. The only published research available (McManus *et al*, 1999) demonstrated that students completing intercalated degrees were more likely show an interest in medical research and less likely to choose general practice as a career option.

Degree awards

To date, 50 students have completed the course, of whom 13% were awarded first-class degrees, and 77% an upper second. The course is always oversubscribed and numbers are limited, to ensure adequate research supervision and small groups for teaching, which results in healthy competition for places.

Challenges of course delivery

Running any degree course has inherent difficulties. Inevitably there will be students who require more intense supervision for either academic or, on occasion, personal difficulties. In addition, however, a few points should be made about the regular challenges, as these may be of interest to anyone considering setting up similar courses.

The challenge of timetabling will be readily identifiable by all. Our unique aspect of delivering themed weeks makes early organisation of timetabling extremely important. There is also an inherent lack of flexibility with the timetable, and it cannot change with, for example, lecturers' other demands or clashes with other streams.

Identifying and securing the commitment of experts able to lead didactic and small-group teaching on a regular basis, with the fixed time commitments mentioned above, have also proved a challenge. Subject matter such as the neurobiology of paraphilias or human sexuality require real commitment in time and preparation from university staff with other competing interests.

Similarly, it can be hard to find research supervisors able and willing to commit to the time needed for adequate supervision.

Finally, difficulties with the research ethics committee can mean projects are delayed or have to be modified without undue delay. Difficulties in obtaining ethical approval for student projects is an ongoing challenge that demands forward planning. This does, however, provide students with 'real world' experience of research.

Implications for psychiatry

Medical students' perceptions of psychiatry can be negative; for example, the (false) perception of psychiatry being unscientific is common. Increasing the scientific profile of psychiatry to larger numbers of students can only help to break down this misperception. Previous research has shown that students taking intercalated degrees showed greater interest in careers in medical research and less interest in general practice than their peers. In addition, intercalated degrees result in higher scores on deep and strategic learning (Cleland *et al*, 2009). Increasing numbers of students will complete an intercalated degree in the coming years. Psychiatry must use this opportunity to counter negative images of the specialty and enhance recruitment of the highest calibre of students to careers in both academic and clinical work. One key question that needs to be answered, and that will form part of a piece of research in its own right, is whether completing an intercalated degree in psychological medicine will increase the likelihood of a student entering psychiatry. The Birmingham course has shown that innovative teaching techniques and the integration of the humanities and neuroscience are attractive to students. The Birmingham course, in addition to, for example, the Cardiff course, should guide those setting up other new intercalated degrees. Factors influencing career choice in medicine have been shown in general studies to be complex and subject to fluctuation: for example, in the USA in the 1970s and 1980s a large increase in the number of doctors choosing psychiatry arose from a therapeutic optimism, enthusiasm for community care and a vast increase in government spending on mental health in response to the needs of Vietnam War veterans (Sierles & Taylor, 1995). It is clear, however, that the quality of medical student teaching also plays a large role (Sierles & Taylor, 1995). Intercalating itself has proven to have a positive influence on future medical school examinations (Cleland *et al*, 2009), demonstrating just one aspect of the positive transferable skills accumulated through this route. Offering students intercalated options relevant to psychiatry, delivered with sound teaching, has the potential to influence career choice. There is, however, a clear need for a formal evaluation of the influence of intercalated degrees on the recruitment of high-calibre students to the specialty.

References

Cleland, J. A., Milne, A., Sinclair, H., *et al* (2009) An intercalated BSc degree is associated with higher marks in subsequent medical school examinations. *BMC Medical Education*, **9**, 24.

Deb, S. & Burns, J. (2007) Neuropsychiatric consequences of traumatic brain injury: a comparison between two age groups. *Brain Injury*, **21**, 301–307.

General Medical Council (2003) *Tomorrow's Doctors* (2nd edn). GMC.

Greeves, A., Best, D., Day, E., *et al* (2009) Young people in coerced drug treatment: does the UK Drug Intervention Programme provide a useful and effective service to young offenders? *Addiction Research and Theory*, **17**, 17–29.

Gregory, R., Roked, F., Jones, L., *et al* (2007) Is the degree of cognitive impairment in patients with Alzheimer's disease related to their capacity to appoint an enduring power of attorney? *Age and Ageing*, **36**, 527–531.

McManus, I. C., Richards, P. & Winder, B. C. (1999) Intercalated degrees, learning styles, and career preferences: prospective longitudinal study of UK medical students. *BMJ*, **319**, 542–546.

Patel, K. & Upthegrove, R. (2009) Self-harm in first-episode psychosis. *Psychiatric Bulletin*, **33**, 104–107.

Pearson, L. J. & Oyebode, F. (2009) Social capital and childhood psychiatric disorders: a cross-sectional study. *Clinical Child Psychology and Psychiatry*, **14**, 183–194.

Sierles, F. S. & Taylor, M. A. (1995) Decline of U.S. medical student career choice of psychiatry and what to do about it. *American Journal of Psychiatry*, **152**, 1416–1426.

CHAPTER 15

Undergraduate experiences of psychiatry: a student view

Fiona Hendry & Vivienne Blackhall

Introduction

At the time of writing this chapter, we were both about to graduate in medicine from the University of Glasgow. We have been exposed to the specialty of psychiatry in a number of guises. These include a 5-week core curriculum placement, two 5-week student-selected components in psychiatric subspecialties and a 1-year intercalated bachelor of science degree in psychological medicine. From our experience, students often feel that they have had inadequate exposure to psychiatry. This may be because many complete only the minimum of 5 weeks in undergraduate training, often confined to one specialty and under the care of one supervisor. This can give an extremely narrowed, skewed view of what psychiatry is all about. Indeed, the specialty is truly suffering from an image problem (Malhi *et al*, 2003) and the misconceptions regarding the specialty harm recruitment. Students are often put off psychiatry because they perceive it to be too far removed from the rest of medicine, with little scientific basis and ineffective treatments (see Chapter 21). In order to challenge these negative perceptions and give students a chance to appreciate psychiatry, we feel that the undergraduate curriculum should be expanded. In this chapter we first argue the case for student-selected components, or modules, as a particularly effective means of doing this. We then comment on our experiences of other exposures to psychiatry.

What are student-selected components?

Student-selected components (SSCs) are elements of the modern medical curriculum recommended by the General Medical Council (2003) in *Tomorrow's Doctors*. During an SSC, students are given an allocated amount of time within the core curriculum usually to study a particular area of medicine at a level greater than is necessarily needed for pre-registration year (General Medical Council, 2003).

The amount of time allocated to SSCs depends on each medical school's individual preference but, according to the General Medical Council (2003), it should be 25–33% of the total curriculum in a traditional 5-year course. It is also recommended that, of the components completed by students, two-thirds should relate directly to medicine. Examples of non-medical SSCs include languages such as French and Spanish. The modules can be based in a laboratory, classroom, research facility or in a clinical environment.

SSCs are one of the only components of the curriculum that promote the development of individuality in what is otherwise a uniform degree. SSCs provide students with the opportunity to develop a self-critical approach to their work. Throughout our undergraduate studies we have been taught the importance of being self-critical in terms of recognising and addressing our weaknesses and limitations.

Students develop and expand upon research, presentation and communication skills during an SSC. Becoming skilled in these areas is crucial for an undergraduate student and proves invaluable in the later years of medical school. Students often wish to undertake audits and research projects and being competent in literature searches and effective presentation makes this far less daunting.

Typically, between one and ten students participate in a particular psychiatry SSC at a time. Clinical SSCs involving such small groups permits students to have more opportunities to interact with patients. This in turn provides more time to practise skills in history taking and examination. There are also more opportunities for students to receive one-to-one teaching and feedback. This allows student supervisors to gain a representative view of the student's ability and thus provide constructive criticism or praise, as is appropriate.

Tomorrow's Doctors (General Medical Council, 2003) also highlights that SSCs enable exploration of particular fields of medicine as potential careers. There is a responsibility, then, for those organising SSCs not only to provide a realistic view of what specialties are about, but also to attract students by running well-organised, interesting and varied placements with enthusiastic supervisors.

SSCs at the University of Glasgow

The SSCs provide a change in pace from the regular curriculum, which students tend to appreciate. The SSCs at the University of Glasgow are 5 weeks in length and can be combined with electives to give a total placement time of 9 weeks. Following a change in the structure of the course in 2009, Glasgow currently offers students the opportunity to choose five SSCs from a large menu, scattered throughout the course (previously the curriculum provided time for seven SSCs), eight of which are related to psychiatry, including community, child and adolescent, and forensic psychiatry, substance misuse, liaison and intellectual disability. In later years of study, students are given the opportunity to propose their own SSCs. In theory this can allow students to explore any facet of medicine they wish. It can, however, be daunting, as it involves a great deal of organisation: finding a supervisor, setting objectives and organising a timetable. This probably appeals to students who already have an interest in a specific branch or subspecialty of medicine, but is less likely to appeal to those who have no experience or appreciation of psychiatry. Further to this, students are far less likely to explore subspecialties within psychiatry, as many are not covered by the core university course and so students remain unaware of their existence.

During our time at the University of Glasgow, we completed two 5-week psychiatry-related SSCs, one in liaison psychiatry and one in addiction psychiatry.

Liaison psychiatry

Five weeks in liaison psychiatry allowed us to appreciate the role of the service. The emphasis on this rotation was on seeing existing in-patients in the hospital, but we were also exposed to out-patient clinics and psychotherapy sessions. The diversity of patients was particularly striking, with individuals of all ages, all walks of life and hugely varying clinical problems presenting to the service. Among these included young motivated males and females dealing with anxiety and depression, helpless individuals in the throes of obsessionality, elderly souls lacking support and looking for a way out and individuals troubled with alcohol and drug misuse.

We saw patients in many stages of treatment and this highlighted the long-term nature of some treatments in psychiatry. As research has shown, students often perceive that treatments in psychiatry lack clinical evidence and that they are ineffective (Feifel *et al*, 1999; Malhi *et al*, 2003). Our time in liaison psychiatry, especially in the out-patient setting, dispelled this misconception. During the SSC we met several patients who were undergoing cognitive–behavioural therapy (CBT). In particular, we remember tracking the progress of one patient with a depressive disorder and comparing his beliefs about himself over time. Initially he had been completely debilitated by his condition, unable to function as a member of society. He was no longer able to attend higher education and had become increasingly introverted. The transformation over time was astonishing; subjectively his affect was brighter and he displayed more confident body language. Diaries detailing his accomplishments each week demonstrated to us and to the patient the treatment's effectiveness and provided evidence that CBT was having a positive effect. He was able to attend university again and had begun once more to socialise. We were also able to appreciate the use of the diaries as an effective teaching tool for students, as they gave solid, meaningful evidence of clinical improvement with treatment. Although psychiatry is generally not the home of 'quick fix' solutions, with the exception perhaps of electroconvulsive therapy, its treatments do work, given time and patience.

An SSC in psychiatry challenges the misconception that treatments are ineffective. Seeing patients progress through treatment allows us to refute any idea that psychiatric disorders are not treatable.

Addiction psychiatry

Addiction medicine afforded us the opportunity to explore an area of psychiatry that has become a huge problem in society. During our time, we were based in academic psychiatry and wrote a literature-based essay examining theories regarding the mechanism of substance addiction. We undertook this SSC in our second year of the undergraduate curriculum, which meant that we became competent in literature searches at an early stage. This stood us in good stead for the remainder of our degree, particularly when completing a research project during our intercalated year.

During the SSC, we met several patients undergoing various biological and psychological therapies for their addiction. We were able to attend outreach clinics in Glasgow, where patients addicted to heroin were monitored and advised on how best to reduce their methadone dose. We also spent time at group therapy sessions, where patients who had stopped drinking spoke about challenges they faced as a result of their actions.

We met individuals from many backgrounds and were able to explore their reasons for taking the substance and how it affected all areas of their lives. The importance of a doctor's ability to evaluate a patient holistically and the multidisciplinary services that are involved in an addicted patient's care became clear during this time.

The SSC also demonstrated the psychological and physical struggle a patient must go through in order to become free from an addiction. Sometimes, individuals affected by an addiction are treated with disrespect, leading to a cycle of mistrust and scepticism between patient and service providers. This SSC illustrated the importance of practising tolerance, empathy and respect when caring for such patients.

During our time spent in addiction medicine we explored bio-psychosocial theories that attempted to explain how addictions develop. We took histories and examined people affected by addictions. We also worked in a multidisciplinary team environment at a relatively early stage in our careers. By doing this, we developed knowledge of how much psychiatry relies on community support and care as well as hospital care.

The importance of SSCs in psychiatry

For those students unsure whether they are willing to invest an entire year's study in psychological medicine in the form of an intercalated degree, SSCs are a good way in which to engage with the specialty. A 5-week block is perhaps sufficient to explore and appreciate a subject without the time commitment of an intercalated bachelor of science degree.

SSCs also afford the opportunity to explore important areas of psychiatry that are not often included in the core curriculum. All doctors should have a basic understanding of psychiatric disorders and of how to assess and take a history from a patient. Every specialty sees patients affected by psychiatric disorders: some specialties are exposed to psychiatric comorbidity more than others, however. For example, it is estimated that 20–25% of children attending primary care or a paediatric hospital have psychological problems (Bernard & Garralda, 1995). Little time is spent on child and adolescent psychiatry within the core course, yet with the significant majority of students pursuing careers in general medicine, teaching and experience within this subspecialty can only work to serve our patients better, although it may not be sensible to expose some children and indeed many other individuals with psychiatric problems to hoards of medical students. For those students who are interested in pursuing a career in psychiatry or a related specialty, an SSC is extremely valuable for allowing access to patients they might not otherwise see.

SSCs are a fantastic way of engaging students in academic psychiatry. As with all areas of medicine, there are constant scientific breakthroughs. Much still remains unknown about the aetiology of many psychiatric conditions; this provides us with a huge opportunity to conduct research and attempt to build upon our knowledge. SSCs can provide a grounding and potential entry into a career in academic psychiatry by highlighting areas suitable for research and allowing students to familiarise themselves with the research process. An SSC provides a student who is keen to pursue psychiatry the opportunity to take part in an audit or small research project. For other students, reading the literature on psychiatric conditions and management options may stimulate an interest in psychiatry that they would otherwise not have had.

SSCs in psychiatry enrich students' basic medical training by allowing them to fill in the missing pieces of the bio-psychosocial jigsaw. We have been taught that the bio-psychosocial model is one that students and doctors alike must appreciate and adopt in order to deliver effective holistic care and to optimise patient outcomes. The importance of the model was demonstrated to us throughout our time spent in psychiatry SSCs. For example, in liaison psychiatry we explored the somatoform disorders and met many patients with such conditions. By definition, these patients present with physical symptoms. What was striking was how their management was impaired by the fact that many physicians either had not contemplated the possibility of such a diagnosis or had done so only very late in the day. As a consequence, patients had difficulty acknowledging a psychological component to their suffering. This was compounded by years of sometimes unnecessary investigations (or even interventions, including surgery) aimed at finding biological cause. It can only help future patients if students are allowed time to explore such disorders, which are extremely common. Improving doctors' understanding of these disorders also has pragmatic benefits for our health service: ensuring that medical and surgical referrals are given only to patients who truly require them will reduce waiting times and costs (Kirmayer, 1988).

Individual psychiatrists can provide insight into the management of an unwell patient more effectively than lectures. In both SSCs we were invited to conferences in order to increase our knowledge and to meet and listen to experts in the field of psychiatry. This has served as great inspiration. As suggested by Maidment *et al* (2004), encouragement by senior doctors during a psychiatric placement can significantly increase interest in the subject, both in its own right and as a potential future career.

Psychiatry is not a specialty where all patients can be assessed and treated by the doctor following a single specific formula. This is one of the most frustrating aspects and yet the most intriguing – psychiatry is a specialty that is led by the patient. As students, we noticed a marked difference between those with physical and psychiatric morbidity; those with physical illness tended to seek medical assistance earlier. A presentation with a psychiatric disorder may be delayed for weeks or even months. This can be due to lack of patient insight. Additionally, a disorder with an insidious onset with non-specific features may not cause concern to the individual's friends and family. Signs and symptoms may be attributed to difficulty coping or life stressors and an element of denial may also exist. Trying to admit, treat and ultimately help patients when they do not recognise they are ill takes skill, determination and the ability to adapt to the situation one is confronted with. Lectures cannot necessarily demonstrate all the techniques needed to glean information from a patient, but watching the experts assess and treat patients can be extremely valuable in terms of skill acquisition.

Various psychiatrists have provided our undergraduate experience of the specialty. They have encouraged us in different ways. One of us has been inspired to consider a career in eating disorders by a consultant who exuded passion and a tireless wish to do what was best for her patients. Another consultant made a lasting impact because of his ability to be frank with his patients and the success this brought. His openness was surprising. Lectures often suggest a soft approach with psychiatric patients. However, patients responded positively to this doctor and often opened up far faster than perhaps would have been expected. This demonstrates that if more students could learn from senior psychiatrists by watching them in practice, they may feel better equipped to cope with psychiatric patients.

In our experience it was often those doctors keenest to transfer their love of psychiatry who taught and developed SSCs. With such a small proportion of students able to pursue psychiatry SSCs at a given time, by expanding the number and range of such SSCs we may encourage more undergraduates to consider psychiatry as a career. Finally, those developing and running SSCs may wish to focus on the transfer of skills needed by all prospective foundation doctors. Oakley & Oyebode (2008) suggested this could include assessment of suicide risk and recognition and ability to treat alcohol withdrawal and delirium.

Other exposure to psychiatry

Core curriculum

For students at the University of Glasgow, teaching in psychiatry begins in the third year. We learned about some of the common conditions in psychiatry, such as depression and schizophrenia. However, this was not followed up with clinical experience of meeting patients until our 5-week core clinical block in either our fourth or fifth year. By way of comparison, we learned about the anatomy and physiology of the major body systems over the first and second year and were introduced to clinical examination of patients early in our second year. We were familiar with performing basic examinations on patients by the end of our third year. The time gap between theoretical teaching in psychiatry and exposure to psychiatric patients contributes to students feeling deskilled and, consequently, apprehensive about meeting psychiatric patients. In order to remedy this, we feel it is important that students are not only exposed early to psychiatric issues but that they also have the opportunity to speak to individuals attending psychiatric services. A psychiatry SSC can be a good way to introduce earlier clinical contact with psychiatric patients and to provide a more complete learning experience.

The 5 weeks we spend in undergraduate psychiatry training is well organised. It is one of few core blocks where we are presented with pre-course reading material (including online resources) and where the lecturers reliably attend for teaching. Despite the curriculum being very full during these 5 weeks, lecturers often face an uphill struggle to teach all the skills necessary to become competent in dealing with the psychiatric patient. This may be particularly important with reference to the management of psychiatric emergencies.

Managing an acute psychiatric emergency is a huge responsibility for any doctor. Inexperienced doctors could find that they alienate a fragile patient from using services through simply using the wrong type of language or approach. Throughout our medical degree we have been continually presented with algorithms for the acute management of a variety of medical and surgical problems. We know these algorithms off by heart. We feel that less importance has been attached to the approach and management of acute psychiatric problems, particularly the kind of emergencies that all doctors have to deal with, often from quite early in their careers. Perhaps curriculum organisers need to find ways of better meeting this need, particularly as community psychiatric services increasingly have developed specialist crisis services to manage emergencies, which means that students have less opportunity to see these on clinical attachments. It may be useful for student doctors to spend time with a local crisis service. This would allow them to observe the specialist service at work and learn how to provide optimum care for patients they may meet in similar scenarios in the future.

Intercalated degrees (see also Chapter 14)

The University of Glasgow provides the opportunity to undertake a year-long bachelor of science in clinical medicine in a number of specialties, including psychological medicine. Both the authors undertook such a degree. Half way through the year we were required to present a current summation of our research project to the year group. We distinctly remember thinking that the psychological medicine module offered the most varied, novel and interesting opportunities for research. We are of course biased in our views, because we chose psychiatry specifically because it interested us, but while many of our colleagues in other modules were repeating research projects that had been conducted in previous years, three out of five of our group were undertaking entirely novel research. The research projects in psychological medicine covered varied topics, including: the understanding of, and attitudes towards, HIV; obsessional symptoms in postnatal women; and clock-watching behaviour in insomnia. We also valued the opportunity to be out talking to and interacting with patients while conducting our research.

We found the BScMedSci truly cemented our interest in psychiatry and made us think about the specialty in a new way. For example, we became more aware that it is difficult to separate psychiatry from the rest of medicine. Also, it is now widely accepted that there is an important biological basis to psychiatric disorders such as psychosis and depression. Moreover, psychiatric disorders can be the result of medical disorders, such as endocrine dysfunction and stroke. Lastly, psychological factors may be important in terms of the aetiology and management of syndromes such as irritable bowel syndrome.

At many medical schools, the focus of learning is biological and sticks to a formula: initially, we learn about anatomy and physiology, and then once this knowledge is established we learn about the pathology, the aberrant structures and functions. It is not easy to fit psychiatry into this formula. This is because although neurobiological factors are crucially important in psychiatry, these are often more difficult to elucidate, given the complexity of the human brain. Also, psychological and social factors may at times be equally important in psychiatry (this is also the case in the rest of medicine but is less often acknowledged). Perhaps by changing the formula to an all-encompassing one we can bridge this perceived gap between specialties. Our experience of both our intercalated degree and our SSCs provided an excellent opportunity in which to do this, as we were able to appreciate the importance of a bio-psychosocial approach to psychiatric disorders.

The importance of good clinical teachers

In our experience, students' contact with their clinical teachers can influence their attitude to a specialty, both for good and for ill. One of our earliest experiences of psychiatrists was very negative. During a conference we met a senior psychiatrist who was heavily critical of the profession, which left us feeling completely demoralised. With such limited contact with psychiatrists as an undergraduate, it is crucial that the specialty is promoted with enthusiasm and a desire to attract the best possible candidates to the profession. We were fortunate to have very positive subsequent experiences to challenge this, but other students may not be so lucky.

Educational supervisors are expected to make sure their student(s) achieve goals set out in the syllabus (Modernising Medical Careers Team & British Medical Association, 2005). Additionally, the General Medical Council (1999) set out criteria that educational supervisors are expected to meet: these include attributes such as enthusiasm, sensitivity to the needs of the training doctor and a commitment to the principles of *Good Medical Practice*. It should therefore be paramount that all supervisors meet the necessary criteria and have the time needed to educate students to the best of their ability.

Some (but not all) of our better experiences came during SSCs. SSCs permit deviation away from traditional teaching methods and can promote the development of a professional teaching relationship with the student(s) and the psychiatrist. This can have a lasting impact on students and either encourage or discourage them. This is the case with all specialties but we believe psychiatry can be particularly influential owing to students, as we have said, having less early exposure clinically and thus meeting far fewer psychiatrists than, for example, physicians or surgeons. Generally speaking, the student experience of psychiatry is governed by mentors. In all specialties we face challenging patients and awkward scenarios. What makes these challenges more manageable and indeed interesting is a focused, capable and engaging tutor.

The need to improve recruitment in psychiatry (see also Chapters 20 and 21)

The proportion of UK graduates committed to a career in psychiatry is estimated to be around 4% (Royal College of Psychiatrists, 2004). There is a concern that this translates into a deficit of psychiatrists compared with the number of available posts (Rajagopal *et al*, 2004). Additionally, a lack of competition may breed a sense of complacency among professionals within the specialty. Potentially, the quality of care delivered to patients could be compromised and advances in research slowed.

Research conducted in the USA has shown that, over the past few decades, there has been a significant decline in the number of first-year medical students considering a career in psychiatry. In the early 1970s Fishman & Zimet (1972) found that 13% of a sample of new US medical students cited psychiatry as their top career choice. Ten years later, Friedman & McGuire (1982) found this had fallen to 11%. Feifel *et al* (1999) found that only 0.5% of their study cohort identified psychiatry as their chosen career and 7.2% as a strong possibility. More encouragingly, an Australian study from 2003 found that psychiatry was the chosen career of 1.4% of first-year medical students, and a strong possibility of 14.5% (Malhi *et al*, 2003).

Further research has examined the attitudes to psychiatry of medical students and doctors, in an attempt to unpick the reasons for such poor interest in a career in the specialty. For example, large studies involving first-year medical students have examined the attractiveness of a career in psychiatry compared with other specialties (Feifel *et al*, 1999; Malhi *et al*, 2003). Psychiatry has been shown to rate consistently poorly in comparison with medicine, surgery, paediatrics, general practice, and obstetrics and gynaecology. In broad terms, these studies identified that students perceived psychiatry to be less attractive because of a lack of scientific evidence, poor job satisfaction, a limited understanding of illnesses and their treatments, and consequently the limited extent to which patients could be helped. Students also perceived their family, colleagues and physicians to have a distinct lack of respect for the specialty. Interestingly, psychiatry was seen to be more attractive in terms of lifestyle, financial reward, having an interesting subject matter and being intellectually challenging.

During our time at medical school, we have of course been exposed to our peers' views, both positive and negative, regarding the specialty. Although these attitudes have not been examined formally, we feel that our anecdotal evidence mirrors many of the myths. Common misconceptions about psychiatry include that it is 'easy', that 'services are ineffective and patients never improve' and that 'psychiatrists are weird'.

Barriers to recruitment

It is important to examine and deal with the barriers that discourage individuals from pursuing a career in psychiatry. Feldmann (2005) suggested that, in relation to medical students, this could be achieved in the following ways:

- increasing the length of placements
- providing varied clinical placements in psychiatric subspecialties
- challenging negative perceptions among medical students by providing them with solid evidence that treatments in psychiatry can be extremely effective (this could be achieved by setting students course work where they are required to perform a literature review to examine the efficacy of certain treatments, and in turn this could be strengthened by a clinical attachment where students have the opportunity to interact with patients who have benefited from said interventions)
- tackling the 'stigma of association' from which psychiatry suffers, by challenging negative attitudes to mental illness.

Psychiatrists should adopt high-profile roles in medical schools. Certainly in our personal experience of medical education, all the clinicians with whom we had early contact were from medical and surgical specialties. Contact with students in their first and second years of study should be made by psychiatrists in order to open their eyes to the specialty.

A sophisticated curriculum should be constructed that involves more than just a placement. As Feldmann (2005) reflected, 'A psychiatry clerkship by itself is inadequate, regardless of length, to stimulate interest in and understanding of our specialty'. This highlights the important role that SSCs, electives and research years play in the undergraduate curriculum.

The Student Psychotherapy Scheme has been shown to improve interest in psychiatry. The scheme allows students to follow the progress of a selected patient receiving psychotherapy. Each week, for 1 year, the student sits in on the psychotherapy session, under senior supervision. The course is currently offered to first-year medical students in the London area. After participating in the scheme, it has been shown that a greater proportion of students consider a career in psychiatry compared with those who do not participate. Although the scheme demands a huge level of commitment from students, psychiatrists and patients, we feel this is balanced by the potential gains. Perhaps a similar scheme should be piloted nationwide and integrated into the curriculum (Royal College of Psychiatrists, 2004). Finally, the Royal College of Psychiatrists has developed a student associate scheme and other initiatives aimed at attracting undergraduates to psychiatry. These are discussed in detail in Chapter 20 and can also be found on the College website (http://www.rcpsych.ac.uk).

Summary

We consider ourselves fortunate that we have both had very positive experiences during our undergraduate psychiatry training. We have been attracted to psychiatry for a number of reasons. First, the quality of the doctor–patient interaction is unlike that in any other specialty that we have experienced. Not only does it afford the luxury of time for history taking, but it also provides the privilege of exploring the thoughts, feelings and lives of many individuals. Many of the patients' stories are fascinating and at times extremely moving. Second, the attitudes and personalities of our tutors heightened our appreciation of the specialty. Although the same can probably be said for all specialties, enthusiastic and charismatic mentors proved to have big pulling power. Third, we enjoy psychiatry simply because we have a genuine interest in psychological processes and psychiatric disorders. Psychiatry may not be to everyone's taste, but for those with an interest or curiosity in the specialty, it is crucial that this interest should be nurtured and explored.

One of us recalls a supervisor during a core clinical attachment telling the story of her father's displeasure at her pursuing psychiatry as a career. He had said that she was 'nothing more than a glorified social worker'. This is but one example, but it is true that psychiatry and indeed other psychosocial vocations are often perceived negatively. In our experience, psychiatry is often seen as the black sheep, not legitimately belonging under the wide umbrella of medicine.

Although many of students' negative perceptions of psychiatry are created before or early in medical training, evidence suggests that existing perceptions can be challenged and changed (Feldmann, 2005). In our experience, a good undergraduate experience (and in our case SSCs in particular) is crucial in achieving this. Psychiatrists need to identify colleagues from all subspecialties with an interest in and flair for teaching who can be involved in creating exciting modules that outline the varied and interesting career options available to students. Psychiatry needs to be placed as early in the curriculum as possible (with patient contact) and be given the same importance by course leaders in the medical school as other specialties. Above all, psychiatry needs to be taught and undertaken by those with a love of the subject. As a science which predominately involves talking and interaction, it is crucial that those with responsibility for training 'tomorrow's doctors' do so with the same enthusiasm and determination that inspired them to enter psychiatry.

References

Bernard, R. & Garralda, M. E. (1995) Child and adolescent mental health practice in primary care. *Current Opinion in Psychiatry*, **8**, 206–209.

Feifel, D., Moutier, C. & Swerdlow, N. (1999) Attitudes toward psychiatry as a prospective career among students entering medical school. *American Journal of Psychiatry*, **159**, 1397–1402.

Feldmann, T. (2005) Medical students' attitudes toward psychiatry and mental disorders. *Academic Psychiatry*, **29**, 4.

Fishman, D. B. & Zimet, C. N. (1972) Specialty choice and beliefs about specialties among freshman medical students. *Journal of Medical Education*, **47**, 524–533.

Friedman, C. T. H. & McGuire, F. L. (1982) A survey of a freshman medical student class: will psychiatry recruit well into the 1980s? *Journal of Psychiatric Education*, **139**, 1003–1009.

General Medical Council (1999) *The Doctor as Teacher*. GMC.

General Medical Council (2003) *Tomorrow's Doctors* (2nd edn). GMC.

Kirmayer, L. J. (1988) *Mind and Body as Metaphors: Hidden Values in Biomedicine. Biomedicine Examined*, pp. 57–92. Kluwer.

Maidment, R., Livingston, G., Katona, C., *et al* (2004) Change in attitudes to psychiatry and intention to pursue psychiatry as a career in newly qualified doctors: a follow-up of two cohorts of medical students. *Medical Teacher*, **26**, 565–569.

Malhi, G. S., Parker, G. B., Parker, K., *et al* (2003) Attitudes toward psychiatry among students entering medical school. *Acta Psychiatrica Scandinavica*, **107**, 424–429.

Modernising Medical Careers Team & British Medical Association (2005) *The Rough Guide to the Foundation Programme*, p. 57. The Stationary Office.

Oakley, C. & Oyebode, F. (2008) Medical students' views about an undergraduate curriculum in psychiatry before and after clinical placements. *BMC Medical Education*, **8**, 26.

Rajagopal, S., Singh Rehill, K. & Godfrey, E. (2004) Psychiatry as a career choice compared with other specialties: a survery of medical students. *Psychiatric Bulletin*, **28**, 444–446.

Royal College of Psychiatrists (2004) 'Tackling the recruitment crisis in psychiatry Student Psychotherapy Scheme encourages medical students to choose psychiatry as a career'. Press release available at http://www.rcpsych.ac.uk/pressparliament/ pressreleasearchive/pr550.aspx

CHAPTER 16

Integration: teaching psychiatry with other specialties

Teifion Davies

Introduction

Psychiatry has not always enjoyed a distinct place in the undergraduate medical curriculum (Davies & McGuire, 2000) and its status remains variable in the current curricula of many of the UK and Ireland's medical schools (Karim *et al*, 2009). Since most UK medical schools emerged from the in-house training courses for physicians and surgeons existing in the major hospitals (the 'teaching' hospitals), perhaps it is not surprising that their curricula replicated the range of specialties available at those hospitals. Specialties that were geographically separated from the great hospitals or were newly developing (e.g. primary care and psychiatry) were less likely to be represented in undergraduate teaching. It was not until the latter part of the 20th century that consideration was given to balancing the medical curriculum with a view to producing omnipotential graduates with the capability of entering a wide range of postgraduate specialties.

As the body of biomedical knowledge increased in both quantity and complexity, so competition increased for time and resources in the curriculum. In the UK, the General Medical Council (1993, 2003, 2009*a*) responded to these pressures on students' time with *Tomorrow's Doctors*, which shifted the balance from 'just in case' learning of facts, regardless of their potential relevance for a newly qualified doctor, to 'just in time' learning, with an emphasis on providing the knowledge and skills necessary for the early years of a clinical career; these ideas, originally from manufacturing, are now firmly established in education. Key to this shift is an increased focus on the patient rather than the specialty, and on developing clinical skills and demonstrating competence in common practical procedures rather than amassing medical knowledge.

As a recent survey of medical schools by the Association of University Teachers of Psychiatry (Karim *et al*, 2009) showed, just over half of medical schools adhere to the traditional medical undergraduate model of teaching psychiatry as a circumscribed block during the latter part of the medical course (the 'clinical' years). Clearly, many psychiatric teachers have been happy to have obtained a block of curriculum time that is their own, to be used as they think fit. Change to a more integrated role for psychiatry in the undergraduate curriculum requires a good deal of effort on the part of curriculum planners and teachers alike.

This chapter first examines the background to curricular integration (what, why and when) and the rationale for integrating psychiatry further into the medical course. It goes on to consider the more practical aspects of how to go about achieving integration.

What is integration?

Integration of a medical specialty into the undergraduate medical curriculum may take many forms. Although usually represented as a dichotomous choice between teaching each specialty in a stand-alone block or the assimilation of all specialties into a homogeneous course, with loss of individual subject identity, the difference between these is a matter of degree, forming as they do the polar extremes of a spectrum (see Fig. 16.1). A transition from block to integrated curricula may involve several stages (Harden, 2000). This spectrum of integration may apply to subjects taught within a single time period (usually a year) without affecting those in earlier or later years of the course (horizontal integration), or to successive years of the course so that the traditional boundary between preclinical biomedical science and clinical medical subjects is blurred (vertical integration).

Integration is regarded as a desirable outcome of medical curriculum planning (Harden, 2000), as it encourages 'deep' and lasting learning about patient-focused problems in a 'real world' context (Dahle *et al*, 2002). This is in contrast to the somewhat procrustean way in which a patient's presentation may be forced to fit into the purview of a single discipline, or split arbitrarily between several disjointed approaches. In this sense, it is

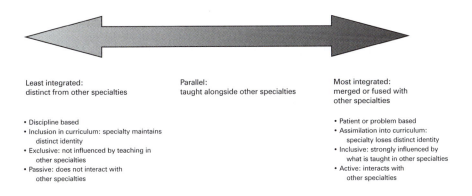

Least integrated:
distinct from other specialties

Parallel:
taught alongside other specialties

Most integrated:
merged or fused with
other specialties

• Discipline based
• Inclusion in curriculum: specialty maintains
   distinct identity
• Exclusive: not influenced by teaching in
   other specialties
• Passive: does not interact with
   other specialties

• Patient or problem based
• Assimilation into curriculum:
   specialty loses distinct identity
• Inclusive: strongly influenced by
   what is taught in other specialties
• Active: interacts with
   other specialties

Fig. 16.1 Spectrum of curriculum integration.

Table 16.1 Traditional block teaching compared with integrated teaching (psychiatry taught with other specialties)

Stand-alone block teaching	Integrated teaching
Traditional in majority of medical schools	Novel approach in minority of medical schools
Fits in well with traditional preclinical–clinical split	Fits well with vertically integrated course
Subject identity preserved: high face validity among clinicians/psychiatrists	Subject identity diminished: high face validity among educationalists
Immediate outcomes: students learn all that is expected in single block	Delayed outcomes: development of skills and knowledge over longer period
Follows unidisciplinary postgraduate model: encourages focus on needs of specialty, such as recruitment into psychiatry as a career	Follows interdisciplinary undergraduate model: encourages focus on needs of all doctors (and their patients) regardless of their specialty
Course management: independent, exclusive, convergent, 'simple'; requires little knowledge of the broader medical curriculum	Course management: interdependent, inclusive, divergent, more complex; requires thorough knowledge of, and engagement with, the broader medical curriculum
Does not conform to requirements of the General Medical Council	Conforms to requirements of the General Medical Council

seen to mirror more closely the everyday practice of medicine, especially when practised in a multidisciplinary setting. Table 16.1 summarises the differences between block and integrated teaching in psychiatry.

Many medical schools employ minor degrees of horizontal integration, teaching a number of medical (e.g. endocrinology, gastroenterology, nephrology) or surgical (e.g. abdominal surgery and urology, or ear, nose and throat and ophthalmology) subspecialties together in such a way as to emphasise their similarities or to maximise available resources (e.g. operating theatre time). More ambitious schemes involve concurrent clinical experience in all specialties – medical, surgical, pathological, and so on – concerned with a particular anatomical region or system. For example, at King's College London School of Medicine (KCLSoM) neurology, general psychiatry and ophthalmology are taught concurrently, with some joint teaching sessions based on shared neural mechanisms in health and disease.

In the simplest forms of vertical integration, 'preclinical' science teaching is illustrated by clinical examples, and clinical teaching revises basic anatomy and physiology or sociology and psychology, depending on the clinical topic. Particular themes (such as ethics) may be followed through the duration of the course in greater or lesser amalgamation with the horizontal topics through which they pass. More elaborate forms of vertical integration might involve basic science teaching being presented in the context of a clinical problem or scenario introduced and directed by a clinician, while clinical experience is supplemented by simulations, demonstrations or prosections to illustrate normal structure and function alongside relevant pathology. Students may be introduced to patients in the earliest years of the course, not merely to have demonstrated to them the clinical features of illness in the region under study, but to learn the clinical skills necessary to elicit those features for themselves. Students in later years may return to the laboratory to study in depth a problem encountered in the ward or clinic.

The essential component of true integration, vertical or horizontal, is collaboration between colleagues working in different clinical or science specialties to devise and deliver a course that meets the educational needs of students and future doctors (Prideaux, 2003). This is in clear contradistinction to teaching a unidisciplinary syllabus regardless of its practical value.

Why integrate psychiatry with other subjects?

Psychiatry is fundamentally a clinical subject, focused on patients and the multidisciplinary services they require, and dependent on interpersonal and communication skills, whose practice cannot be learned in a lecture theatre. Thus, it should be ideally suited to the new curricular structures that arise from the General Medical Council's requirements (1993, 2003, 2009*a*). However, a number of factors affect the delivery of teaching and uptake of learning in psychiatry courses: allocation of time in the undergraduate curriculum; disagreement about the purpose of undergraduate psychiatry teaching; organisation of mental health services within the National Health Service (NHS); and negative images of psychiatry.

Psychiatry in the medical curriculum

Curriculum content provokes much argument, as specialists in all subjects see their specialty as pre-eminent. Allocation of curriculum space may be caricatured as a macho competition between traditional 'heavyweights' (i.e. medicine, surgery, obstetrics and gynaecology, and possibly psychiatry), with little concern about balanced educational outcomes. However, distorted and disproportionate curriculum content benefits nobody: an undergraduate medical curriculum must be designed to meet the learning needs of future doctors in all specialties (Prideaux, 2003). Balancing the territorial claims of different specialties is fraught with difficulties: should teaching time be allocated according to general practice consultation rates, prevalence, mortality rates, or burden of disability of disease, or with a view to producing 'well rounded' junior doctors? Given the requirement of the

General Medical Council (1993, 2003, 2009a) that undergraduate medical education is aimed broadly at producing junior doctors with a wide range of basic skills and professional abilities, any specialty must earn its place in the curriculum by showing its benefits to the widest range of doctors (and their patients).

The World Health Organization has estimated that mental disorders comprise five of the top ten causes of years lived with disability, and produce about 22% of the total disability, worldwide (Mathers & Loncar, 2006). As the bulk of psychiatric presentations take place in non-psychiatric settings (general practice, accident and emergency departments, general hospital wards and clinics; Davies & Craig, 2009), all future doctors need adequate instruction in the recognition and initial management of psychiatric problems. For this reason above all others, psychiatry has a crucial position in undergraduate medical teaching. However, to be effective in achieving this goal, medical students must be taught to consider psychiatric morbidity (whether primary, secondary or coincidental) *at the same time* as they assess the disorders of other specialties.

Purpose of undergraduate psychiatry

Similar questions may be asked, in essence, of the purpose of undergraduate psychiatry: is it intended to meet the needs of all future doctors, or merely those who plan (or can be persuaded) to specialise in psychiatry? The answer to this question is crucial, since undergraduate psychiatry has more in common with other undergraduate medical subjects than with its postgraduate version (see Table 16.2); for instance, it will be taught by specialists to students the majority of whom will not enter the teachers' specialty. This has important implications for psychiatrists who wish to teach undergraduate students and postgraduate trainees identically. Undergraduate teaching must take account of the milder presentations and wide range of comorbidity encountered in non-psychiatric settings, as well as the shorter time for assessment that may be available. Schizophrenia and bipolar affective disorder, disorders that characterise much of postgraduate psychiatry, are much less common in the general medical encounter than anxiety, depression and adjustment disorders.

Psychiatry within the National Health Service

In the UK, all of the traditional medical specialties that contribute to the undergraduate curriculum have been squeezed and constrained by changes in the NHS, within which the bulk of undergraduate teaching and clinical experience occur. The 'general hospital' has evolved so that some specialties (e.g. ophthalmology and otolaryngology) are not represented at all hospital sites. In-patient stays are briefer and many common complaints (varicose veins are a frequently cited example), the core of undergraduate medicine,

Table 16.2 Differences between postgraduate and undergraduate psychiatry

	Postgraduate/specialist psychiatry	Undergraduate/generalist psychiatry
Context of clinical practice	Secondary, specialist setting	Primary, non-specialist setting
Presenting circumstances	Self-presentation rare; patients usually pre-screened and referred (e.g. by general practitioners or police)	Self-presentation or coincidental presentation common; patients not pre-screened nor referred by other agency
Typical assessment	Long, focused on confirmation and delineation of psychiatric morbidity	Brief (as part of broader assessment of non-psychiatric morbidity); focused on initial ascertainment
Typical disorders	Usually well defined, meeting formal diagnostic criteria (schizophrenia; bipolar disorders; personality disorders)	Often less well defined, symptomatic or subsyndromal (anxiety; depression; adjustment disorders; cares of life)
Characteristics of disorders	Lower prevalence; greater severity; biomedical complexity	Higher prevalence; lower severity; psychosocial complexity
Clinical management	Secondary management or advice to generalist	Initial management or referral to specialist
Numbers of trainees/students	Small number of trainees	Variable, but possibly large number of students
Medical skills	Maintaining basic medical skills	Gaining basic medical skills
Careers of trainees/students	>90% will become or remain psychiatrists	>90% will not become psychiatrists

are managed in primary care or by day-case treatment, so limiting further the student's opportunities for direct contact with affected patients.

The reorganisation of psychiatric services has paralleled the changes in other branches of medicine, with the development of 'functional' teams dealing with a limited range of psychiatric problems (often severe mental illness, SMI), or multidisciplinary community services with no associated in-patient facilities and an emphasis on non-medical 'mental health' needs of patients (St John-Smith *et al*, 2009). The net result of these changes has been to distance psychiatrists – both geographically and conceptually – from other doctors, and to make them appear to students as non-medical and deskilled.

Psychiatry's negative image

Members of the general population, including school students (Pinfold *et al*, 2003), hold predominantly stigmatising attitudes to psychiatric illness. Medical students are not immune to these influences in their prevailing culture, although surveys of their attitudes towards psychiatry, psychiatrists and psychiatric patients in the UK (Dogra, 2009) and elsewhere (Pailhez *et al*, 2005; Tonge, 2005) suggest that they do not hold these views as firmly as those around them. Nonetheless, the background negativity to all things psychiatric appears to exert a disproportionate effect on the students' responses to experiences in their psychiatry clinical placements (Goldacre *et al*, 2004; Lambert *et al*, 2006; see also Chapters 20 and 21).

Regaining lost ground

Students approve of courses that equip them for their early years in medical practice, and for this reason give greater support to integrated than to traditional psychiatry courses (Oakley & Oyebode, 2008). While the two course structures have a similar impact on choice of psychiatry as a postgraduate career, positive attitudes to psychiatry gained during the course decline less rapidly following problem-based or integrated learning than after traditional block teaching (Maidment *et al*, 2004). Newly qualified doctors identify 'visibility' of psychiatrists in prominent teaching roles throughout the curriculum as promoting a positive view of psychiatry (Goldacre *et al*, 2004), and encouragement from senior (i.e. consultant) psychiatrists as exerting a significant influence on choice of psychiatry as a career (Maidment *et al*, 2004) (see Box 16.1).

Integration offers an opportunity to reassert psychiatry's centrality to medicine and to affirm the psychiatrist's medical role, by placing psychiatrists as equals alongside teachers from other medical specialties. The need for mental health services to take a holistic view of the patient's mental and physical health provides many opportunities to contextualise psychiatry as a branch of medicine. Several aspects of the clinical encounter in the psychiatric out-patient clinic or community mental health centre – such as hand-washing, relevant physical examination (including blood pressure measurement), choosing and explaining the results of tests and investigations, venesection – emphasise the links between mental and physical healthcare. Thus the psychiatrist models good medical management, and the student may perform the interventions under his or her supervision. The educational impact is

---

Box 16.1 Factors that give students a positive experience of psychiatry

- 'Visibility' of psychiatrists in teaching
- Welcome and encouragement received in psychiatry placements
- 'Acceptability' of psychiatrists to their medical colleagues
- Effective 'can do' behaviour

Based on Goldacre *et al* (2004); Maidment *et al* (2004).

greatest when the psychiatrist is the initiator of medical interventions, rather than merely following the advice or directions of another medical specialist. Indeed, it highlights the psychiatrist's versatility in applying a bio-psychosocial approach in medicine as well as within the multidisciplinary mental health team.

Since it is not dependent on a single ('once and for all') teaching block, the integrated psychiatry course is less vulnerable to the vagaries of NHS structural changes, or to the negative effects of a poor-quality placement. By contributing to basic biomedical and social science teaching, psychiatrists can emphasise the scientific and evidence-based nature of their subject. Finally, by taking a prominent role in course design and direction, psychiatrists disseminate their professional skills, demonstrate their effectiveness in leadership and increase the visibility of psychiatry.

What should be taught?

It should be clear from the foregoing that psychiatry courses must provide education in attitudes, skills and knowledge ('ASK') that is enduring and will benefit future doctors in all medical specialties (Prideaux, 2003), a view endorsed by final-year medical students (Oakley & Oyebode, 2008). Recent recommendations from the Royal College of Psychiatrists provide a practical syllabus for the psychiatric component of all undergraduate medical courses (Dogra, 2009; see also Chapter 3).

A common concern among psychiatrists is that integrating psychiatry into the broader medical course will involve a 'dumbing down', a reduction in psychiatric knowledge expected of the students. This concern is unfounded, or should be, as the content of undergraduate psychiatry – the psychiatric syllabus – should not be diminished by integration. The fundamental change required by integration is one of form rather than content (a distinction that should be familiar to psychiatrists). Indeed, integrating throughout the entire duration of the course gives opportunities to repeat, review and reassess knowledge and skills learned at an earlier stage.

When should psychiatry be taught?

The brief answer to this question is: all over the curriculum – like a rash! Integration of psychiatric teaching works best when it is the norm for the medical course as a whole. Attitudes of students towards psychiatry and mental disorder tend to deteriorate throughout the traditional course, improve briefly following a single psychiatric placement, but decay again afterwards (Baxter *et al*, 2001). Psychiatric skills are also lost once the traditional placement is completed (Oakley & Oyebode, 2008). Thus, many psychiatry courses appear too late in the medical curriculum to be effective in changing attitudes and promoting lasting skills. Earlier is better; integrated throughout the medical course is best. Early contact with patients should aim

193

to overcome fears and stigma, and generate interest; skills and knowledge learned early and practised and tested repeatedly are most enduring.

How should psychiatry be integrated into the curriculum?

If it is to work properly, integration requires a considerable amount of work and has implications at all levels of the medical course. No single specialty should be allowed to dominate the process of integration, and as that would amount to an external take-over, with critical content being 'orphaned' (i.e. not seen as the responsibility of any teacher) or overshadowed by the other major specialties that retain their exclusive curricular time. This is exactly the outcome most feared by psychiatry teachers who wish to hold on to a traditional psychiatry block in the curriculum. Not surprisingly, this is also the major objection to integration held by teachers in other medical specialties, and psychiatrists who propose integration may experience the stiffest opposition from outside psychiatry.

Each medical school and its undergraduate course is at a different stage of curriculum development (Harden, 2000), so there cannot be a single recipe that meets every set of local circumstances. For this reason we must consider first a suitable model for integration of psychiatry, and then a general strategy that could apply to any undergraduate course but that can be modified to suit the local situation. Finally, we look at some examples of specific tactical steps to achieve integration. (The needs of psychiatrists who aim for an overall leadership role in medical curricula are beyond the scope of this chapter; for them, a formal qualification in teaching and learning, or at least attendance at courses on curriculum management, is likely to provide the best route.)

Helical curriculum (see also Chapter 2)

While several approaches to curricular integration might be considered – from merely distributing distinct components of a psychiatry syllabus through successive years, to repeating the same topics in different years – the helical curriculum (Dance, 1967; Kurtz et al, 2005) has a particular appeal for psychiatry (Fig. 16.2). Developed as an approach to learning communication skills, this model permits students to revisit similar topics at successive stages in their education. At each successive stage of the course, students revise and build on existing subject-specific knowledge and skills to extend their ability to understand, analyse and apply their learning. New knowledge and skills acquired at each successive stage are partial, that is, they can be utilised only by incorporating learning from earlier stages, and at each stage issues are raised that cannot be resolved until later stages.

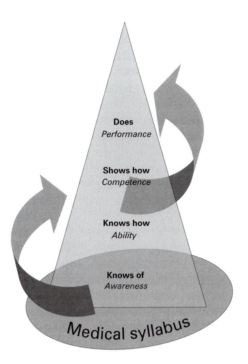

Fig. 16.2 Relationship of helical curriculum to Miller's hierarchy.

This model (Fig. 16.2) mirrors the process of acquisition of knowledge (Bloom, 1965) and demonstration of clinical skills (Miller, 1990) that inform much of both undergraduate and postgraduate assessment (see also Chapter 2 on Miller, p. 22). From the practical point of view, this reinforces for the student the currency of previous learning (and goes a long way towards answering the student's question 'Is what I'm studying now relevant to my future needs?').

Table 16.3 shows how a psychiatric topic (schizophrenia) might be covered comprehensively in an integrated helical curriculum.

Strategic planning

The most descriptive term to apply to the process of developing an integral but integrated role for psychiatry is 'constructive engagement': committing a little to gain a great deal. This raises questions immediately about engaging with what, and how. As noted, every undergraduate medical school course is at a different stage of development, so psychiatry must engage with whatever exists locally. Traditional block- or year-based courses do not encourage subject teachers to understand the overall curriculum, but for any degree of integration this is essential if glaring gaps as well as fruitless repetition are to be avoided. In any case, regardless of course structure,

Table 16.3 Example of psychiatric topic (schizophrenia) followed through a fully integrated (helical) curriculum

Year or phase of course	Vertically integrated psychiatric topic (here, schizophrenia)	Horizontally integrated subjects
1	Concept of mental illness	Ethics, rights Concept of disease; philosophy of mind Legal context of medical practice
2	Biology of schizophrenia Psychosocial aspects of mental illness	Neuroscience Psychology Sociology applied to medicine
3	Diagnosis and treatment of schizophrenia	Adult general medicine (including psychiatry)
4	Schizophrenia at different ages Emergency management and crisis care	Old age medicine (including psychiatry) Child and adolescent medicine (including psychiatry) Emergency medicine (including psychiatry)
5	Management of schizophrenia	Primary care and community services (including mental health services)

the General Medical Council (2009*b*) has criticised teachers at UK medical schools for knowing too little about the curricula in which they teach.

The main stages in developing a strategic plan for integration are listed in Box 16.2. If such a plan does not exist, then the first stage is to create a psychiatry course team that mirrors the year, stage or phase structure of the overall undergraduate course, a sort of 'shadow cabinet'. Specific members of the team should aim to become thoroughly familiar with each level of the undergraduate course, its assessment processes and its programme of student-selected components (SSCs, previously known as special study modules, SSMs), even if there is no current psychiatry content at a particular level. For many medical courses this might be achieved by starting small, getting to know those specialties that have existing or potential temporal (taught in the same year block), spatial (taught at the same hospital campus), or conceptual (other 'neurosciences', Davies & McGuire, 2000; but also primary care) links to psychiatry. At least one designated member of the team, perhaps its leader, must have a broader role in understanding the overall medical curriculum and its learning outcomes, and the competing demands of many apparently dissimilar specialties for the student's time and attention. Similarly, at least one member, again probably the leader, will need to take on the role of negotiating any proposed changes with the medical school authorities.

Box 16.2 Stages in developing a strategic plan for integration

- Take decision to integrate (academic/departmental level)
- Establish strategic course team
- Allocate curriculum tasks within team (both overview of existing curriculum and knowledge of specific stages)
- Agree aims and objectives for integration, and learning outcomes for the new stages of the curriculum
- Liaise with medical school authorities to set date for implementation (usually start of academic session or year)
- Take leadership of new course and manage change
- Disseminate information, initially through discussion of ideas, later by focused training sessions
- Manage dissent
- Allow for concurrent running of both 'old' and 'new' curricula
- Monitor progress and maintain momentum

Setting up a course team may appear a daunting prospect. Relatively few clinicians or academics come to curriculum design and management 'fully formed', but many will have been teachers who wish to take some control of the course in which they teach. Psychiatrists, experts as they are in managing complex bio-psychosocial problems and working with multiprofessional teams and diverse agencies, have many of the negotiating skills and organisational abilities to take an active part in managing the structure and content of the curriculum. Current course leaders will know, generally, who is willing and able to take on a management role in the team; local policies and practices will determine whether candidates can be invited to join or whether a formal recruitment process will be needed. However, given the clinical pressures on psychiatrists, there will need to be a formal negotiation with employers (whether NHS trusts or university departments) to ensure members of the course team are allocated adequate time in their job plans for the tasks they will undertake (minimum of one programmed activity, or PA, in the current job planning jargon).

As soon as practicable, the team should meet to agree its aims and objectives (see Box 16.3) and to set a practical timescale for their delivery. This will involve reviewing the existing medical syllabus and curriculum structure, and producing a 'curriculum map' that indicates opportunities for the inclusion of psychiatry learning (see 'Tactical steps', below). This must be coupled with an analysis of the current psychiatry course to see what components can be delivered in a new niche without losing any of the attitudes, skills and knowledge that comprise the current psychiatry block. In many instances, local structures and initiatives might already be in place that could form the basis of best practice, to be shared and disseminated

---

Box 16.3 Aims and objectives of an integrated psychiatric course

Aims

- To mould and guide the formation of students' attitudes to psychiatry and psychiatric patients
- To demythologise psychiatry and in so doing to destigmatise psychiatric patients – and psychiatrists – in the eyes of all students and doctors
- To inculcate a psychiatric approach in the assessment of all patients and in the clinical practice of all doctors
- To ensure early recognition and initial management of psychiatric morbidity in all clinical settings
- To ensure mental disorder is not 'someone else's problem'

Objectives

- To introduce psychiatric knowledge and skills early in a student's medical education
- To make explicit the bio-psychosocial evidence base of psychiatric practice
- To revisit, review and reassess psychiatric knowledge and skills repeatedly throughout the medical course
- To embed psychiatric skills in the clinical procedures of all other specialties

---

across the whole course (general hospital or general practice liaison services are often cited as examples).

The next stage is to set learning outcomes (Bloom, 1965; Atherton, 2009) and appropriate assessment standards (Miller, 1990) for the distributed, integrated psychiatry content. This will involve a shift from assessing all psychiatry knowledge and skills at the end of a traditional teaching block to assessment in stages appropriate to cumulative development of those same attributes. Final assessment of 'psychiatry' cannot take place until completion of the cumulative elements of the integrated course. This should ensure a place for psychiatry in the student's final qualifying examinations, so reinforcing the critical role of psychiatry in the new doctor's practice.

The course team must take leadership of the new course and manage the process of change (Hayes, 2006). Some aspects of this are relatively straightforward: the course team must keep every teacher fully informed of the emerging strategy by clear written briefings or newsletters, or by holding regular meetings. Dissenting views will need to be heard and unforeseen problems addressed as part of 'work in progress'. Part of this process will involve reassurance that psychiatry is not disappearing from the curriculum but is being disaggregated and distributed, that while form is changing to meet the functional requirements of new doctors the content has been preserved. When a final strategy emerges, it must be disseminated through clear but firm guidance to teachers at each level of the curriculum: reference to a new curriculum map should ensure each teacher knows his or her role in the overall course, and that cherished topics are being covered. At this stage, discussion meetings should be superseded by 'teaching the teachers' sessions to disseminate information. In due course, all local initiatives will be informed by, and will have to conform to, the overall strategy for psychiatry – to avoid the lack of standardisation criticised by external regulators (General Medical Council, 2009b).

Some teachers in traditional block courses will feel devalued, disempowered or disenfranchised by the proposed changes and the course team will need to manage their responses. Most will be won over by a combination of argument and persuasion; others will accept change provisionally on a try-it-and-see basis. A small number may refuse to take part, and the course team should have a contingency plan to support or replace these teachers, and this might involve discussion with their NHS employer. Critically, a new teaching strategy should not be allowed to fail because teachers insist on going their own way.

Finally, a start date must be set and adhered to. Although some tactical changes (see below) may be made simultaneously at several levels of the curriculum, the overall integration strategy requires that a new undergraduate curriculum begins with a new intake of undergraduate students, and is rolled out progressively as that cohort passes through each stage of the medical course. In effect, two courses, following the 'old' and the 'new' curricula, will run concurrently for one complete cycle of medical education (5 years for a standard medical undergraduate programme). Steps will be needed to ensure students (and their teachers) on the old block course are not disadvantaged. Equally, the rearrangement of psychiatry topic teaching may mean that some teachers have a double workload for a short time as the same topic is taught to two cohorts of students at different phases of their education.

Once the changes begin to be implemented, the course team must meet regularly to review and monitor the process of change (Harden, 2000) and to maintain its momentum as it runs through the full course (Hayes, 2006). Clearly, this is an iterative process and the course team will need to incorporate feedback from teachers and other outcomes such as assessment results into their forward planning. The strategy will evolve, although if well prepared it should not undergo major upheaval, and the sequence of planning, discussion, training and implementation will become an established cycle.

Tactical steps

The tactical steps that may be taken to integrate psychiatry into the medical curriculum must flow from the overall strategy adopted by the psychiatry course team (Table 16.4). Some are general, in that they relate to the manner in which psychiatrists approach teaching their specialty; others are specific to a stage or phase of the undergraduate course (Box 16.4).

Table 16.4 Strategic and tactical approaches to integrating psychiatry must be coordinated

Strategy	Tactics
Top down: decisions taken and managed by course team at departmental level, taking account of overall medical curriculum	Bottom up: may be initiated and implemented by individuals, based on local circumstances, but must meet strategic objectives
Group or team of psychiatrists sharing tasks in a coordinated manner	Individual psychiatrists working with 'local' colleagues
Exert influence over entire curriculum; sharing good practice	Influence local; establishing good practice
Benefits long term, diffuse and indirect	Benefits may be localised in time and space, but specific and direct

General steps

These relate to the behaviour and approach of the psychiatric teachers. They are important because they affect the student's experience of psychiatry and thus its image as a medical specialty. Failure to present a positive image cannot be compensated for by integration or any other form of course structure. Given the factors that discourage students from an interest in psychiatry, or from considering psychiatry as a career, the approach of individual teachers is of prime importance. Teachers should ask themselves 'What stands out from my medical education: what I was taught, or who taught me?' Psychiatric teachers should be enthusiastic about teaching, welcoming and accessible to students when they join a placement, and positive about their specialty. At the very least, they should avoid whingeing to students about pressures on the psychiatrist. Psychiatry is a medical specialty and part of the undergraduate curriculum, so teachers should emphasise the similarities of psychiatric history taking, examination and clinical inference to their equivalents in the general medical assessment, rather than their differences (Davies & Craig, 2009).

Box 16.4 Useful tactical questions to ask about each stage of the curriculum

- Is psychiatric research contributing to basic biomedical science teaching?
- Is there a psychiatric component of this medical topic?
- Are psychiatrists involved in teaching this topic?
- How are the psychiatric aspects of these disorders being covered?
- When is the mental health of patients (e.g. with non-psychiatric disorders) being considered?

Psychiatric patients, too, should be empowered by their psychiatrists to take a positive role in teaching. Many patients, although reticent about disclosing their personal experiences to students, can be persuaded to do so if they see a benefit for themselves in facilitating an understanding of their problems in the doctors they will meet in future years (see Chapter 12). Some may be encouraged to become 'standardized patients' or 'patient educators' who take part in formal teaching sessions outside their regular clinic attendances.

Specific steps

Specific interventions may be classified roughly according to the stages of a student's undergraduate medical education (Dogra, 2009):

- pre-selection
- selection
- early (preclinical) years
- later (clinical) years, including preparation for medical practice
- student-selected components (SSCs)
- self-directed learning and self-assessment materials
- examinations and assessments
- career planning.

Interventions at the pre-selection stage might involve 'outreach' visits and talks at local schools, or hosting school student visits or 'taster sessions' at the psychiatric clinic or to the mental health team. This raises the profile of psychiatry and the expectations of the students about the experiences they will gain at medical school. Participation in the selection process is also important, especially in shortlisting and interviewing, as evidence suggests that selectors might be biased towards candidates who share their attitudes and aspirations (the 'like-me effect': Byrne, 1971; Rand & Wexley, 1975; Edwards et al, 1990).

Contributions to all components of the early, preclinical, years of the course will build on the psychological bias often shown by new students but lost gradually if not reinforced. Psychiatric research provides many cutting-edge examples of the scientific basis of medicine (e.g. imaging, genetics, psychopharmacology) and these may be incorporated into basic biomedical teaching. Examples from clinical psychiatry will show students the relevance of the neuroscience, pharmacology and psychology they learn in the lecture theatre. This will be reinforced by early contact with psychiatric patients (perhaps as patient educators); such contact also helps to combat stigmatising attitudes to patients and promote both intellectual and clinical interest in their problems.

Every patient, presenting with whatever condition, has mental health needs. Thus, the clinical years of the medical course provide psychiatry with the greatest number of opportunities for integration and for a focus on the whole patient. General hospital liaison psychiatry provides a ready model of psychiatry being practised alongside other specialties, and contributing to the management of patients with non-psychiatric problems. However, because most liaison psychiatry services are small in size, they cannot provide an experience for large numbers of students and so other opportunities must be sought. Many medical specialties recognise the need for psychological input in the management of chronic disease (e.g. diabetes, stroke, pain) and these should be incorporated into the available psychiatry placements (or developed as SSCs – see below and Chapter 15). The psychiatric subspecialties that already exist in the medical curriculum may be realigned with their medical equivalents: for example general and community psychiatry may be taught alongside general practice, or neurology, or other adult medical topics; child psychiatry fits well with paediatrics; and old age psychiatry complements geriatric medicine.

All undergraduate courses allocate 20–30% of curricular time for SSCs, permitting in-depth study of a topic of the students' own choosing. SSCs provide an ideal vehicle for promotion of the content and values of psychiatry (see Chapter 15). The range of settings of psychiatric practice – from community teams and hospital liaison services to specialist clinics, research laboratories and secure forensic units – provides potential topics of interest for students at all stages of learning.

Psychiatrists may enhance the students' learning experience by providing a coordinated set of course-related materials for self-directed learning and self-assessment. These should be easily accessible to students at all stages of the curriculum, either in paper format or, better, as e-learning materials accessible from the medical school's learning-based website (see Chapter 6). Learning materials may take the form of interactive scenarios, or more traditional lecture notes, to provide core information on psychiatric disorders as a supplement to regular reading lists and to flesh out topics encountered in clinical placements. Self-assessment exercises are a popular aid to revision, and they work best if the online system keeps a cumulative record of the student's performance. Students may use their self-assessment records to facilitate formative feedback and guidance from their tutors.

Assessment drives and focuses learning (see Chapter 5), so psychiatrists and psychiatry should be prominent at each level of assessment that students must attempt. This will include providing questions for inclusion in written examinations, and ensuring that psychiatric disorders and their treatments are included in the differential diagnoses that students must consider to pass an examination. Clinical examinations (whether objective structured clinical examinations, OSCEs, or other forms) are particularly compelling drivers to learning, and psychiatrists should be available to devise and examine in these. The status of the psychiatrist as a doctor can be reinforced by examining students in non-psychiatric clinical subjects (this is rarely as testing for the psychiatrist as many fear). Again, the earlier in their education students encounter psychiatric examinations and the more years in which they are examined, the more likely psychiatry is to become entrenched in their clinical practice.

Students are encouraged increasingly to consider and review their career aspirations as they pass through their undergraduate education. Clearly, the undergraduate psychiatry course should contribute to promoting psychiatry as a career choice, but the widely held view that this is achieved by piling on more 'teaching' is mistaken. The critical element is the demeanour of psychiatrists themselves – who teaches, rather than what is taught – as positive, 'can do', effective doctors. This positive image can be enhanced substantially by running a regular series of talks on aspects of psychiatry by famous, interesting, or provocative psychiatrists chosen for their charisma and appeal to students. Many academic psychiatric faculties will have members of staff who can present their research and its clinical applications enthusiastically to a general audience.

Summary

This chapter has reviewed the rationale for developing a psychiatric curriculum that is fully integrated into the entire undergraduate medical course. Integration represents a potent method of exerting the influence of psychiatry over the attitudes, skills and knowledge to be acquired in a medical undergraduate course. The strategic stages and tactical steps to be taken to achieve integration have been outlined. While there are many obstacles to integration, none is insurmountable, and integrated courses are increasing in number and are well received by students. The onus lies with psychiatrists who know the importance of their specialty to have confidence that integration does not weaken that importance but strengthens it, for the benefit of psychiatry, of all future doctors and of their patients.

References

Atherton, J. S. (2009) *Learning and Teaching: Bloom's Taxonomy*. Available at http://www.learningandteaching.info/learning/bloomtax.htm

Baxter, H., Singh, S. P., Standen, P., *et al* (2001) The attitudes of 'tomorrow's doctors' towards mental illness and psychiatry: changes during the final undergraduate year. *Medical Education*, **35**, 381–383.

Bloom, B. S. (1965) *Taxonomy of Educational Objectives*. Longman.

Byrne, D. (1971) *The Attraction Paradigm*. Academic Press.

Dahle, L. O., Brynhildsen, J., Behrbohm Fallsberg, M., *et al* (2002) Pros and cons of vertical integration between clinical medicine and basic science within a problem-based undergraduate medical curriculum: examples and experiences from Linköping, Sweden. *Medical Teacher*, **24**, 280–285.

Dance, F. (1967) Toward a theory of human communication. In *Human Communication Theory: Original Essays* (ed. F. Dance), pp. 288–309. Holt Reinhart Winston.

Davies, T. & Craig, T. (2009) Mental health assessment. In *ABC of Mental Health* (2nd edn) (eds T. Davies & T. Craig), pp. 1–6. Wiley-Blackwell.

Davies, T. & McGuire, P. (2000) Teaching medical students in the new millennium. *Psychiatric Bulletin*, **24**, 4–5.

Dogra, N. (2009) *Report of the Scoping Group on Undergraduate Education in Psychiatry.* RCPsych.

Edwards, J. C., Johnson, E. K. & Molidor, J. B. (1990) The interview in the admission process. *Academic Medicine,* **65,** 167–177.

General Medical Council (1993) *Tomorrow's Doctors* (1st edn). GMC.

General Medical Council (2003) *Tomorrow's Doctors* (2nd edn). GMC.

General Medical Council (2009a) *Tomorrow's Doctors: Outcomes and Standards for Undergraduate Medical Education.* GMC.

General Medical Council (2009b) *UK Medical Schools – Quality Assurance Results.* GMC.

Goldacre, M. J., Turner, G. & Lambert, T. W. (2004) Variation by medical school in career choices of UK graduates of 1999 and 2000. *Medical Education,* **38,** 249–258.

Harden, R. M. (2000) The integration ladder: a tool for curriculum planning and evaluation. *Medical Education,* **34,** 551–557.

Hayes, J. (2006) *The Theory and Practice of Change Management* (2nd edn). Palgrave Macmillan.

Karim, K., Edwards, R., Dogra, N., *et al.* (2009) A survey of the teaching and assessment of undergraduate psychiatry in the medical schools of the United Kingdom and Ireland. *Medical Teacher,* **31,** 1024–1029.

Kurtz, S., Silverman, J. & Draper, J. (2005) *Teaching and Learning Communication Skills in Medicine* (2nd edn). Radcliffe Publishing.

Lambert, T. W., Goldacre, M. J. & Turner, G. (2006) Career choices of United Kingdom medical graduates of 2002: questionnaire survey. *Medical Education,* **40,** 514–521.

Maidment, R., Livingston, G., Katona, C., *et al* (2004) Change in attitudes to psychiatry and intention to pursue psychiatry as a career in newly qualified doctors: a follow-up of two cohorts of medical students. *Medical Teacher,* **26,** 565–569.

Mathers, C. D. & Loncar, D. (2006) Projections of global mortality and burden of disease from 2002 to 2030. *Public Library of Science Medicine,* **3,** e442.

Miller, G. E. (1990) The assessment of clinical skills/competence/performance. *Academic Medicine,* **65** (suppl.), S63–S67.

Oakley, C. & Oyebode, F. (2008) Medical students' views about an undergraduate curriculum in psychiatry before and after clinical placements. *BioMed Central Medical Education,* **8,** 26.

Pailhez, G., Bulbena, A., Coll, J., *et al* (2005) Attitudes and views on psychiatry: a comparison between Spanish and US medical students. *Academic Psychiatry,* **29,** 82–91.

Pinfold, V., Toulmin, H., Thornicroft, G., *et al* (2003) Reducing psychiatric stigma and discrimination: evaluation of educational interventions in UK secondary schools. *British Journal of Psychiatry,* **182,** 342–346.

Prideaux, D. (2003) ABC of learning and teaching in medicine: curriculum design. *BMJ,* **326,** 268–270.

Rand, T. M. & Wexley, K. N. (1975) A demonstration of the Byrne similarity hypothesis in simulated employment interviews. *Psychological Reports,* **36,** 535–544.

St John Smith, P., McQueen, D., Michael, A., *et al* (2009) The trouble with NHS psychiatry in England. *Psychiatric Bulletin,* **33,** 219–225.

Tonge, B. J. (2005) Some Australian reflections on problems with recruitment into the profession of psychiatry. *International Psychiatry,* issue 10, 8–9.

CHAPTER 17

Teaching the teachers in a cross-cultural setting: the Scotland–Malawi Mental Health Education Project

Johannes Leuvennink

Introduction

It has long been accepted that consultants are appointed to posts in the National Health Service (NHS) with an expectation that they will immediately take the lead in teaching medical students, general practitioner trainees and specialists in training. It is often the case, however, that they will have had little formal supervision or training in teaching and assessment methods. This chapter describes the Scotland–Malawi Mental Health Education Project, an innovative project that provides higher trainees in Scotland with the opportunity to prepare, deliver and examine an undergraduate psychiatry course, while supporting the development of psychiatric capacity in a low-income country.

Background to the project

Ever since the travels of the Scottish Presbyterian pioneer and medical missionary Dr David Livingstone (1813–73), Scotland and Malawi have had strong cultural and educational links. Malawi is a sub-Saharan African country with a population of around 14 million and a per capita gross domestic product of US$312. The health of the Malawian people has suffered under the burdens of poverty, a devastating HIV/AIDS epidemic (the adult prevalence was 14.4% in 2003), a lack of health workers owing to attrition and emigration, and a lack of training resources. This has given rise to a human resource emergency in the health sector (Kauye & Mafuta 2006; Kauye, 2008).

In 2005, the Scottish and Malawian governments established the Scotland–Malawi Partnership (see http://www.scotland-malawipartnership.org), the purpose of which was to support Malawi in areas of medical and social development. The International Development Unit of the then Scottish executive (now the Scottish government) and the Ministry of Health in Malawi identified appropriate areas of focus for the initiative.

These included teaching and training for all cadres of health workers, clinical support (after discussion with Malawian counterparts to ensure appropriateness and cultural sensitivity) and provision of clinical supplies and equipment. A specific priority area identified was support for teaching at undergraduate and postgraduate levels at the College of Medicine, Malawi's only medical school.

Mental health services in Malawi are provided mainly at three psychiatric hospitals – Zomba Mental Hospital (333 beds) in Zomba in the south, a small mental health unit in Lilongwe in the central region (30 beds) and the charity-funded St John of God Hospital in the north (50 beds) – amounting to a total of just over 400 in-patient psychiatric beds for the entire population. At Zomba Mental Hospital, there is one consultant psychiatrist, one other doctor (a medical officer), four clinical officers, one occupational therapist, 25 trained nursing staff and approximately 100 ward attendants. In the absence of sufficient psychiatrists, clinical officers (who have a 3-year medical training) provide much of the clinical service in the psychiatric units. At district level, mental healthcare is provided by psychiatric nurses, who are often also expected to work as general nurses and midwives. Community mental health services are underdeveloped and largely run by psychiatric district nursing staff. Some clinical officers are currently receiving higher training in psychiatry (as part of a bachelor of science degree) at St John of God College of Health Sciences, with the aim that they will bolster district-level services.

Taking the opportunity offered by the Scotland–Malawi Partnership, four Scottish psychiatrists with enthusiasm for teaching and supporting Malawi came together in response to a request from Malawi's only psychiatrist (Dr Felix Kauye) to help provide undergraduate psychiatric teaching at the College of Medicine. They recognised that such a project could meet two identified needs: first, the need of the College of Medicine to provide high-quality undergraduate psychiatric teaching to its expanding student intake; and second, the need for higher trainees in psychiatry in Scotland to gain experience in teaching and examination techniques before they become consultants.

Malawian undergraduate psychiatry teaching

The College of Medicine is based in Blantyre, Malawi's main commercial centre, about 1 hour's drive from Zomba. Around 50–60 medical students qualify per year. Psychiatric training in the undergraduate medical curriculum is of particular importance as, after their medical qualification, the graduates will often work in environments with limited access to specialist psychiatric care. Many spend time working as district health officers, in which role they are responsible for the administration of a district health service, including psychiatric provision in the community. Secondary care psychiatric services are usually not able to provide direct medical input at district level, as they are mainly based at the in-patient units.

The undergraduate psychiatry curriculum is mainly taught in a teaching block in the fourth year of undergraduate training. A clear need was expressed for external support for the teaching and assessment of medical students in psychiatry. There was already support provided by volunteers from Norway as well as, on occasion, from Scotland, but the sustainability of this input was uncertain, putting the consistency of undergraduate psychiatric training at risk.

Scottish psychiatric trainees' teaching skills

Trainees in psychiatry usually are able to become involved in teaching duties. This may include participation in clinical teaching to undergraduate medical students during their psychiatric placements. Occasionally, they may also take on teaching duties to other trainees or to other disciplines. It is, however, very often the case that such teaching activities are not well coordinated and supervised.

The Royal College of Psychiatrists has for some time identified the need to provide trainees with opportunities to improve their teaching skills. This could be achieved through a variety of ways, including attendance at 'teaching the teachers' courses, doing formal training in medical education and, most importantly, providing teaching under supervision, which allows trainees to gain competence in a variety of teaching modalities, as well as examination and assessment techniques and giving feedback to students.

A combination of teaching needs at the Malawi College of Medicine, the training needs of Scottish psychiatric trainees and the context of the wider Scotland –Malawi Project created the opportunity for the initiative described in this chapter.

Establishing the project

The group developed the project with Dr Felix Kauye, who welcomed the initiative. Dr Kauye was pivotal throughout in overseeing and guiding the teaching and assessments. From its inception, the project had as its aim to be governed by the specific needs in Malawi, rather than a perceived need from Scotland. A steering group was formed that comprised four Scottish psychiatrists (Professor Douglas Blackwood, Dr Johannes Leuvennink, Dr Leonie Boeing and Dr Robert Stewart, who at that stage worked as a specialist registrar in Manchester), who were later joined by Dr Ben Baig, clinical lecturer and honorary specialist registrar at the University of Edinburgh. Henceforth, the project became known as the Scotland–Malawi Mental Health Education Project (SMMHEP).

The activities of the project

The College of Medicine curriculum

During the first 3 years of SMMHEP's support to Malawi (2007–09), the teaching programme consisted of a 3- to 4-week block of theory teaching based at the College of Medicine in Blantyre followed by a 2- to 3-week block of clinical teaching based at Zomba Mental Hospital. At the end of this block, written and clinical examinations are taken.

Through the activities of the volunteer trainees, the range of teaching methods has expanded and improved each year. The theory block now includes formal lectures, visits to a street children project and a rehabilitation unit, and a group presentation mini-project, where the volunteers supervise student-guided projects that are presented later in the course. In 2009, topics chosen by the students included 'Mental health aspects of palliative care' and 'Students' stress coping strategies at the College of Medicine'. During the clinical teaching, volunteers act as tutors to groups of about eight students and focus on clinical and presentation skills and safe management of common psychiatric presentations. The teaching takes place on the acute and rehabilitation wards at Zomba Mental Hospital, where many of the in-patients experience florid psychotic symptoms. The students themselves act as interpreters for the volunteers when needed.

The undergraduate psychiatry curriculum and teaching programme in Malawi is currently under review and SMMHEP is providing some input into that review.

Table 17.1 gives an example of a part of the teaching timetable with SMMHEP volunteer input.

Assessment structure

Scotland–Malawi Mental Health Education Project volunteers actively partake in the assessments of the undergraduate students, including setting and marking the written examination in accordance with the Malawi College of Medicine guide and under the supervision of Dr Felix Kauye. The assessment structure consists of the following:

- continuous assessment (60%)
    - logbook (attendance, knowledge, skills, attitudes – tutor assessed)
    - written long case
- written examination (40%)
    - multiple-choice questions (MCQs, in both true/false and single best answer format)
    - short answers (two out of three)
- pass/fail and distinction oral examinations.

Table 17.1 Three sample weeks from the fourth-year undergraduate psychiatry module at the College of Medicine, Malawi

Day	Morning	Afternoon
Week 1 – *Introduction to psychiatry*		
Monday	Introduction to the module Broad introduction to mental disorder and classification Aetiology of mental disorder – the bio-psychosocial approach	Mental health services in Malawi Culture and psychiatry
Tuesday	Psychiatric history Mental state examination Psychopathology	Psychopathology
Wednesday	Groups A and B – Zomba Mental Hospital Groups C and D – role-play/presentation preparation	
Thursday	Groups C and D – Zomba Mental Hospital Groups A and B – role-play/presentation preparation	
Friday	Delirium Introduction to treatments in psychiatry Introduction to psychopharmacology	Personal study
Week 2 – *Major mental disorders*		
Monday	Mood disorders	Mood disorders
Tuesday	Schizophrenia	Schizophrenia
Wednesday	Group A – Limbe health centre Group B – general medical ward Group C – Zomba Mental Hospital Group D – district general hospital	Presentation preparation Presentation preparation Presentation preparation
Thursday	Group B – Limbe health centre Group C – general medical ward Group D – Zomba Mental Hospital Group A – district general hospital	Presentation preparation Presentation preparation Presentation preparation
Friday	Neuropsychiatry, including HIV/AIDS, neurosyphillis and cerebral malaria Suicide	Private study
Week 5		
Monday	Division into groups Introduction to tutors and wards	Ward work/tutorial
Tuesday	Ward work/tutorial	Ward work/tutorial
Wednesday	Electroconvulsive therapy Ward work/tutorial	Ward work/tutorial
Thursday	Ward work/tutorial	Ward work/tutorial
Friday(Blantyre)	Mental health law/forensic psychiatry Community psychiatry/rehabilitation Psychiatric emergencies	Private study

This specific teaching block ran from 26 January to 13 March 2009. Weeks 1–4 covered theory, taught to four of groups of 12 students. Week 5–7 covered clinical teaching, delivered to six groups of 8 students. Morning sessions were 8 a.m. to noon in weeks 1 and 2, and 9.30 a.m. to noon in week 5; afternoon sessions were 2 to 5 p.m. in weeks 1 and 2, and 1.30 to 4 p.m. in week 5.

Student presentations

In an attempt to include an aspect of student-directed learning, and to develop understanding of mental health issues in a specifically Malawian context, students are asked to work in groups to prepare presentations. Topics can be decided by the students. Examples include:

- suicide in Malawi – legal aspects, stigma and meaning
- the use of cannabis in Malawi
- psychosocial interventions in HIV services available in Malawi
- religion and mental disorder.

The presentations can include case studies, literature reviews and the results of interviews with professionals. Time is allocated during the theory weeks and presentations are made in the final week of the clinical placement. Tutors are available to facilitate if needed.

From 2010, SMMHEP has assisted in the introduction of structured problem-based learning sessions (see Chapter 9 on problem-based learning).

Recruitment of volunteers

Each year, SMMHEP obtains information on the specific weeks and numbers of students requiring clinical teaching in order to plan the Scottish side of recruitment. Usually, SMMHEP looks to recruit five higher trainees in psychiatry from the four deaneries in Scotland, and one consultant psychiatrist from Scotland to support and supervise the trainees while in Malawi, in addition to his or her own input into the teaching programme.

Recruitment is initiated through members of the SMMHEP steering group at the Royal College of Psychiatrists' Scottish Division meetings, during which information is provided by means of a verbal update and call for volunteers; these meeting have on occasion featured a stall providing information leaflets, posters and photographs, with a SMMHEP member. Members of the steering group and previous volunteers have also given presentations to the Scottish Division on its work and how volunteers benefited from this as a training experience. Presentations are also given at local psychiatric service departmental education meetings and regional postgraduate training meetings. In September 2008, SMMHEP hosted a one-day conference in Edinburgh. The purpose of this was: first, to inform stakeholders, including employers, trainers and potential trainee volunteers, about the project; second, to share our experience and process with similar projects in other medical fields in Scotland; and third, to host all involved in the project, past and present, as members and owners of a network. The Scotland–Malawi Mental Health Education Project is very fortunate to have had, during each year of recruitment, significantly more potential volunteers interested in taking part than were required. We therefore had to shortlist candidates by requesting them to submit brief resumés with an exposition of their level of experience and training needs. Trainees in their final year of higher training are usually given priority.

Planning the visits

The next stage is the planning of the teaching programme, in terms of topics, modes of teaching and content. All volunteers take topics, as governed by the curriculum supplied to SMMHEP each year, and they then prepare lectures, small-group tutorials and role-play sessions on these. The work of previous volunteers enables the project to make use of teaching materials from earlier years, including presentations, references, audiovisual materials and other material in the teaching 'bank'.

The process of clinical tuition during the students' clinical placement is discussed in detail. These discussions include preparation for different methods of clinical teaching, such as small-group teaching, student-directed teaching, case presentations and discussions, and ward-based teaching. Also discussed are issues around the use of patients during small-group teaching, aspects of confidentiality, respect and autonomy. Emphasis is put on cross-cultural aspects of teaching. Sensitivities related to perceptions of illness, mental illness, the place of religion in Malawian society and any similar issues, often brought to light by previous volunteers or Dr Kauye in Malawi, are discussed in preparation. The volunteers are also advised on giving feedback to the students.

Supervision of trainees

Before they leave for Malawi, a number of preparatory meetings are held with the trainee volunteers and the Scottish consultant psychiatrist who will be attending the teaching block in Malawi. They are supervised by members of the SMMHEP steering group, who are consultant psychiatrists in the NHS in Scotland. The trainee volunteers are supervised in the following areas:

- design of the teaching programme, including the presentation by trainees of the main content of their lectures
- design of and preparation for clinical teaching, including the use of small-group discussions, student-directed learning, case presentations, and so on
- design of examinations
- giving feedback to students.

The activities in Malawi – the lecture series, interaction with Malawian students and patients, final preparation, execution and marking of the examination, and feedback to students – are supervised by Dr Kauye, a Scottish consultant psychiatrist volunteer and Dr Robert Stewart, a member of the steering group who has coordinated each teaching block as honorary lecturer at the College of Medicine (and who was recently appointed a full-time lecturer there).

Finally, trainee volunteers are expected to provide members of the steering group with a formal report on their activities, learning points and competencies attained and any pitfalls to be considered by future volunteers. The volunteer trainees are also expected to give presentations to their own departments, regional postgraduate meetings and/or meetings of the Royal College of Psychiatrists. These have met with much enthusiasm and interest for involvement by potential volunteers. The volunteers are furthermore expected to incorporate these reports and competencies into their training portfolio.

Practical arrangements

As the project develops and experience is gathered through feedback, SMMHEP is increasingly able to advise new volunteers on practical arrangements in preparation for their work in Malawi, for example on personal safety, immunisations, culturally sensitive dress code and behaviour, and flight and transport arrangements. Accommodation arrangements vary from year to year and SMMHEP is also in the process of securing more consistent transport arrangements within Malawi.

Feedback on the project

College of Medicine

The College of Medicine regards the project as having been of great benefit to the institution. It believes that the high-quality teaching will lay the foundation for the later development of postgraduate training in psychiatry.

Each year, structured feedback on the course has been sought from the students themselves. Although not afraid to point out areas in need of improvement, their feedback has been very positive. For example, in 2009, 85% of the students rated the tutors as good or excellent. A second measure of evaluation from the relevant medical students was the circulation of an 'Attitudes to psychiatry' questionnaire. This was given to the students prior to the course and then again after the final examination; it has been used in the UK as a standardised way of measuring attitudes to psychiatry (Calvert *et al*, 1999). It was evident that students viewed psychiatric patients and psychiatric practice itself with much more esteem following the course.

Psychiatric trainees

Trainee volunteers consistently report this experience as invaluable in a number of areas of learning and development. They find that they benefit greatly from peer development. This relates to working as a group to deliver the teaching and assessments. They value the opportunity to share skills, observe others teach, share good practice and learn from each other's experiences where they encountered any problems such as issues with language, culture or mode of teaching. They also gain experience in using multimedia equipment in teaching and designing presentations and in lectures using these.

They often report on the benefits of having taken part in developing culturally relevant teaching. Five examples follow:

- There is a lesser focus on primary progressive dementia, as the average life expectancy in Malawi is 40 years, and more emphasis on acquired cognitive disorders, such as HIV-related dementia, given the high incidence of this infection in the population.

- Suicide is illegal in Malawi and there is a suspicion that it is therefore underreported. No reliable statistics are currently available, although a nationwide anonymous system for reporting suspected completed or attempted suicide was introduced in 2009. Volunteers are able to discuss the practical and ethical implications of the legal prohibition of suicide with Malawian health workers and students. This offers valuable exposure to the human rights implications of legislation surrounding mental disorder at a global level, and encourages reflection on UK practice.

- When teaching on eating disorders, the influence of culture on attitudes to body shape and image are emphasised, and the impact of urbanisation upon such attitudes in Malawi is discussed.

- Few psychotropic medications are available in government services in Malawi. The infrastructure is also such that medications requiring careful monitoring (e.g. lithium and clozapine) are not available for prescription to the majority who may benefit from them. Therefore, in their teaching, volunteers focus on those medications that are available, but do make students aware of other relevant pharmacological treatments used elsewhere.

- Religion plays a large part in the lives and culture of Malawians, including those of the medical students. The main religions are Christianity and Islam. The sometimes blurred line between psychotic illness and religious experience is a topic of considerable debate among the students. Many Malawians also believe in witchcraft and traditional healing, which affects the optimal delivery of psycho-education regarding mental illnesses and the role of medication. These issues are covered in detail in the teaching.

Trainee volunteers also experienced the need always to remain sensitive to any possible perception that they were imposing British values, morals and standards on Malawian students. Trainees often reported that they thought the students in Malawi were very alert to any such suggestion.

One higher-trainee volunteer in 2009 wrote as follows in her feedback report:

The project has offered us a unique experience in the organisation and application of an entire undergraduate psychiatry curriculum, from planning the lectures, to calibrating the pass mark in the assessments and participating in the pass/fail and distinction vivas. It has given us an understanding of the philosophy underpinning undergraduate education and an appreciation of how to translate the standards that we have in the UK into an international setting. The intensity of the work, the sense of ownership and culpability for the quality of the teaching that working in a small group afforded is an experience that I think would be difficult to find in our practice in the UK. The clinical work at Zomba Mental Hospital gave us experience of the practice of psychiatry in a developing country without the rich resources available in the UK. We were able to appreciate how the cultural context of the patient affects their psychiatric presentation. It would have been difficult without the students to achieve such an in-depth insight, as the language barrier would have precluded effective communication. Overall I think that involvement in SMMHEP has provided me with skills not only in teaching but also in educational administration, team working and transcultural psychiatry that will continue to be of use to me throughout the rest of my higher training in psychiatry and into my consultant practice.

Publications resulting from the project

The project provides volunteers with opportunities to pursue special areas of interest through audits, for example, and questionnaires on medical students' attitudes to psychiatry and how these can change after a teaching block. Volunteers are also encouraged to publish their feedback where appropriate (Beaglehole *et al*, 2008).

The examination taken by the Malawian undergraduate students was repeated with a group of Scottish students as a quality assurance measure. In an attempt to quantify the educational quality of undergraduate psychiatry teaching by Scottish psychiatrists to medical students at the College of Medicine, Malawi, the following study was performed. After the undergraduate psychiatry course was delivered to 57 medical students in Malawi in 2006, mainly by SMMHEP volunteers, an MCQ examination was sat by the students. The same MCQ examination was also sat by medical students at the University of Edinburgh, as a mock examination, just prior to their own examination. The results showed that there were no significant differences between the performance of the Edinburgh students in the Malawian mock examination and their own examination, which suggests the Malawi MCQ examination is of a standard comparable to the Edinburgh University examination. Furthermore, 84% of the Malawian medical students scored over 60%, the hypothetical pass by UK university standards (Baig *et al*, 2008).

Ensuring the sustainability of the project

Any such project involving international collaboration, requiring human resources, financial resources and a variety of permissions regularly needs to review processes and requirements, to secure the sustainability of the project and its original goals.

Ensuring that the needs of Malawi are met

Close collaboration is essential with the Ministry of Health (through Dr Kauye), the College of Medicine and management at the relevant hospitals. The project, in its execution, aims always to be directly in line with the requirements and expressed needs in Malawi. The feedback from the medical students in Malawi and Dr Kauye is used to amend, enhance and generally continue to improve the input.

Of relevance, in terms of the sustainability and consistency of the project, as well as in the interest of ensuring the longer-term development of mental health capacity, is that there is a large degree of political stability in Malawi.

Maintaining the focus of the project

From the outset, the SMMHEP steering group was aware of the great need in Malawi for mental health services, not only service provision, but also for the training of other disciplines (including clinical officers and nursing staff). The Malawian psychiatric services wanted to modernise the electroconvulsive therapy (ECT) service, to develop the forensic psychiatric service and to organise more local research. Although the temptation is always there to help where one can, it was essential for the sustainability and governance of SMMHEP that all volunteer psychiatrists remain primarily focused on undergraduate psychiatric teaching. The volunteers are not registered with the Malawian Medical Council and therefore are not allowed to perform any clinical duties. Although other 'spin-off' projects have been initiated, they do not impinge upon the main focus of SMMHEP.

Quality assurance

Quality assurance is achieved through supervision and feedback, as outlined above. A repetition of the examination to the Malawian students reassuringly confirmed a similar standard of knowledge required to pass and achieve merit (see Chapter 18).

Finance

Since the inception of the project, volunteer psychiatrists have generally agreed to fund a proportion of their own expenses. The Scotland–Malawi

Mental Health Education Project was, however, fortunate to have been given a financial grant by the Tropical Health and Education Trust (THET) to support its initial setting up and a grant from the then Scottish executive. Further grants were also awarded to the project, one of which was for the related ECT project. This resulted in training of multidisciplinary teams in modernisation of the ECT service and promoting audit processes for quality assurance. The Scottish government awarded a grant in 2008 in order to support the project for a further 3 years. The Scotland–Malawi Mental Health Education Project is also grateful for private donations and grants awarded. In 2008 the project became a formal Scottish charity, the trustees being members of the SMMHEP steering group. This financial support not only allowed for travel and accommodation expenses, but also for sending teaching materials to support the undergraduate training, including textbooks and training DVDs.

Other support for the project

The viability of the project has depended on the support of those institutions closely related to its workforce.

The Scottish government

The International Development Unit of the Scottish government continues to support SMMHEP and similar projects. Its activities include linking projects with authorities in Malawi and establishing links between all similar Malawi initiatives across Scotland's NHS. It guided a link with Voluntary Service Overseas (VSO) Malawi, in order to ensure 'dovetailing' between NHS link activities and volunteers working under the VSO umbrella. Moreover, in the early stages of the Scotland–Malawi Partnership it was essential that the then Scottish executive raise the awareness of projects (and its support for them) at NHS Scotland. Through workshops and other means, the Scottish executive's expectation that professionals within NHS Scotland would take such initiatives and execute partnerships with Malawi was communicated.

Royal College of Psychiatrists

The main benefit to the Scottish side of the project was in terms of the opportunity to 'teach the teachers how to teach'. The further benefit was the development of awareness of and sensitivity to cross-cultural aspects of teaching psychiatry and observing psychiatry being practised in such an environment. These are now considered to be very important competencies for British psychiatrists to achieve during their training years. Both Professor Dinesh Bhugra (initially as Dean and subsequently as President of the Royal College of Psychiatrists) and the Scottish Division of the College have supported the project. It was acknowledged that this training experience is both important and valid, especially during the years of higher training in psychiatry. This view was also supported by College tutors and educational supervisors. This support was strengthened by the degree of supervision for the trainee volunteers, in both the preparation and delivery of the teaching programme and examinations.

NHS Education for Scotland (NES) and Scottish deaneries

The Medical Director of NES and the Scottish postgraduate deans, regional psychiatric advisers to the deans and higher-training programme directors were apprised of the project at an early stage. They supported the initiative and trainees have been allowed periods of leave where this experience was considered appropriate to their training needs, while their salaries were protected (although approval does require annual renewal). Trainees have been able to negotiate leave as study leave, often combined with a period of annual leave. Another option, where a large part of the experience includes research projects, combined with study and/or annual leave, is to take these as blocks of protected 'special interest' sessions or research sessions. Individual trainees have also been allowed to accredit this experience, where prospectively agreed by the Postgraduate Dean of the Royal College of Psychiatrists and the Postgraduate Medical Education Training Board (PMETB), as valid 'out of programme' experience counting towards a certificate of completion of training (CCT). In 2008, one Scottish deanery, after careful appraisal of the project, its aims, supervision arrangements and outcomes to date, approved the experience of trainees as 'within programme experience' for up to three higher trainees per year, allowing for up to 5 weeks' involvement in Malawi. The rest of the teaching block (i.e. the residual 3 weeks) could then be taken as a combination of study and annual leave. Other Scottish deaneries are also considering this approval.

Local services

The medical directors in the health boards in Scotland were appraised of the project and it met with their support. Although trainees from more than one health board are involved in the project at any one time, it was found that the project and the trainees' periods of absence from their local NHS duties did not significantly impinge on service provision.

Summary

The SMMHEP continues to have as its main focus undergraduate medical student psychiatric tuition, delivered mainly by Scottish higher-trainee volunteers. Its ultimate aim is to support the psychiatric education of larger numbers of professionals in Malawi, in order that the country can become more self-sufficient in the delivery of psychiatric education. A number of other projects have developed from SMMHEP, including an ECT education project, and training of clinical officers during the psychiatry BSc course at the St John of God College of Health Sciences.

It is hoped that many of the trainees who have taken part in the undergraduate teaching will maintain links with SMMHEP and may participate in its expanding activities. Through this they will continue to develop their educational skills and cross-cultural experience, and play a part in helping Malawi achieve self-sufficiency in mental health clinical and training capacity.

The Royal College of Psychiatrists is keen to improve its links with its International Divisions. This project, carried out by members of the Scottish Division of the College, is an example of a means of doing this which brings benefits to both College members and the wider international medical community.

Acknowledgements

We sincerely thank the following for their involvement in and support for SMMHEP, and acknowledge that they are all vitally important for the success of the project:

- those people living with mental disorders in Malawi, who on every occasion were agreeable to support the process of clinical tuition for students
- medical undergraduate students in Malawi, without whom this opportunity for our trainees to gain such experience would of course not have arisen; they are thanked for their agreeability throughout the teaching and their subsequent invaluable feedback
- staff of the College of Medicine, Blantyre and Zomba Mental Hospital, who have been generous in their attitudes to and support for our volunteers
- the Scottish government (previously the Scottish executive), with special thanks to Dr Elizabeth Grant for her guidance and help to establish initial links with relevant groups involved in similar projects
- NHS Education Scotland (NES), the Scottish postgraduate deaneries; the Royal College of Psychiatrists, with specific reference to its Scottish Division and its chair during the first few years of the project, Dr Tom Brown; College tutors; NHS Scotland Health Boards
- volunteers to the project since 2006; SMMHEP steering group members and trustees (also for their suggestions in relation to this chapter).

The Scotland–Malawi Mental Health Education Project (SMMHEP) is a registered Scottish charity (SC039523), and can be contacted through its website, http://www.smmhep.org.uk

References

Baig, B. J., Beaglehole, A., Stewart, R. C., *et al* (2008) Assessment of an undergraduate psychiatry course in an African setting. *BMC Medical Education*, **8**, 23.

Beaglehole, A., Baig, B. J., Stewart, R., *et al* (2008) Training in transcultural psychiatry and delivery of education in a low-income country. *Psychiatric Bulletin*, **32**, 111–112.

Calvert, S. H. S., Sharpe, M., Power, M., *et al* (1999) Does undergraduate education have an effect on Edinburgh medical students' attitudes to psychiatry and psychiatric patients? *Journal of Nervous and Mental Disease*, **187**, 757–761.

Kauye, F. (2008) Management of mental health services in Malawi. *International Psychiatry*, **5**, 29–30.

Kauye, F. & Mafuta, C. (2006) Country profile: Malawi. *International Psychiatry*, **4**, 9–11.

CHAPTER 18

International undergraduate teaching

Benjamin Baig

Introduction

Few clinical disciplines can be subject to as much cultural variation as psychiatry. The social, cultural and spiritual shaping of clinical psychiatry varies widely between countries. The recognition of mental health issues may be highly related to political climate and level of economic development. While every undergraduate medical student requires competency in managing diabetes or orthopaedic trauma, the need to include anorexia nervosa or somatoform disorders on the curricula of medical schools may be seen as variable. If prominence in undergraduate medical curricula purely reflected local disease epidemiology, this would be in part understandable. Yet a major concern with psychiatric illness is the limited acceptance of the considerable prevalence of many illnesses owing to sociocultural barriers.

It is with this background that undergraduate teaching of psychiatry in an international context is discussed in this chapter. The focus here is on the following questions:

- In designing a curriculum in a non-Western country, are there core aspects of psychiatry that are generalisable or should curricula be based on indigenous models of mental health?
- Where the apparent prevalence of mental illness is low or unknown, how much emphasis should be placed on psychiatry in an undergraduate curriculum?
- Where many forms of unusual or aberrant behaviour are managed as social or spiritual problems, to what extent should a psychiatric paradigm be taught?
- When teaching undergraduate psychiatry in a different culture, what ideological and practical challenges are faced by both local and foreign educators?

The Scotland–Malawi Mental Health Education Project (Chapter 17) is one of many initiatives that link high- and low- to middle-income countries in terms of undergraduate psychiatric teaching. Some of the questions above are discussed in relation to teaching medical students in Malawi and with reference to other available literature.

The importance of psychiatry in medical curricula

The shape of psychiatric teaching in undergraduate medicine may well reflect the perceived importance of mental illness within a given culture. The paucity of psychiatric services and clinicians could easily prevent the establishment of psychiatric issues at the heart of medical training. Table 18.1 presents some gross indicators of psychiatric services in selected countries, which may be taken to represent Europe, Africa, South Asia, South East Asia and South America.

Only limited epidemiological data exist as to the prevalence of all mental illnesses in low- to middle-income countries. International studies indicate that the lifetime risk of schizophrenia is similar around the world. Evidence suggests that in sub-Saharan Africa the prevalence of schizophrenia, bipolar disorder and postnatal depression is in fact similar to that in high-income countries (Odejide et al, 1989; Stewart, 2007). General epidemiological surveys in primary care have indicated that as many as 30% of patients attend health services primarily for a mental health problem (Murthy & Khandelwal, 2007). Suicide is illegal in many countries, thus a true estimate is difficult to establish, but international studies in low-income countries rarely estimate fewer than 10–20 suicides per 100 000 population per year (Dzamalala et al, 2006). This figure is similar to that in the UK, which approximates to 16 per 100 000 per year. Dementia related to HIV infection is an increasing problem in sub-Saharan Africa that often goes unrecognised. The prevalence of HIV/AIDS is high in the region, with 25% of women of child-bearing age being HIV positive. Life expectancy has been seriously affected by the HIV epidemic and has fallen to 41 years.

In Malawi, the College of Medicine was set up in 1991 and many initiatives have supported medical education in the past 15 years, but an on-going concern has related to teaching in mental health (Broadhead & Muula, 2002). Before 2005, the undergraduate psychiatry module was delivered

Table 18.1 International comparison of psychiatric service provision (figures per 100 000 population)

	UK	Malawi	India	Vietnam	Chile
Psychiatrists	11	0	2	3.2	4
Psychiatric nurses	104	2.5	0.05	0.3	1.1
Psychologists	9	0	0.03	0.06	15.7
Psychiatric beds	58	4	2.5	6.3	12.7

Source: World Health Organization (2005).

at times by a single lecturer and provided variable clinical experience for students. Several attempts have been made to design a sustainable psychiatry teaching programme in Malawi (Herzig, 2003). Presently, the undergraduate medical degree in Malawi contains a 6-week clinical training placement in psychiatry. There is no discrete psychiatric department in the medical school and psychiatric teaching falls under the umbrella of community health. The lack of an academic department, combined with limited funding and research activity, may well reduce the importance of psychiatry within the curriculum. The same cannot be said for communicable diseases, which are understandably well supported by collaborating institutions from high-income countries. However, there are several reasons why psychiatry should be as prominent within the curriculum as the latter conditions. As noted above, the prevalence of major mental illness is in fact similar to that in high-income countries. Furthermore, as Malawi becomes more economically developed, it is possible that the prevalence of mental illness will mirror that in Europe. The increasing burden of HIV-related illness means that African doctors have to be able to treat HIV-related psychiatric sequelae, including dementia and delirium, which would be vastly more prevalent than in Europe.

A second major issue concerning the place of psychiatry in Africa relates to the globalisation of mental health. The 'brain drain' of health professionals from low-income to high-income countries has led to a need for a more global medical training. The huge demand for psychiatrists in countries like the UK, Australia and New Zealand leads to regular migration of trained psychiatrists from India, for example, to these countries. Medical schools in Africa may well not receive accreditation from the World Health Organization without due prominence being given to psychiatry on their syllabus, as has been noted in Nigeria (Desjarlais *et al*, 1995).

A final issue relating to the importance of psychiatry in the curriculum is that many locally trained doctors, while not specialising in psychiatry, will work in the community and be expected to manage mental illness with little specialist support. This situation pertains to India, where emphasis has been placed on reforms in undergraduate psychiatry by increasing the amount of training, making psychiatry an independent subject and revising the psychiatry curriculum (Murthy & Khandelwal, 2007). Today, however, as many as 25–30% of medical colleges in India do not have independent departments of psychiatry. The exposure of medical students to mental disorders is limited to some visits to the mental hospitals, but reported inhumane conditions there discourage medical students rather than developing their interest in mental health. The syllabus prescribed by the Medical Council of India devotes only 20 lectures to psychiatry and specifies only a 2-week posting of 3 hours a day in psychiatry (Murthy & Khandelwal, 2007).

Therefore, while it is understandable that psychiatry training may feature less in low- to middle-income countries, there are strong arguments as to why it must be comparable in significance to undergraduate programmes in high-income countries.

The psychiatric paradigm

While a Westernised medical model represents a workable paradigm to physical illness in most cultural contexts, the same cannot be said for psychiatric problems. Broadly speaking, a Westernised view of psychiatric illness hinges on a deterministic bio-psychosocial concept of disease, albeit subject to cultural variations, and psychotic phenomena (as defined by ICD–10 or DSM–IV, say) are broadly, though not exclusively, described by brain biology. The experience of 'hearing voices' or a belief in 'possession' in an African context may be seen very differently. While there exist many subcultures within Africa, it is widely accepted that an individual may experience demonic possession, for instance. In this situation, it is the view held by some that traditional healers and not psychiatrists may hold the key to treatment and management. It is with great caution that a Westernised psychiatric paradigm can or should be used in this situation. Should undergraduate psychiatric teaching focus on unusual perceptual experience and thought content in association with neurotransmitter metabolism and neuroimaging? Conversely, can Westernised models of psychosis be challenged by transcultural and spiritual paradigms? Such questions illustrate the limitations of a psychiatric paradigm within an African undergraduate curriculum. Unlike cardiology or paediatrics, a psychiatric medical educator must be sensitive to the limits of acceptable explanatory models.

A further example of this relates to suicide. Owing to religious attitudes, suicide is widely considered a sin; moreover, those who complete suicide are subject to restrictions in inheritance laws and burial rites. Suicide risk assessment nonetheless remains an essential part of psychiatric practice. In the UK, up to 90% of completed suicides relate to an undiagnosed or insufficiently managed mental illness. It is difficult when performing a suicide risk assessment simultaneously to attribute a moral dimension to the patient's thoughts or behaviour. From experience in Malawi, many African medical students, however, would appear to feel that suicide does have a strong moral component and there can be no doubt that such an opinion might flavour an assessment.

Core psychiatric teaching

In 1988 the Edinburgh Declaration stipulated a universal basis for under-graduate medical teaching (Walton & Gelder, 1999). The World Health Organization presently accredits medical schools throughout the world based on their educational standards and content of the curriculum, irrespective of possible cultural variations between countries.

As noted above, the practice and theory of clinical psychiatry is subject to more cultural variation than are other medical specialties. As such, an important question arises as to how universal psychiatric teaching may be. Are there core elements that should exist in all psychiatric curricula, or should each medical school tailor its syllabus to the cultural context in which psychiatry is locally practised?

When looking at the priorities of medical education in countries where resources are severely restricted, authors in both Africa and Asia have noted several important principles (Broadhead & Muula, 2002; Murthy & Khandelwal, 2007):

- Medical curricula should be firmly based on community and public health, to reflect the medical problems of the country.
- To increase the effectiveness of undergraduates in identifying and managing common mental and behavioural health problems in the community, quality training must be provided at undergraduate level.
- Joint teaching by different departments, especially in the basic medical sciences, allows for more economic and flexible use of staff and teaching facilities.
- If possible, the clinical disciplines should be introduced to students during their study of basic medical sciences.
- Wide access to information should be provided, and self-learning should be encouraged. Teachers must be encouraged to enhance their teaching skills by application of newer technology, such as audiovisual media, computers and the internet (on which, see Chapter 6).
- Research is needed in low-income countries to generalise this evidence and then guide reforms in mental healthcare.

With regard to psychiatry in Malawi, Herzig (2003) noted several key features for a psychiatric curriculum:

- Teaching sessions should present the economic evidence that justifies expenditure on basic mental healthcare for even the poorest nation (Blue & Harpham, 1994; Desjarlais et al, 1995).
- Coverage of psychopharmacology should be limited to the few basic drugs that are cheap, have a long shelf life, and are widely available.
- Mental health should be framed within the community medicine teaching programme.
- Some sessions should be taught in community settings – school, police station, social welfare department, centre for people with intellectual disabilites – to introduce students to the potential for (mental) health education to community groups.

In an African context, there can be no doubt that community medicine plays an essential part in psychiatric care. Furthermore, it is clear that the limitations in psychopharmacology necessitate some focus on available medication. However, there are arguments against this. The advent of globalisation has led to the large-scale economic migration of healthcare professionals. Furthermore, the process of economic development has led to a transitional epidemiology of psychiatric illness. An example of this is the prevalence of eating disorders. While anorexia nervosa was, historically, more common in high-income countries, its prevalence appears to be increasing in Black south African populations, in parallel with the spread of both economic prosperity and Western culture (Szabo & Allwood, 2004; Le Grange *et al*, 2006). Core psychiatry – pharmacology, genetics, neuropsychiatry, classification of illness and biological treatment – could be therefore be seen as generalisable (Walton, 1999). Indeed, the new medical graduates in Africa today will probably face a different kind of psychiatric presentation by the end of their careers.

An African psychiatry syllabus must also highlight psychiatric aspects of HIV.

Culture-bound syndromes

Culture-bound syndromes are recurrent geographically specific patterns of aberrant behaviour and troubling experience which may or may not relate to the nosological structure of international psychiatric classificatory systems. Such syndromes are considered as illnesses indigenous to a culture that are not recognised outwith it. The inclusion of these in DSM–IV marks an acknowledgement of globalised psychiatry. The high levels of migration require clinicians across the world to recognise not only cultural variations but also non-Westernised models of psychiatric diagnostic systems. DSM–IV goes on to describe these as having localised, folk, diagnostic categories that frame coherent meanings for certain repetitive, patterned and troubling sets of experiences and observations.

A parallel view is that certain disorders, such as anorexia nervosa or even paranoid schizophrenia, can be seen as themselves culture-bound syndromes of the Westernised or developed world (Lee, 2002). Here, international classificatory systems would fall under the definition of a social construct.

The criteria for a culture-bound syndrome include: the syndrome's categorisation as a disease in the culture (i.e. it does not represent a voluntary behaviour or false claim); widespread familiarity with it in the culture; and its frequent recognition and treatment by the folk medicine of the culture. Ultimately, the existence of such syndromes throws doubt over the validity of a comprehensive classificatory system and over whether such a system can ever be exhaustive. This raises the issue of the extent to which these syndromes should feature on an undergraduate curriculum. Indeed, in the case of anorexia nervosa, have we, as Westernised medical educators, assumed that our culture-bound syndromes are more important than those of other cultures?

Assessment methods and their limitations

Medical education in Africa is evolving from didactic teaching to incorporate community-based education, problem-based learning and integrated teaching (Horton, 2000; Banda & Yikona, 2001). This process has been facilitated through external aid funding from resource-rich countries. However, when resources are limited, the cost-effectiveness of lecture-based teaching and examinations based on multiple-choice questions (MCQs) may prove paramount (Sims, 1997).

In spite of the many initiatives that have supported medical education in Africa, it has often been difficult to measure the standard of education delivered. While many of the African medical schools are accredited with the World Health Organization, it is difficult to assess how the standard of individual undergraduate courses compares with their equivalents in high-income countries.

Challenges for the medical educator

Medical education in low- and middle-income countries has historically been supported by foreign medical educators. How should such educators modify aspects of teaching? A student cohort in Africa may differ in several ways from one in the UK. It can be noted that a medical education remains a privileged one. Just as in high-income countries, a large proportion of medical students come from parents of social class I. Such certainly appears to be the case in Malawi. Students studying medicine at the University of Malawi will be among the highest academic achievers in Malawi. Of the medical students, around 70% are male and those on the psychiatry course have an average age of 21.7 years. As in the UK, they are required to have high secondary educational achievements: at least six O-level passes, including English and mathematics, and three A-level passes with a grade of at least C in biology, chemistry and one other science subject. Some 90% of the students are from Malawi, with the remainder mostly coming from Zimbabwe, South Africa, Mozambique and India. All students are expected to speak English. All the Malawi students will also be fluent in Chichewa (the official language of Malawi, along with English).

Within medical education, certain resources are required to create a good teaching and learning environment. In the Malawian context the availability of rooms for teaching can be limited. Lecturers needed to provide their own audiovisual equipment (such as computers and projectors). An important development in medical education has been the introduction of the internet as a learning resource. It can be noted that the College of Medicine, University of Malawi, now has a computer laboratory, which students may use for online learning. It has been possible to provide a copy of all presentations on a teaching website, such that the students may use this to review lecture material. Of note, the lack of availability of photocopying facilities has required handouts for lectures to be brought from the UK. While UK medical schools now have the capacity to mark MCQ examinations by machine, this has to be done by hand in Malawi. Such limitations may shape the future of examination design.

At the time of the writing, the psychiatry curriculum at the College of Medicine consists of 2 weeks of theoretical teaching in the third year followed by a 5-week psychiatry placement and assessment in the fourth year. The third-year programme includes a basic introduction to psychiatry. The fourth-year course consists of 2 weeks of lectures and tutorials, following which the students receive a theoretical examination. The theoretical teaching is followed by a 3-week clinical attachment in which students acquire clinical skills. At the end of the clinical attachment there is a final clinical oral examination. The final mark is derived from the grades from the theoretical examination, clinical attachment (which includes attendance, participation and clinical skills), clinical oral examination and a clinical case report written during the clinical attachment. The examination which the students sit after their 2-week period of theoretical teaching consists of MCQs and three short-essay questions.

Medical educators in all cultures must be sensitive to cultural variations when teaching. As discussed above, views on issues such as the role of spirituality, sexuality and witchcraft must be taken into account when teaching psychiatry.

As discussed in Chapter 17, the Scotland–Malawi Mental Health Education Project has now 5 years of experience in training doctors in Malawi. This work has provided a unique opportunity to contribute to a developing health system while offering an important training experience for those involved. Lessons can be learnt about the development of a curriculum to match need, the preparation of lectures that were captivating and informative, and the importance of conveying succinct messages during clinical teaching. The exposure to a range of illnesses rarely seen in the UK, such as HIV-associated psychosis and cerebral malaria, was educational.

The experience of a psychiatric hospital in a low-income country can be seen as intimidating by both student and teacher. The lack of resources, the nature of quite severe and often only partially treated mental illness combined with a low nurse:patient ratio can easily lead to perceived threats to the personal safety of medical students. The lack of suitable interviewing environments and even the lack of chairs make the experience of learning history taking and mental state assessment more difficult. Furthermore, while the medical students themselves may speak fluent English, it is likely that most patients will not. The opportunity to demonstrate psychiatric practice through a second language has limitations. In these environments, clinical educators must be aware that the standards and practices may vary from those in the UK. An example of this would be the use of chemical and physical restraint with agitated patients. In the psychiatric hospital in Malawi (Zomba Mental Hospital), on occasion agitation has been managed through the use of seclusion rooms, which can be devoid of bedding, light and toilet facilities. While it may be easy to deplore this practice, the reality of how a limited nursing staff workforce manages a large agitated population should not be prematurely judged by those who have experience only of working in a Western context. The environment at Zomba Mental Hospital highlights the challenges of working in an undeveloped health system.

An important question relating to educational practice concerns standards. What should a medical educator expect from a group of students in a different culture and context? To gain accreditation from the World Health Organization, a medical school needs to have universal educational measures, but how can these be translated into comparable standards in psychiatry? In looking at this question, it can be argued that an MCQ examination, focusing on core theoretical knowledge, is comparable in any country, yet the measurement of clinical skills is harder to define, given language, culture and resource-related issues (Baig *et al*, 2008).

Ultimately, a medical educator, in an international context, must balance validated educational objectives against the local clinical and educational reality.

Summary

In low- and middle-income countries, mental health is less recognised and mental health staff are often inadequately trained (Saraceno *et al*, 2007). A further issue in the delivery of healthcare relates to the 'brain drain' of professionals (Kirigia *et al*, 2006; Muula & Panulo, 2007). The establishment of medical schools in such countries has had a positive effect in encouraging locally trained physicians to work in their home country (Broadhead & Muula, 2002). The advantages of local training of medical professionals, and the difficulties posed by scarce resources, mean that there is a need for high-income countries to support education delivery in low- and middle-income countries.

There is a need for the globalisation of medical education. With the large-scale migration of healthcare professionals, the changing epidemiology of psychiatric illness and global inequalities in healthcare, it is clear that an undergraduate psychiatric syllabus must be universal yet culturally sensitive and practically relevant. Above all, it is wrong to assume that knowledge transfer should always flow from high-income to low-income countries. In psychiatry, more than in many other specialties, clinicians, educators and academics have much to learn from diverse educational practices and the cultural variability of illness presentation.

References

Baig, B. J., Beaglehole, A., Stewart, R. C., *et al* (2008) Assessment of an undergraduate psychiatry course in an African setting. *BMC Medcial Education*, **8**, 23.

Banda, S. & Yikona, J. (2001) Medical education. *Lancet*, **358**, 423.

Blue, H. & Harpham, T. (1994) The World Bank World Development Report 1993: Investing in health. *British Journal of Psychiatry*, **165**, 9–12.

Broadhead, R. L. & Muula, A. S. (2002) Creating a medical school for Malawi: problems and achievements. *BMJ*, **325**, 384–387.

Desjarlais, R., Eisenberg, L., Good, B., *et al* (1995) *World Mental Health: Problems and Priorities in Low-Income Countries*. Oxford University Press.

Dzamalala, C. P., Milner, D. A. & Liomba, N. G. (2006) Suicide in Blantyre, Malawi (2000–2003). *Journal of Clinical and Forensic Medicine*, **13**, 65–69.

Herzig, H. (2003) Teaching psychiatry in poor countries: priorities and needs. A description of how mental health is taught to medical students in Malawi, Central Africa. *Education for Health*, **16**, 32–39.

Horton, R. (2000) North and south: bridging the information gap. *Lancet*, **355**, 2231–2236.

Kirigia, J. M., Gbary, A. R., Muthuri, L. K., *et al* (2006) The cost of health professionals' brain drain in Kenya. *BMC Health Services Research*, **6**, 89.

Le Grange, D., Louw, J., Russell, B., *et al* (2006) Eating attitudes and behaviours in South African adolescents and young adults. *Transcultural Psychiatry*, **43**, 401–417.

Lee, S. (2002) Socio-cultural and global health perspectives for the development of future diagnostic systems. *Psychopathology*, **35**, 152–157.

Murthy, R. S. & Khandelwal, S. (2007) Undergraduate training in psychiatry: world perspective. *Indian Journal of Psychiatry*, **49**, 169–174.

Muula, A. S. & Panulo, B., Jr (2007) Lost investment returns from the migration of medical doctors from Malawi. *Tanzania Health Research Bulletin*, **9**, 61–64.

Odejide, A. O., Oyewunmi, L. K. & Ohaeri, J. U. (1989) Psychiatry in Africa: an overview. *American Journal of Psychiatry*, **146**, 708–716.

Saraceno, B., van Ommeren, M., Batniji, R., *et al* (2007) Barriers to improvement of mental health services in low-income and middle-income countries. *Lancet*, **370**, 1164–1174.

Sims, P. (1997) A medical school in Zambia. *Journal of Public Health Medicine*, **19**, 137–138.

Stewart, R. C. (2007) Maternal depression and infant growth: a review of recent evidence. *Maternal & Child Nutrition*, **3**, 94–107.

Szabo, C. P. & Allwood, C. W. (2004) A cross-cultural study of eating attitudes in adolescent South African females. *World Psychiatry*, **3**, 41–44.

Walton, H. & Gelder, M. (1999) Core curriculum in psychiatry for medical students. *Medical Education*, **33**, 204–211.

World Health Organization (2005) *Mental Health Atlas*. WHO.

CHAPTER 19

Teaching with simulated patients and role-play

John Eagles & Sheila Calder

Introduction

Simulated patients (SPs) are now very widely used in the teaching and assessment of medical students and of doctors. In psychiatric teaching, SPs have been rather less widely used than in many other medical specialties, partly because of the complexities in the plausible portrayal of psychiatric presentations. Nonetheless, teaching in our specialty with SPs is likely to become more prevalent and thus, notably for younger psychiatrists, it should be helpful to become familiar with the background provided by this chapter, especially in tandem with hands-on experience.

At the outset, some clarification of terms may be helpful. A *simulated patient* is an umbrella term for anyone who participates in a medical encounter for educational and/or assessment purposes, and this simulation may or may not involve the simulator's own medical history, symptoms or signs. SPs range from relatively untrained community volunteers through to professional actors. A *standardised patient* is a simulated patient who is specifically trained to produce consistent history, symptoms and signs, as required in student assessments. In *role-play*, which overlaps with patient simulation, participants are essentially untrained (in fact they are usually the medical students themselves) but their performance is often guided by background details of the role they are asked to play.

The chapter covers the following: historical background; whether, in psychiatric teaching, SPs should be actors; the practical aspects of teaching with SPs and what can be taught using them; the authors' experience in Aberdeen; assessment and research using SPs; role-play; and the advantages and disadvantages of SPs.

Historical background

There are three good reviews of early developments in the use of SPs for teaching and assessment, by Barrows (1993), Wallace (1997) and

Ainsworth *et al* (1991). Howard Barrows is recognised as the 'father' of this innovation, and he first used the technique in 1963 (Wallace, 1997). In his first post as a neurologist in Los Angeles, he coached a young woman to present with abnormal neurological findings and then to report on the performances of his students. Colleagues greeted his ideas with general scepticism (Barrows, 1993) and in non-medical circles his practices were vaguely ridiculed, for example attracting press coverage with the headline 'Hollywood Invades USC Medical School' (Wallace, 1997). Barrows persevered, however, continuing to develop techniques at the University of Southern California before moving to continue his work at McMaster University in Ontario in the early 1970s. He extended his use of SPs to postgraduate clinics for general practitioners and introduced further innovations such as the 'time-in/time-out' technique. Barrows (1993) described his early efforts as a 'relatively lonely undertaking' but both he and Wallace (1997) accord credit to the pioneering efforts of Paula Stillman in Arizona. From the early 1970s, she used simulated mothers as a technique to teach interviewing skills, and she and Barrows together appear to have been the figures most instrumental in helping the medical establishment to become more receptive to the use of SPs.

By the 1970s, SPs were being used for formal student assessments. The first objective structured clinical examination (OSCE) was probably conducted in the Scottish city of Dundee, by Ronald Harden and colleagues (Harden *et al*, 1975). As reviewed by Adamo (2003), the use of SPs in student assessments has since mushroomed, especially during the 1990s, so that by 2003/04, 94 of 126 American medical schools were using SPs in their clinical examinations (Barzansky & Etzel, 2004). Concomitantly, there has been a huge increase in their use in teaching, with refinements of methodology, including research involving SPs; these advances were underlined in 2001 when the Association of Standardized Patient Educators (ASPE, http://www.aspeducators.org) was established in the USA to advance SP methodology and research and to set standards of practice.

In less than five decades, the use of SPs has moved from a ridiculed 'lonely undertaking' to a fairly pivotal position in the education of medical students in most higher-income countries.

Simulated patients: need they be actors?

For students to be taught or examined adequately, SPs must be credible and realistic. Most community volunteers, from their own experience of illness and their own encounters with health services, will be able to portray straightforward physical illnesses in a plausible manner, given appropriate instructions and training. At risk of being slightly precious, even common psychiatric conditions, such as depression or anxiety, are much more difficult for lay people to enact plausibly. Not only is it necessary to be able to deliver a psychiatric history authentically, but SPs need to enact emotional symptoms and distress at an appropriate and credible level. This is quite a skilled enterprise. Despite the disadvantages of cost (see below) we therefore feel that trained professional actors are the optimal SPs with whom to teach psychiatry to medical students. We accept, of course, that circumstances may dictate practice, and no doubt gifted amateurs (perhaps with additional training and scrutiny) will often do an adequate job.

Practical aspects of teaching with SPs

Some of the practicalities of teaching medical students using SPs are also touched upon below, when advantages and disadvantages of the teaching method are reviewed.

With regard to individual teaching topics, as ever it is necessary to be clear about the aims and objectives of the session in the first instance. Careful attention to the SP's 'script' is required to address these objectives. Once the SP has become familiar with the script of the character, rehearsal (optimally with the script writer) of the teaching session is required with feedback to the SP on performance. Following subsequent 'live performances' with the students, students and staff should reflect on the SP's contribution and relevant comment can be relayed to the SP with the expectation of an ever improving performance. For example, a 'depressed' SP can be advised on the degree of psychomotor retardation that is helpfully illustrative without demoralising the student and causing the session to proceed too slowly.

Feedback from the SP to the students (see further below) is often helpful. Experienced SPs will be interviewed by many students and become well practised in identifying good and poor aspects of students' communication skills.

Didactic teaching will very often occur in tandem with interactive SP scenarios, in a combination of theory and practice. Opinion varies on whether it is better to do the didactic teaching before or after the interaction with the relevant SP. Carter *et al* (2006) randomised the order for students in Louisville of a lecture on peripheral vascular disease first or an interview with the SP first. The students perceived the 'SP second' format as having more value and (not surprisingly) the 'SP second' students performed better when interacting with the SP. As a general rule, doing something well is probably a better learning experience, and for this reason a 'didactic teaching first, SP interaction second' model is probably preferable.

Some authors (e.g. Stafford, 2005) emphasise the need for students to 'de-role' after SP encounters and role-play, by identifying the ways in which the role-player differs in reality from the character of the assumed role. Maybe this should indeed be routine, but perhaps if it is necessary then the roles expected of students may be deemed rather too intricate and stressful.

Writing roles for patients can be difficult and time-consuming. While it may be a less relevant technique in psychiatry than in some other specialties, Rosenbaum & Ferguson (2006) and Nestel *et al* (2008) describe giving experienced SPs a lead role in writing their own scenarios, based on a real occasion when they sought, or thought of seeking, healthcare. This technique can apparently lead to very realistic scenarios, while saving staff time and effort.

While their model relates to volunteer SPs across a range of specialties, the tips given by Ker *et al* (2005) on developing and maintaining a bank of SPs are valuable. These include the need to have identified and dedicated staff in charge of the enterprise, the need to identify costs and to budget accordingly at the outset, the desirability of developing SP recruitment policies and the need for regular training, recognition and feedback for SPs.

What can be taught using SPs?

The short answer to this question is 'almost anything' (Boxes 19.1 and 19.2). Instead of attempting to list topics exhaustively, the aim here is, by providing examples and references, to trigger readers' ideas as to how SPs might be helpfully deployed with their own medical students.

Two of the overriding considerations in planning the psychiatric topics one might teach using SPs are, first, convenience and availability and, second, the feasibility of teaching a topic with a real patient. For reasons of convenience and availability, much psychiatric teaching still takes place in hospital settings, where patients are not only less numerous than they used to be but

---

Box 19.1 Examples from the literature of the teaching uses of simulated patients in psychiatry

- Introduction to psychotherapy with emotionally difficult patients (Trudel, 1996)
- Consulting with patients seeking benzodiazepines or opiates (Taverner *et al*, 2000)
- SPs with schizophrenia for whole-class teaching of mental state examination (Birndorf & Kaye, 2002)
- Introduction of junior medical students to delirium to aid integration of psychiatric, physical and psychosocial concepts (Chur-Hansen & Koopowitz, 2002)
- International videoconferencing to illustrate transcultural psychiatry (Ekblad *et al*, 2004)
- 'Clinging, somatising' SPs to address personality disorders and counter-transference (Ghatavi & Waisman, 2006)
- An SP with post-herpetic neuralgia to illustrate psychiatric–physical comorbidity (Leila *et al*, 2006)
- Investigation of stigmatising attitudes to psychiatric illness among medical students (Roberts *et al*, 2008)

Box 19.2 Pertinent examples from the literature of the teaching of non-psychiatric topics with simulated patients

- Presenting and discussing a medical error with a simulated patient (Halbach & Sullivan, 2005)
- Empathic and effective death disclosure (Quest *et al*, 2002)
- Illustration of ethical dilemmas (Tysinger *et al*, 1997)
- Sexual history taking and HIV counselling (Haist *et al*, 2004)
- Addressing domestic violence (Haist *et al*, 2003)
- A 'standardised family' to aid understanding of family dynamics and community orientation (Clay *et al*, 2000)
- A standardised hospitalisation experience for medical students (Wilkes *et al*, 2002)
- Choosing and prescribing medication (Vollebregt *et al*, 2006)
- Risk-taking adolescents (Blake *et al*, 2006)
- Assessing the suitability of an elderly patient for discharge from hospital (Williams *et al*, 2006)
- Fostering awareness of racial disparities in healthcare (Beach *et al*, 2007)

---

also less representative of the patients the students will subsequently see in the course of their (mostly non-psychiatric) careers. Thus, very common conditions, such as anxiety and mild/moderate depression, which nearly all practising doctors will encounter frequently, cannot generally be found among current in-patient populations. Most teachers will encounter logistic difficulties in arranging, and ensuring the attendance of, representative out-patients to assist with student teaching. Recruiting, training and paying SPs overcomes these problems.

With regard to feasibility, a significant (and possibly growing) proportion of our patients may not wish to be seen by medical students. Furthermore, those patients who are willing may be atypical of the people students will subsequently encounter. Many of our patients, for very understandable reasons, including stigma, confidentiality and embarrassment, will not wish to be 'practised on' by students. SPs address these difficulties elegantly. Indeed, they can portray psychiatric presentations that are clinically important but would never be seen by students, such as reluctant historians with hidden alcohol problems (Eagles *et al*, 2001*b*) or patients seeking benzodiazepines or opiates for misuse (Taverner *et al*, 2000).

The latter example leads into another broad area of relevance to student teaching. In the course of undergraduate training, students interview real patients but go no further than this: they do not enter the realms of making a diagnosis and sharing it with the patient, far less formulating and discussing a management plan. Thus, to give a psychiatric example, it can be very formative for a student to interview a 'depressed' SP, to share the diagnosis with her and then to discuss with her the merits of possible management strategies. Teaching basic psychotherapy skills (Trudel, 1996; Coyle *et al*, 1998) with SPs is another example.

Non-psychiatrists have used SPs in several ways which may have relevance to our own teaching (see Box 19.2). One clear linking theme is that of communication skills, and this is an area in which SPs are used extensively. Experienced SPs are often more than passive participants in such teaching, since they can 'come out of role' at the end of the session to give students valued feedback on their skills (Eagles *et al*, 2001*a*). Specific communication tasks such as breaking bad news are often undertaken and this can be done to promote interprofessional learning (Wakefield *et al*, 2006). Teaching communication skills not infrequently extends into counselling and in North America it seems common to use SPs to teach motivational interviewing skills (e.g. Brown *et al*, 2004). This often focuses on smoking cessation, but the skills are germane to psychiatry and perhaps UK medical schools might consider deploying SPs in this way.

Students rarely see more than one patient at a time in an interview and so their first professional exposure to a family can be daunting. A 'standardised family' (Clay *et al*, 2000) can be used to teach family dynamics and communication, and again this is perhaps an area that undergraduate teaching might address during psychiatry attachments. It is also of interest that adolescents can be trained to be proficient SPs (Blake *et al*, 2006), since this is an age group to which students may be less exposed during their psychiatric attachments.

The use of actors in Aberdeen

Our use of actors as SPs in Aberdeen has been covered elsewhere (Eagles *et al*, 2007). This section is therefore brief; the intention is to give an illustration of the use of SPs in one psychiatric teaching curriculum.

In 1996 we contacted Aberdeen Actors, a professional group who had done similar work with social workers. Detailed scripts were discussed and rehearsed, and have been modified over subsequent years in response to students' and tutors' feedback. New scenarios have been developed as the curriculum changed and when our teaching committee agreed that changes would be advantageous educationally.

Most performances are live, but some have been recorded and the recordings are currently deployed mainly during the introductory course which students receive in their third year. During the tutorials in students' main clinical attachments, actors are interviewed, usually by students in groups of about 16, in tandem with didactic teaching on the same topics as the actors' scenarios. These topics include hypomania, schizophrenia, alcohol misuse, managing aggression, obsessive–compulsive disorder, anxiety and depression. In their final year, psychiatrists and general practitioners (GPs) have a joint teaching week and during this there are five half-day sessions on life crisis/depression, drug misuse, dementia, somatisation and adolescent eating disorders. The scenarios, again interspersed with didactic teaching and open discussion, illustrate the development of a disorder and its management. For example, with a student playing the part of her GP, a lady is seen in primary care on three occasions: first with stress following a difficult incident at work; then after she has developed depression of sufficient severity to merit treatment; and in a final consultation that addresses suicide risk and psychiatric referral when the patient has become even more unwell.

At the end of the sessions, actors often come out of role and give feedback to students on their interviews. It was this aspect of the sessions, in a study of different methods of teaching about alcohol misuse, that gave rise to students rating sessions using actors as superior to sessions using videotaped interviews with an actor or real patients with drinking problems (Eagles *et al*, 2001*a*).

The costs of Aberdeen's teaching with actors is not prohibitive. During the first few years they were higher, owing to the increased time required for scripting, rehearsals and related discussions, but thereafter costs stabilised. In the academic year 2008–09, we conducted a total of 107 live actor sessions at a total cost of £8587.

Students enjoy the sessions and find the actors to be convincing. Indeed, we adopted a routine policy of informing students that they had interviewed an actor after a student gave a dressing down to an 'alcoholic' actor she encountered in a local hostelry. The issue, though, of exactly when students should be told has proved contentious, and teachers in Aberdeen differ in their practice. Some feel more comfortable informing students at the beginning of a session that they will see an actor, while others feel it is better to proceed with what the students may perceive to be a 'real' interview before telling them that they were speaking with an actor. On balance, we feel that it is better practice to inform students before the interview.

Assessment using SPs

As mentioned above, Howard Barrows was using SPs for informal assessments of students in the 1960s. By the mid-1970s, SPs were being used in OSCEs, and their subsequent use in these was reviewed by Adamo (2003). In psychiatric OSCEs, the student's task with an SP will include taking a history in a focused area, educating or counselling the SP and starting a new treatment. In an examination setting it is of course all the more important that the SP is skilled, plausible and consistent; and thus perhaps it is preferable that they are professional actors.

The SPs will often act as assessors themselves in either a formative or a summative role. The ratings of SPs have been shown to correlate satisfactorily with the independent ratings of medical examiners made either live (Kilminster *et al*, 2007) or against audio transcripts (Luck & Peabody,

2002). Lurie *et al* (2008) found that, while different actors depicting the same scenario scored students differently, this gave rise to only a small proportion of the total variance in scores if these were combined across an adequate number of cases. It does seem legitimate and appropriate, therefore, for SPs to take on an assessment role.

Unannounced SPs are an interesting innovation. As an example, Kahan *et al* (2004) describe unannounced SPs presenting to general practice trainees during routine surgeries in Toronto with alcohol-induced insomnia or hypertension in order to assess the trainees' skills in detection and counselling. Rethans *et al* (2007) have reviewed the use of unannounced SPs in clinical practice.

Research using SPs

Partly because medical teaching is complex, it has not been widely researched. Some of these complexities can, though, be ameliorated by the use of SPs. Notably, standardised patients can be used across different sites, for example to assess the acquisition of clinical skills (Hauer *et al*, 2005), with collaborative projects yielding sufficient numbers of students to produce meaningful results and to detect more subtle differences than could be found with smaller numbers of taught students. SPs also provide an excellent way in which to assess the merits of different teaching methods, for example in the area of alcohol misuse (Eagles *et al*, 2001b; Lee *et al*, 2008). Hook & Pfeiffer (2007) used SPs to demonstrate that Connecticut students' communication skills had benefited following the transition from one teaching curriculum to another. It is also possible to tease out biases in attitudes and practices; for example, Wilson *et al* (2002) found that doctors had more positive attitudes to females than to males who presented with an alcohol problem.

The use of unannounced SPs to assess the clinical skills of doctors may become more common in both assessment and research, although Rethans *et al* (2007) bemoan the quality of research design in such studies conducted to date. Indeed, writing on behalf of the ASPE, Howley *et al* (2008) criticise the general standard of SP research reports, largely on the grounds of being insufficiently detailed, thus giving rise to difficulties in replicating the study or in knowing if the findings justify the conclusions. In summary, research with SPs has considerable potential, as yet largely untapped, to inform the development of medical teaching methods.

Role-play

The essential difference between teaching using SPs and role-play is that with SPs the learner is playing the part of herself or himself as a clinician, whereas in role-play he or she may well be acting the part of a patient

(McNaughton *et al*, 2008). This difference is taken up below, after a brief review of role-play in medical education.

From their perspective in Queensland, Joyner & Young (2006) offer useful suggestions for the use of role-play with medical students. These include the need for adequate preparation, such as the provision of good information for both the 'doctor' and the 'patient' before the role-play commences. Especially for the 'patient', whose role is less clear, a good 'script' is essential. All students should be involved, either directly or as active observers, to ensure a group learning process develops. It is helpful to specify the ground rules at the outset, usually including the freedom to decline roles and a reminder that initial feedback should be positive. Muskin & Stevens (1990) stress the importance of trusting relationships among the students and between tutors and students if role-play is to work well and it may thus be best to avoid it in 'one off' group teaching sessions.

There are many published accounts of the use of role-play in the medical literature, but not of its use in psychiatric teaching. It does seem to be effective and well received in areas such as the acquisition of skills in counselling for smoking cessation, especially when role-plays are conducted among postgraduates. With less-experienced learners, however, SPs have been evaluated more positively than role-play, even where there was no difference in the clinical skills acquired by students using the two methods, as Papadakis *et al* (1997) describe for first-year medical students in San Francisco. Nestel & Tierney (2007) surveyed 284 medical students in London about their perceptions of role-play. Students rated opportunities for observation, rehearsal, realistic roles and relevance to their current curriculum as helpful factors. Unhelpful factors included role-plays that evoked strong emotions (which may have psychiatric relevance) and any aspect that contributed to a lack of realism.

It would be possible to characterise role-play as the cheap and easy alternative to the use of trained SPs, but this would be only partly fair. When students portray a patient, this can constitute an excellent learning opportunity, by placing them for a time 'in the patient's shoes' and thus fostering empathy and a broader understanding of patient–doctor relationships. One possibly slightly extreme example in this area comprises medical students personally undergoing a 'standardised hospitalisation' in Los Angeles (Wilkes *et al*, 2002). The students tend to emerge from the experience with enhanced respect for the caring and attentive attitudes of nursing staff, while feeling upset by the distance and coldness they perceived from the medical staff.

Role-playing in psychiatric teaching may also have an intangible effect on medical students' perceptions of our profession. While a surgeon may be deemed empathic for suggesting that a student play the part of an apprehensive man contemplating a vasectomy, when a psychiatrist asks a student to portray one of our patients, which will usually be emotionally challenging, we may risk the epithet of 'typical touchy feely shrink'. While this should perhaps not concern us unduly, it is appropriate to be mindful of our image within the medical profession in terms of students' attitude formation and recruitment into the specialty (see Chapters 20 and 21).

Advantages of SPs

Several advantages of using SPs in teaching have been touched upon earlier and these are summarised below.

- *Safeguards patients*. SPs avoid the possible mistreatment of real patients in learning situations and protect them against 'novice practice' (Du Boulay & Medway, 1999).
- *Credible and realistic*. Well-trained SPs cannot be readily distinguished from real patients.
- *Confidentiality*. Not only with live performances, but also with videos and videoconferencing, there are no concerns about patient confidentiality.
- *Reassuring for students*. Emotionally sensitive areas (e.g. sexual histories, domestic violence) can be approached with greater confidence. The possibility that this confidence may be false is mentioned below under 'Disadvantages'.
- *Assessments*. These uses of SPs have been described above.
- *Availability*. While it can be problematic to locate real patients who will be involved in teaching, SPs are 'available at any time and available in any setting' (Barrows, 1993).
- *Flexibility in teaching sessions*. The session can be taken in different directions, for example after 'freezing' or utilising the time-in/time-out technique.
- *Curriculum planning*. Teachers can timetable sessions with confidence around specific clinical scenarios using cases at the most appropriate level of complexity.
- *Specific types of patients*. Students can see SPs when it would not be possible or appropriate to see the equivalent real patient (e.g. those seeking opiates, evasive problem drinkers).
- *Non-student areas of practice*. Students can enact scenes that they could not otherwise experience until after graduation (e.g. counselling, explaining management plans).
- *Feedback to students*. Experienced SPs can give valuable feedback to students about their communication skills.
- *Advantages to SPs*. As well as enjoying the sessions and gaining altruistic satisfaction (and/or money), SPs become more knowledgeable about their own health and healthcare system.

Disadvantages of SPs

Perhaps partly since papers about SPs will tend to be written by enthusiasts for the technique, and the authors of this chapter share that enthusiasm, we identified many fewer disadvantages than advantages. Indeed, we found only three disadvantages identified in the literature, these being cost, SP stress and authenticity.

Cost

Compared with role-playing or real patients, SPs are more expensive to deploy in teaching, even though patients may have to be paid expenses, especially if they are out-patients. Actors clearly cost the most, and teaching costs are described for Aberdeen above; for a day's work in an OSCE a trained actor might be paid in the region of £75, their hourly rate being about £12.50.

The relevant question about cost is whether this is money well spent. In Galway, Kelly & Murphy (2004) conducted an analysis of teaching costs in a communication skills course for fifth-year students. Their SPs cost €960, which was 10.7% of the total cost of the course, being essentially dwarfed by the cost of other staff. Given the millions of pounds spent nationally on student teaching, from both university and National Health Service sources (see Chapter 22), it may be felt that SPs constitute a very small proportion thereof and a cost-effective use of resources.

SP stress

Bokken et al (2004) found that 73% of their SPs in the Netherlands experienced stress symptoms, albeit mild, in relation to their roles. Following subsequent focus groups among 35 SPs, Bokken et al (2006) reported that negative effects were usual, but mild and transient and did not detract from SPs' enjoyment of their roles. Stress was increased by a high number of consecutive performances (as in OSCEs), among less-experienced SPs and when giving feedback. Emotionally complex roles (as in psychiatry) were deemed to be more stressful. Teachers should be aware of these possible stresses.

Authenticity

While junior students may not differentiate SPs from real patients, plausibility may be more limited for experienced learners. In the study by Kahan et al (2004) of unannounced problem drinkers, 47 out of 104 simulated consultations were detected by trainee general practitioners.

When students are aware that they are interviewing an SP, it is possible that they may be inappropriately relaxed and confident. It is not impossible that this could spill over into their dealings with real patients.

This point relates to a broader and more philosophical/ethical issue, on which Hanna & Fins (2006) and Wear & Varley (2008) have developed similar arguments. The power dynamics in an interaction between a student doctor and a real patient differ from those in an interaction between a student doctor and an actor; 'patients' in the latter scenario are not worried or dependent and, indeed, they may well be in the role of assessing or giving feedback to the medical learner. Hanna & Fins (2006) worry that there is a risk of producing 'simulation doctors', while Wear & Varley (2008) express concerns that students may come to rely upon 'formulaic and superficial behaviors', and point out that 'real empathy is not a simulation'. We feel that these points are well made, and a reminder that the advantages of SPs must not diminish the need for students to spend time interviewing and assessing genuine patients with psychiatric disorders.

Summary

In a psychiatry teaching curriculum, there is a great deal to be said for integrating the use of SPs with real patients. Instigating this type of teaching is challenging and time-consuming, but we feel that the effort diminishes subsequently and is very worthwhile in terms of teaching quality.

It seems highly probable that teaching with trained SPs will continue to become more common in teaching psychiatry to medical students. Standardised patients may be used in uniform national assessment of students. Collaboration and sharing of resources between teaching centres can be facilitated through SPs, either live, through videos or by video-conferencing. The rather flimsy evidence base underpinning much student teaching can also be addressed by the use of SPs in appropriate research.

Acknowledgements

We are grateful to Angela Girling for providing background information about local teaching and for her efforts in coordinating SP teaching. Bill Dick of Aberdeen Actors has been a very constructive and enthusiastic collaborator. The secretarial work for this chapter was done by Lana Hadden.

References

Adamo, G. (2003) Simulated and standardized patients in OSCEs: achievements and challenges 1992–2003. *Medical Teacher*, **25**, 262–270.

Ainsworth, M. A., Rogers, L. P., Markus, J. F., *et al* (1991) Standardized patient encounters: a method for teaching and evaluation. *JAMA*, **266**, 1390–1396.

Barrows, H. S. (1993) An overview of the uses of standardized patients for teaching and evaluating clinical skills. *Academic Medicine*, **68**, 443–451.

Barzansky, B. & Etzel, S. I. (2004) Educational programs in US medical schools, 2003–2004. *JAMA*, **292**, 1025–1031.

Beach, M. C., Rosner, M., Cooper, L. A., *et al* (2007) Can patient-centered attitudes reduce racial and ethnic disparities in care? *Academic Medicine*, **82**, 193–198.

Birndorf, C. A. & Kaye, M. E. (2002) Teaching the mental status examination to medical students by using a standardized patient in a large group setting. *Academic Psychiatry*, **26**, 180–183.

Blake, K. D., Gusella, J., Greaven, S., *et al* (2006) The risks and benefits of being a young female adolescent standardised patient. *Medical Education*, **40**, 26–35.

Bokken, L., Van Dalen, J. & Rethans, J.-J. (2004) Performance-related stress symptoms in simulated patients. *Medical Education*, **38**, 1089–1094.

Bokken, L., Van Dalen, J. & Rethans, J.-J. (2006) The impact of simulation on people who act as simulated patients: a focus group study. *Medical Education*, **40**, 781–786.

Brown, R. L., Pfeifer, J. M., Gjerde, C. L., *et al* (2004) Teaching patient-centered tobacco intervention to first-year medical students. *Journal of General Internal Medicine*, **19**, 534–539.

Carter, M. B., Wesley, G. & Larson, G. M. (2006) Lecture versus standardized patient interaction in the surgical clerkship: a randomized prospective cross-over study. *American Journal of Surgery*, **191**, 262–267.

Chur-Hansen, A. & Koopowitz, L. (2002) Introducing psychosocial and psychiatric concepts to first year medical students using an integrated biopsychosocial framework. *Education for Health*, **15**, 305–314.

Clay, M. C., Lane, H., Willis, S. E., *et al* (2000) Using a standardized family to teach clinical skills to medical students. *Teaching and Learning in Medicine*, **12**, 145–149.

Coyle, B., Miller, M. & McGowan, K. R. (1998) Using standardised patients to teach and learn psychotherapy. *Academic Medicine*, **73**, 591–592.

Du Boulay, C. & Medway, C. (1999) The clinical skills resource: a review of current practice. *Medical Education*, **33**, 185–191.

Eagles, J. M., Calder, S. A., Nicoll, K. S., *et al* (2001*a*) Using simulated patients in education about alcohol misuse. *Academic Medicine*, **76**, 395.

Eagles, J. M., Calder, S. A., Nicoll, K. S., *et al* (2001*b*) A comparison of real patients, simulated patients and videotaped interview in teaching medical students about alcohol misuse. *Medical Teacher*, **23**, 490–493.

Eagles, J. M., Calder, S. A., Wilson, S., *et al* (2007) Simulated patients in undergraduate education in psychiatry. *Psychiatric Bulletin*, **31**, 187–190.

Ekblad, S., Manicavasagar, V., Silove, D., *et al* (2004) The use of international video-conferencing as a strategy for teaching medical students about transcultural psychiatry. *Transcultural Psychiatry*, **41**, 120–129.

Ghatavi, K. & Waisman, Z. (2006) Teaching medical students about personality disorders and psychotherapeutic principles: a resident pilot initiative. *Academic Psychiatry*, **30**, 178–179.

Haist, S. A., Wilson, J. F., Pursley, H. G., *et al* (2003) Domestic violence: increasing knowledge and improving skills with a four-hour workshop using standardized patients. *Academic Medicine*, **78**, S24–S26.

Haist, S. A., Griffith III, C. H., Hoellein, A. R., *et al* (2004) Improving students' sexual history inquiry and HIV counselling with an interactive workshop using standardized patients. *Journal of General Internal Medicine*, **19**, 549–553.

Halbach, J. L. & Sullivan, L. L. (2005) Teaching medical students about medical errors and patient safety: evaluation of a required curriculum. *Academic Medicine*, **80**, 600–606.

Hanna, M. & Fins, J. J. (2006) Power and communication: why simulation training ought to be complemented by experiential and humanist learning. *Academic Medicine*, **81**, 265–270.

Harden, R. M., Stevenson, M., Downie, W. W., *et al* (1975) Assessment of clinical competence using objective structured examination. *BMJ*, **i**, 447–451.

Hauer, K. E., Hodgson, C. S., Kerr, K. M., *et al* (2005) A national study of medical student clinical skills assessment. *Academic Medicine*, **80**, S25–S29.

Hook, K. M. & Pfeiffer, C. A. (2007) Impact of a new curriculum on medical students' interpersonal and interviewing skills. *Medical Education*, **41**, 154–159.

Howley, L., Szauter, K., Perkowski, L., *et al* (2008) Quality of standardised patient research reports in the medical education literature: review and recommendations. *Medical Education*, **42**, 350–358.

Joyner, B. & Young, L. (2006) Teaching medical students using role play: twelve tips for successful role plays. *Medical Teacher*, **28**, 225–229.

Kahan, M., Wilson, L., Liu, E., *et al* (2004) Family medicine residents' beliefs, attitudes and performance with problem drinkers: a survey and simulated patient study. *Substance Abuse*, **25**, 43–51.

Kelly, M. & Murphy, A. (2004) An evaluation of the cost designing, delivering and assessing an undergraduate communication skills module. *Medical Teacher*, **26**, 610–614.

Ker, J. S., Dowie, A., Dowell, J., *et al* (2005) Twelve tips for developing and maintaining a simulated patient bank. *Medical Teacher*, **27**, 4–9.

Kilminster, S., Roberts, T. & Morris, P. (2007) Incorporating patients' assessments into objective structured clinical examinations. *Education for Health: Change in Learning and Practice*, **20**, article 6.

Lee, J. D., Triola, M., Gillespie, C., *et al* (2008) Working with patients with alcohol problems: a controlled trial of the impact of a rich media web module on medical student performance. *Journal of General Internal Medicine*, **23**, 1006–1009.

Leila, N. M., Pirkko, H. E. P., Eija, K., *et al* (2006) Training medical students to manage a chronic pain patient: both knowledge and communication skills are needed. *European Journal of Pain*, **10**, 167–170.

Luck, J. & Peabody, J. W. (2002) Using standardised patients to measure physicians' practice: validation study using audio recordings. *BMJ*, **325**, 679–683.

Lurie, S. J., Mooney, C. J., Nofziger, A. C., *et al* (2008) Further challenges in measuring communication skills: accounting for actor effects in standardised patient assessments. *Medical Education*, **42**, 662–668.

McNaughton, N., Ravitz, P., Wadell, A., *et al* (2008) Psychiatric education and simulation: a review of the literature. *Canadian Journal of Psychiatry*, **53**, 85–93.

Muskin, P. R. & Stevens, L. A. (1990) An AIDS educational program for third-year medical students. *General Hospital Psychiatry*, **12**, 390–395.

Nestel, D. & Tierney, T. (2007) Role-play for medical students learning about communication: guidelines for maximising benefits. *Medical Education*, **7**, 3.

Nestel, D., Tierney, T. & Kubacki, A. (2008) Creating authentic simulated patient roles: working with volunteers. *Medical Education*, **42**, 1122.

Papadakis, M. A., Croughan-Minihane, M., Fromm, L. J., *et al* (1997) A comparison of two methods to teach smoking-cessation techniques to medical students. *Academic Medicine*, **72**, 725–727.

Quest, T. E., Otsuki, J. A., Banja, J., *et al* (2002) The use of standardized patients within a procedural competency model to teach death disclosure. *Academic Emergency Medicine*, **9**, 1326–1333.

Rethans, J.-J., Gorter, S., Bokken, L., *et al* (2007) Unannounced standardised patients in real practice: a systematic literature review. *Medical Education*, **41**, 537–549.

Roberts, L. M., Wiskin, C. & Roalfe, A. (2008) Effects of exposure to mental illness in role-play on undergraduate student attitudes. *Family Medicine*, **40**, 477–483.

Rosenbaum, M. E. & Ferguson, K. J. (2006) Using patient-generated cases to teach students skills in responding to patients' emotions. *Medical Teacher*, **28**, 180–182.

Stafford, F. (2005) The significance of de-roling and debriefing in training medical students using simulation to train medical students. *Medical Education*, **39**, 1083–1085.

Taverner, D., Dodding, C. J. & White, J. M. (2000) Comparison of methods for teaching clinical skills in assessing and managing drug-seeking patients. *Medical Education*, **34**, 285–291.

Trudel, J. F. (1996) Simulated patients for the teaching of basic psychotherapeutic techniques: a practical guide. *Annales de Psychiatrie*, **11**, 14–18.

Tysinger, J. W., Klonis, L. K., Sadler, J. Z., *et al* (1997) Teaching ethics using small-group, problem-based learning. *Journal of Medical Ethics*, **23**, 315–318.

Vollebregt, J. A., Van Oldenrijk, J., Kox, D., *et al* (2006) Evaluation of a pharmacotherapy context-learning programme for preclinical medical students. *British Journal of Clinical Pharmacology*, **62**, 666–672.

Wakefield, A., Cocksedge, S. & Boggis, C. (2006) Breaking bad news: qualitative evaluation of an interprofessional learning opportunity. *Medical Teacher*, **28**, 53–58.

Wallace, P. (1997) Following the threads of an innovation: the history of standardized patients in medical education. *Caduceus*, **13**, 5–28.

Wear, D. & Varley, J. D. (2008) Rituals of verification: the role of simulation in developing and evaluating empathic communication. *Patient Education and Counseling*, **71**, 153–156.

Wilkes, M., Milgrom, E. & Hoffman, J. R. (2002) Towards more empathic medical students: a medical student hospitalization experience. *Medical Education*, **36**, 528–533.

Williams, B. C., Hall, K. E., Supiano, M. A., *et al* (2006) Development of a standardized patient instructor to teach functional assessment and communication skills to medical students and house officers. *Journal of the American Geriatric Society*, **54**, 1447–1452.

Wilson, L., Kahan, M., Liu, E., *et al* (2002) Physician behaviour towards male and female problem drinkers: a controlled study using simulated patients. *Journal of Addictive Diseases*, **21**, 87–99.

CHAPTER 20

Undergraduate medical education and recruitment to psychiatry

Tom Brown, John Eagles & Clare Oakley

Introduction

For some time now, both in the UK and elsewhere, concern has been expressed over the recruitment and retention of psychiatrists (Pidd, 2003). The Royal College of Psychiatrists' annual census over many years has demonstrated consultant vacancies of 10–15%. Goldacre *et al* (2005), in a substantial national survey of career choice, found that 4–5% of doctors graduating in the UK from 1974 to 2000 chose psychiatry as a career. This is not enough to meet workforce demands. Changes in the methods and content of undergraduate teaching and indeed in the demography of the medical student population (more females) have had no effect on this. In a survey of Scottish psychiatrists, Brown *et al* (2007) highlighted that a positive undergraduate experience was in the top five factors that consultants rated as being important in attracting them to psychiatry. Moreover, when asked what should be done to improve recruitment, improving undergraduate teaching was seen to be crucial. Similarly, Goldacre *et al* (2005) highlighted that undergraduate experience of teaching influences career choice. A number of studies have looked at various aspects of the undergraduate experience in relation to career choice; in this chapter we summarise these and draw some conclusions of possible relevance to those engaged in the important task of teaching medical students.

Selection of medical students

Brockington & Mumford (2002) highlighted the fact that psychiatry's recruitment problems may even start with factors influencing the selection of medical students, in that selection procedures favour applicants with a background in biological sciences rather than social sciences. They further note that a number of studies suggest that those with humanities or social science backgrounds are overrepresented in psychiatry training programmes (e.g. Donnan, 1976). This bias may be reinforced by the biological bias of medical education. Brockington & Mumford quote a US study (Silverman *et al*, 1983) which demonstrated that Boston medical students failed to recognise and attend to the relevance of psychosocial factors in the assessment of patients with chest pain and abdominal pain.

Pidd (2003) suggests the targeting of medical students 'with positive attitudes to psychological approaches'. She also speculates that the introduction of graduate entry training in some medical schools may draw in people of more diverse backgrounds and with more interest in psychological approaches; as yet this remains to be demonstrated, at least in terms of increasing recruitment to psychiatry.

Medical students' attitudes to psychiatry

A number of studies in the past decade or so have looked at the attitudes of medical students to psychiatry. Feifel *et al* (1999) surveyed 223 medical students at three US medical schools in the first 2 weeks of their undergraduate careers. The survey assessed their perceptions of careers in various specialties, not only psychiatry. It is of interest to note that these students valued highly aspects of the practice of medicine that may be seen as important in psychiatry, including a 'desire for interpersonal contact', 'helping patients', 'attractive lifestyle' and 'challenging work'. Nonetheless, the students consistently viewed psychiatry as less attractive than the other specialties they were asked about (internal medicine, family practice, paediatrics, surgery, and obstetrics and gynaecology). Worryingly, over 25% of the students even at this early stage in training (the first 2 weeks of medical school) had 'ruled out' psychiatry as a possible career. Psychiatry ranked worse than the other specialties on nearly all aspects on which the students were surveyed, such as job satisfaction, interest, intellectual challenge, lifestyle and helpfulness to patients. An important finding was that the students perceived that psychiatrists were less respected than other doctors by their classmates, by other doctors themselves and even by their own families. This perception that psychiatry is stigmatised within the medical profession was strongly supported by our own survey of Scottish psychiatrists (Brown *et al*, 2007), in which the single most important factor adversely affecting medical students' attitudes to psychiatry was judged to be the attitude of other medical professionals. At a recent meeting of over 100 Scottish psychiatrists, one of us (TB) asked for a show of hands in response to the question 'Were your family upset or embarrassed or disappointed by your choice of psychiatry as a career?' Around half of the audience put their hands up. Stigma in society at large and within the medical profession appears to be a real problem here.

Malhi *et al* (2003) in Australia replicated the US study by Feifel *et al* with broadly similar results. They surveyed 655 first-year medical students at six medical schools. Although the Australian students felt psychiatry was both interesting and intellectually challenging, they rated it as less attractive than the other specialties (the same specialties as Feifel *et al* incuded in their US study). Importantly, the students felt that psychiatry appeared not to build on the undergraduate curriculum and to lack a scientific basis. Malhi *et al* point out the irony of this latter finding, claiming that psychiatry has been 'avowedly scientific in recent times ... it is increasingly biological and for many at risk of "biologism"'. They point out our clear failure to demonstrate the scientific basis to students. This is clearly one area where the perceptions of students lack a factual basis and these perceptions persist into the early postgraduate years (see Chapter 21). Challenging this view is surely one of the tasks to be tackled in changing attitudes to psychiatry.

Wigney & Parker (2007) surveyed more senior Australian medical students, and invited them to detail why doctors would be less likely to choose psychiatry as a career. Their questionnaire had a negative bias, as it explicitly set out to explore why students would *not* choose psychiatry as a career, but nonetheless their findings are of great interest. Issues around treatability of patients, under-funding of psychiatric services and the 'unscientific' nature of psychiatry emerged as important. Similarly, stigma, 'including within the medical profession', was highlighted as a key issue. They conclude that if we wish to attract high-quality trainees, we need to focus on providing a positive and exciting undergraduate experience for students; they finish with the telling statement that 'currently medical students, like canaries in the mine, are sending a perturbing signal'.

The role of undergraduate exposure to psychiatry

A number of studies have examined the role of undergraduate teaching in relation to attitude formation and change, and recruitment to psychiatry. Broadly speaking, these studies have addressed three questions:

- Can attitudes to psychiatry be changed by undergraduate teaching?
- What aspects of undergraduate teaching encourage students to pursue a career in psychiatry?
- Are the teaching methods we use important?

McParland *et al* (2003) examined the attitudes of 379 medical students to psychiatry before and after an 8-week attachment (during the fourth year of the course). They demonstrated that their attitudes improved during the attachment, as did the numbers interested in pursuing psychiatry as a career. Interestingly, this was unrelated to how the students actually performed on the attachment. They concluded that undergraduate teaching was an important influence on career choice for psychiatry.

These conclusions are broadly supported by other studies (e.g. Holm-Peterson *et al*, 2007), although there is considerable debate as to whether these improved attitudes are sustained or whether they weaken with the passage of time. Baxter *et al* (2001) followed up a group of final-year medical students 1 year after their psychiatry attachment and showed that post-attachment improvement in attitudes to psychiatry decayed significantly during the final year. Similarly, Maidment *et al* (2004) demonstrated that although a positive post-attachment attitude predicted intent to pursue psychiatry as a career, such improved attitudes decayed over time and were less evident in their cohort of 223 newly qualified doctors (the same cohort as in the McParland study cited above).

Manassis *et al* (2006) argue a more subtle case from their work with Canadian medical students. They looked at the influence of a number of factors on medical students' career choice, including pre-existing interest in psychiatry, pre-psychiatry clerkship exposure to psychiatry, psychiatry clerkship experiences and so-called 'enrichment activities' designed to attract students to psychiatry. These activities included electives, career nights, dinner with a psychiatry speaker and some research scholarships. They predicted that those with low initial interest in psychiatry as a career might be influenced principally by enrichment activities rather than the psychiatric clerkship. Respondents ranked initial (pre-clerkship interest) as the most important factor in career choice. Those with low initial interest were most influenced by the clerkship itself (contrary to the authors' prediction) rather than by the enrichment activities. Enrichment activities were, however, not unimportant, merely less important. Of these activities, electives were rated as particularly important. It is of interest to note that in this study negative experiences of other specialties and income considerations were also ranked as influential, particularly by those with a low initial interest. Manassis *et al* concluded that 'different groups take different career paths in psychiatry' and suggested that those with low initial interest may be pushed in the direction of psychiatry because of negative experiences of other specialties as well as a positive clerkship experience.

It is of relevance to ask what it is about undergraduate experiences of psychiatry that acts as both 'push' and 'pull' factors, driving some students away from psychiatry and attracting others to it. Our reading of the literature leads us to conclude that interpersonal and experiential aspects of the undergraduate attachment are more important in terms of recruitment to the specialty than are teaching methods *per se* (on which, see below). That is not to say that the latter are unimportant in delivering the goals of the curriculum, but merely to argue that in terms of recruitment to psychiatry other factors may be more important.

A number of authors have highlighted the importance of encouraging students with interest in and/or aptitude for psychiatry. Maidment *et al* (2004) suggested that 'encouragement during medical school from senior doctors' increased the numbers of students wishing to pursue a career in psychiatry. It is of note in this study that 'senior doctors' included both consultants and specialist registrars. We would argue that perhaps not enough attention has been paid to the importance of undergraduate teaching and the acquisition of teaching skills during training in psychiatry. Not only should better teaching itself enhance recruitment, but better teachers are likely to become more enthusiastic encouragers and recruiters.

McParland *et al* (2003), in their study of fourth-year medical students, noted that positive change in their attitudes correlated with encouragement from consultants and also having direct involvement in patient care, especially when students saw patients respond well to treatment. Of their sample, 74% reported that they had been encouraged by someone during the attachment and those reporting such encouragement showed a greater intention to pursue psychiatry as a career. Eagles *et al* (2007), discussing the impact of undergraduate teaching on recruitment in psychiatry, also highlighted the importance of good role-models and the quality of clinical contacts with patients.

The importance of teaching methods

A number of studies have attempted to assess the importance of teaching methods in the undergraduate curriculum in terms of enhancing recruitment to psychiatry. In this section we review some of these. The focus of this review is *not* on the effectiveness of these teaching methods in successfully delivering the curriculum but on improving recruitment to psychiatry.

Manassis *et al* (2006) highlight inconsistency in previous research in this area. They conjecture that the duration of exposure to psychiatry may be less important than the nature of the exposure, and, indeed, their own study provides some support for this (see above). It is clear, however, that what they mean by the 'nature' of the exposure does not primarily relate to teaching methods used during attachments but more to interpersonal and experiential aspects of the exposure. For example, their study found that psychiatry electives and clerkships were influential in improving attitudes, but what they highlight about these is that both involve 'a high degree of contact with clinicians and patients in the field'.

The Maidment *et al* (2004) study discussed above included students who had a problem-based learning (PBL) curriculum and compared them with those who had a more traditional curriculum. There was no difference between the groups in terms of attitude to psychiatry (attitude improved in both groups). This confirms the findings of earlier authors (e.g. Singh *et al*, 1998) who similarly found no difference in attitude between students who had experienced PBL curricula and those in traditional curricula.

It is perhaps the case that the actual experience of students is not primarily determined by the method of teaching. McParland *et al* (2003) certainly reported that students in the two cohorts (PBL versus traditional curriculum) reported no differences in their experience in the attachment in terms of encouragement received, involvement with patients and seeing patients recover, all factors that we have already argued may be crucial in terms of both attitude formation and recruitment. It is also noteworthy that in this study students' performance in examinations was unrelated to career intention or to change in attitudes.

Other factors of importance

Self-assessment of aptitude for psychiatry appears to be important in governing career choice in medical students and newly qualified doctors. In the study by Goldacre *et al* (2005), 70% of those choosing psychiatry felt that self-assessment of aptitudes and skills was an important factor in their career choice. This was highly statistically significantly different from those choosing other careers. This was also deemed important in Wigney & Parker's (2007) study of Australian medical students, in which perceived 'lack of personal skills' was rated as a reason for not pursuing a career in psychiatry. Those authors stated that some students disliked the level of interpersonal contact and skills required to do psychiatry. Some felt that attributes like sensitivity and empathy were 'difficult to master'. The same students also perceived psychiatry as emotionally demanding and feared a 'contamination' effect, with patients seeming to 'suck the happiness out of you'.

Students' reactions to mental illness and to those who are mentally ill appear to act as a 'push' factor for some students but a 'pull' factor for others in relation to psychiatry. Dein *et al* (2007) and Brown *et al* (2007) surveyed consultant psychiatrists and asked them why they had chosen psychiatry as a career. In the Dein *et al* study, 36% highlighted empathy for patients with mental disorders as an important influence in career choice. In Brown *et al*'s survey, 83% highlighted 'interest in and concern for the mentally ill' as an important influence and 65% stated they were 'more interested in people than diseases'.

A number of authors have highlighted that medical students often perceive psychiatry to be different, unscientific and not integrated with the rest of the medical curriculum (e.g. Brockington & Mumford, 2002; Wigney & Parker, 2007). This has led to calls for psychiatry teaching to be more integrated with the teaching of other specialties. Brockington & Mumford suggest that liaison psychiatry clerkships may be of value, a view echoed by Oakley & Oyebode (2008). Oakley & Oyebode surveyed medical students before and after their psychiatry attachment. The survey considered the relevance of psychiatry to the rest of their careers. The students felt that awareness of the presentation of psychiatric illness in general practice and in general hospitals was important and felt these were useful settings in which to learn psychiatry. Although this survey was not about recruitment, it certainly suggests that students may be more engaged by psychiatry if it is taught more in general practice and in general hospital settings. This may also address the questions of relevance and scientific basis, at least to some degree.

When do medical students make career choices?

Brockington & Mumford (2002) have argued that career goals at medical school may not necessarily predict later career choice and that student choices are unstable and subject to change. They acknowledge, however, that preference to psychiatry may be more enduring than for other specialties. Goldacre *et al* (2005) demonstrated that choices made in the early postgraduate period, by contrast, are fairly enduring. Two-thirds of those whose sole first choice was psychiatry in their pre-registration house officer year and four-fifths of those whose first choice was psychiatry 3 years after graduation were working in the speciality 10 years after graduation. In broad terms, studies have shown that about a quarter to a third of doctors choose their specialty before or during undergraduate training, with the rest choosing usually during the early postgraduate years. Targeting both the undergraduate period and the early postgraduate years seems crucial if we are to improve recruitment (see Chapter 21 for a discussion on the importance of foundation years programmes).

The Royal College of Psychiatrists' initiatives

We have argued in this chapter that undergraduate experience of psychiatry is of considerable importance in influencing not only medical students' attitudes to psychiatry but also their career choice. This was highlighted for us by our own survey of Scottish psychiatrists (Brown *et al*, 2007), in which consultants in response to an open question regularly highlighted the importance of undergraduate teaching (for good or for ill) in influencing recruitment. Our response to this was to set up the Scottish Division Undergraduate Student Teaching And Recruitment Group (S-DUSTARG) in 2003. This group has, among other things, encouraged review of the undergraduate psychiatry curricula in Scotland, supported the Scottish Division Malawi Project (see Chapter 17), organised conference sessions and undergraduate teaching (at College meetings), organised a conference to train trainees in teaching methods, and published papers on undergraduate teaching (e.g. Brown *et al*, 2007; Eagles *et al*, 2007). As yet we have no data to indicate whether or not this has improved recruitment to psychiatry but it seems a reasonable place to start, in the light of what we have discussed above.

More recently, at a UK level, the Royal College of Psychiatrists has launched a number of initiatives aimed at undergraduate medical students. In December 2008, the College launched the new Student Associate grade, an initiative that had been proposed by the Psychiatric Trainees' Committee (PTC). While the grade was initially intended for medical students, it was quickly found that foundation doctors were also a key group to engage, and therefore they were also encouraged to join the College. The aim of the

Student Associate grade is now to allow medical students and foundation doctors to learn more about a career in psychiatry and to have access to opportunities that will demonstrate the exciting and interesting nature of training in psychiatry. It is free for any UK medical student or foundation doctor to join and the benefits include a free annual conference, a summer school, electronic subscriptions to *The Psychiatrist* (formerly the *Psychiatric Bulletin*) and *British Journal of Psychiatry*, and regular e-newsletters produced by an editorial team of Student Associates in collaboration with the PTC. There is also a dedicated section of the College website that contains personal perspectives of trainees and consultants, information about prizes and bursaries offered by the College and a range of useful information about choosing psychiatry as a career. At the time of writing there were nearly 1000 Student Associates registered with the College. Hundreds of these students have been actively involved through attending the conference or summer school, and contributing to the website or newsletter. Crucially, two Student Associates have been co-opted on to the PTC, highlighting that they are valued by the College.

This collaboration has promoted the development of psychiatry student societies in medical schools across the UK. These societies are led by the students with the support of local trainees and more senior psychiatrists. They meet for film nights, careers evenings and talks by prominent psychiatrists. Importantly, events aimed at examination revision have been able to attract students who may not already be interested in psychiatry to attend and find out more. In less than a year the number of such medical school societies has increased from 1 to 20, demonstrating the enthusiasm to tackle these issues locally. The key to the success of this strategy seems to be the close working relationship between the Student Associates and the trainees on the PTC. Owing to their proximity on the career pathway, it is perhaps easier for students to relate to trainees. While it is too early for a formal evaluation of this scheme, it seems clear that it has helped raise the profile of psychiatry within those 20 medical schools and built a national network of students who are enthusiastic about psychiatry.

Summary

High-quality undergraduate exposure to psychiatry invariably improves medical students' attitudes to it and also increases students' at least stated intention to pursue a career in the specialty. Both relate more to experiential aspects of the attachment (including contact with and encouragement from senior doctors and also patient contact) rather than to specific teaching methods. Unfortunately, the improvements in attitudes seem to decay over time. Also, psychiatry is often perceived as unscientific and remote from the rest of medicine. Critical comments from other doctors may be very important in this regard (Brown *et al*, 2007; see also Chapter 21). It is likely that some of this decay of positive attitudes can be addressed by regular exposure to psychiatry over the 5-year curriculum rather than in one block (as argued by Baxter *et al*, 2001). Timing of psychiatry within the foundation-year programme is also important in this regard (see Chapter 21).

Given the importance of the undergraduate experience, we argue that a number of factors need to be addressed at that stage to increase the likelihood of enhancing recruitment to psychiatry. These include:

- identifying interested students and offering them encouragement and support (utilising the new student societies in medical schools)
- dealing with stigma within the medical (and allied) professions
- integrating the teaching of psychiatry with that of other specialties (consideration should be given to teaching psychiatry in general practice and exposing more students to liaison psychiatry)
- demonstrating to undergraduate medical students that psychiatry does have a scientific basis and that patients in psychiatry are as treatable as those in other areas of medicine
- improving the teaching skills of psychiatric trainees
- considering aptitudes for psychological and social aspects of medicine in the selection of medical students.

The seminal work of Goldacre *et al* (2005) has highlighted that the numbers of medical students entering psychiatry are too low to meet demands. We have an urgent need to address the above issues if this situation is to be improved and more students are to choose the challenging and exciting career of psychiatry.

References

Baxter, H., Singh, S. B., Standen, P., *et al* (2001) The attitudes of tomorrow's doctors towards mental illness and psychiatry: changes during the final undergraduate year. *Medical Education*, **35**, 381–383.

Brockington, I. & Mumford, D. (2002) Recruitment into psychiatry. *British Journal of Psychiatry*, **180**, 307–312.

Brown, T. M., Addie, K. & Eagles, J. M. (2007) Recruitment into psychiatry: views of consultants in Scotland. *Psychiatric Bulletin*, **31**, 411–413.

Dein, K., Livingston, G. & Bench, C. (2007) 'Why did I become a psychiatrist?' Survey of consultant psychiatrists. *Psychiatric Bulletin*, **31**, 221–230.

Donnan, S. P. D. (1976) British medical undergraduates in 1975: a student survey in 1975 compared with 1966. *Medical Education*, **10**, 341–347.

Eagles, J. M., Wilson, S., Murdoch, J. M., *et al* (2007) What impact do undergraduates experiences have upon recruitment into psychiatry? *Psychiatric Bulletin*, **31**, 70–72.

Feifel, D., Moutier, C. Y. & Swerdlow, N. (1999) Attitudes towards psychiatry as a prospective career among students entering medical school. *American Journal of Psychiatry*, **166**, 1397–1402.

Goldacre, M. S., Turner, G., Faztz, S., *et al* (2005) Career choices for psychiatry: national surveys of graduates of 1974–2000 from UK medical schools. *British Journal of Psychiatry*, **186**, 158–164.

Holm-Peterson, C., Vinges, H. J. & Eyrd-Hansen, D. (2007) The impact of contact with psychiatry on senior medical students' attitudes towards psychiatry. *Acta Psychiatrica Scandinavica*, **116**, 308–311.

Maidment, R., Livingston, G., Katona, C., *et al* (2004) Changes in attitude to psychiatry and intention to pursue psychiatry as a career in newly qualified doctors: a follow-up of 2 cohorts of medical students. *Medical Teacher*, **26**, 565–569.

Malhi, G. S., Parker, G. B., Parker, K., *et al* (2003) Attitudes towards psychiatry among students entering medical school. *Acta Psychiatrica Scandinavica*, **107**, 424–429.

Manassis, K., Katz, M., Lofchy, J., *et al* (2006) Choosing a career in psychiatry: influential factors within a medical school programme. *Academic Psychiatry*, **30**, 325–329.

McParland, M., Noble, L. M., Livingstone, G., *et al* (2003) The effect of a psychiatric attachment on students' attitudes to and intention to pursue psychiatry as a career. *Medical Education*, **37**, 447–454.

Oakley, C. & Oyebode, F. (2008) Medical student views about an undergraduate curriculum in psychiatry before and after clinical placements. *BMC Medical Education*, **8**, 26.

Pidd, S. A. (2003) Recruiting and retaining psychiatrists. *Advances in Psychiatric Treatment*, **9**, 405–413.

Silverman, D., Gartell, N., Aronson, M., *et al* (1983) In search of the biopsychosocial perspective: an experiment with beginning medical students. *American Journal of Psychiatry*, **140**, 1154–1159.

Singh, S. P., Baxter, H., Standen, P., *et al* (1998) Changing the attitudes of 'tomorrow's doctors' towards mental illness and psychiatry: a comparison of two teaching methods. *Medical Education*, **32**, 115–120.

Wigney, T. & Parker, G. (2007) Medical student observations on a career in psychiatry. *Australia and New Zealand Journal of Psychiatry*, **41**, 726–731.

CHAPTER 21

Choosing psychiatry: factors influencing career choice among foundation doctors in Scotland

Premal Shah, Tom Brown & John Eagles

Introduction

Despite substantial change in undergraduate medical education over the past two or three decades, in terms of student demographics, teaching methods and curriculum content, this has had little effect on recruitment into psychiatry in the UK, the rate remaining consistently at 4–5% of British medical graduates (Goldacre *et al*, 2005).

It is well established that undergraduate experience is of primary importance in influencing career choice (see Chapter 20), but when and why medical students become dissuaded from choosing psychiatry, having been at worst neutral before admission to medical school (Maidment *et al*, 2003), has still to be elucidated. A number of studies (e.g. Malhi *et al*, 2002; Brown *et al*, 2007) suggest that several factors operate during the undergraduate years that may reduce the likelihood of a student choosing psychiatry as a career. However, few inferences can be drawn from these studies, as they either offer 'expert opinion' (i.e. views from within the profession) or are surveys overtly conducted by psychiatrists, which may have influenced respondents.

While undergraduate experience may shape the basis of career choice, postgraduate experience appears to act as an important modifying influence; traditionally, psychiatry gained recruits within the early postgraduate years, which suggests that the balance of influencing factors changes, perhaps owing to positive and negative practical work experiences, opportunity or personal circumstance (Goldacre & Lambert, 2000). This is partly reassuring ,though concerns have been raised recently about the impact that the more streamlined specialist training scheme may have on psychiatric recruitment. On the one hand, limiting potential experience by requiring an earlier specialty choice may reduce postgraduate gain. Alternatively, foundation programmes could improve recruitment, through trainees working in specialties that they may not otherwise have considered as a career.

It is therefore important to establish which factors encourage and discourage trainees into and from psychiatry, when these become influential and whether foundation experience improves recruitment. Establishing these factors should help to guide changes within the undergraduate and early postgraduate years that are required to improve psychiatric recruitment.

Survey method

As part of the Royal College of Psychiatrists' 'Images of Psychiatry' campaign in 2007, the Scottish Division Undergraduate Student Teaching And Recruitment Group (S-DUSTARG) was funded by the College to conduct a cross-sectional survey of foundation trainees in Scotland. This survey examined their career intentions at key times and the factors that may have influenced those intentions. The study was carried out in partnership between NHS Education Scotland (NES) and S-DUSTARG, to allow relevant data to be available to other medical specialties and in order to minimise response bias.

An initial questionnaire was assembled by the research team, using questions derived from previous surveys, relating to potentially important influencing factors. This was revised in light of comments from S-DUSTARG and after an online pilot survey of foundation doctors.

The final questionnaire was delivered, completed and analysed entirely electronically. Data collection was anonymous (i.e. not linked to the respondent) and protected using industry-standard encryption and security. Further, to ensure unbiased responses, the questionnaire invitations were sent out on behalf of NES alone, blinding potential respondents to the involvement of psychiatrists. After their (anonymised) demographic data had been gathered, trainees were asked to rank ten types of specialty (anaesthetics, accident and emergency, general medical specialties, surgical specialties, laboratory specialties, general practice, radiology, paediatrics, psychiatry, obstetrics and gynaecology) in order of career preference. They also chronologically listed the six specialty posts of their foundation programme. Trainees were then presented with 31 potential factors that might have influenced them when they considered a particular specialty group. For both top- and bottom-ranked choices, trainees indicated whether each factor had had a positive, negative or no influencing effect. The same list was presented when trainees were asked to consider a middle-ranked specialty choice. Trainees who did not place psychiatry as their top or bottom choice were asked to consider psychiatry as the middle-ranked specialty.

All foundation year 2 trainees (FY2s) in Scotland were sent electronic invitations containing the survey's web-link at the beginning of March 2008 (nearing the end of the fifth of their six posts), and a universal electronic reminder was sent 2 weeks later. The survey was open for 4 weeks, this being chosen to coincide with the period between the trainees' specialty training application submission and any interviews, in order to give a 'snapshot' of the trainees before the results of their interviews were known. The same procedure was applied to all foundation year 1 trainees (FY1s) in Scotland at the beginning of September 2008, this period being chosen to capture opinions minimally influenced by work experience.

Survey responses

In total, 359 FY1s responded to the survey conducted 2 months into their first foundation post. None was currently in psychiatry. In total, 311 FY2s responded to the survey conducted in the middle of their second-last foundation post. It is important to note that a third of the FY2s with a foundation psychiatric posting were still to experience it (i.e. it was to be the last of their six foundation posts).

Ranking of psychiatry

As Fig. 21.1 shows, while only 7 of the 359 FY1s (1.9%) placed psychiatry as their top choice, a significantly greater proportion of FY2s (15/311, 4.8%, $\chi^2 = 4.33$, $P = 0.037$) did so. Overall, 16.1% of FY1s and 17.9% of FY2s placed psychiatry in their top three. A significantly greater proportion

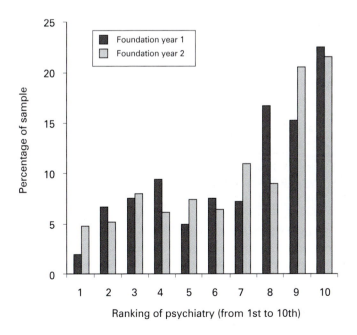

Fig. 21.1 Ranking of psychiatry as a career choice.

257

of FY1s who were going to have psychiatry as part of their foundation programme placed psychiatry as their top choice compared with those who were not (4/59 *v.* 3/300; $\chi^2 = 8.85$, $P = 0.003$), suggesting that those who had already decided on a psychiatric career chose foundation programmes with psychiatry. However, and perhaps importantly, 16% (12/75) of FY2s who had psychiatry as part of their programme placed it as their first choice compared with 6.8% (4/59) of FY1s who were going to have psychiatry ($\chi^2 = 2.67$, $P = 0.1$), suggesting that foundation psychiatric experience may have increased the proportion selecting psychiatry. There was no difference in the proportion placing psychiatry as their top choice among FY1s and FY2s with no foundation psychiatry – 3/300 (1%) *v.* 3/236 (1.3%), respectively.

Factors influencing career preferences

We assumed that FY1s' views on influencing factors represented the sum effect of their undergraduate experience, as they had been in post for only a month, whereas we assumed that FY2s' views also incorporated the effect of almost 2 years of foundation work experience.

Top choice of specialty

When considering their top specialty choice (whatever it may have been), the most common and consistent positive influences for both FY1s and FY2s were:

- finding the patients or work interesting (95% of FY1s and 97% of FY2s)
- having an aptitude for the specialty (93% and 96%)
- seeing role-models in the specialty (90% and 93%)
- amount of patient contact (88% and 89%)
- encouragement from seniors (87% and 89%)
- team-working ethos (84% and 86%)
- general pace of the specialty (79% and 85%)
- morale among seniors (75% and 74%).

The most common negative influence was the amount of paperwork (42% of FY1s and 39% of FY2s).

Undergraduate teaching, another important positively influencing factor, was less positively influential and more negatively influential in the FY2s – 82% of FY1s and 75% of FY2s said it had a positive influence, with 4% and 10% indicating a negative influence. Postgraduate teaching in the subject was a significantly more positively influencing factor among the FY2s (70% *v.* 60%; $\chi^2 = 10.7$, $P = 0.005$).

The influence of the perceived patients' prognosis did not differ between FY1s and FY2s – only 6.5% and 4.5%, respectively, indicated that it had a negative influence, whereas 57% and 62% indicated it was a positive influence. This was the similar for the scientific basis of the specialty – 3.2% of FY1s and 2.4% of FY2s found it a negatively influencing factor, while 63% and 69% found it a positive influence. Interestingly, 17% of FY1s and 14% of FY2s found comments by other specialists to have had a negative influence, although 41% and 40%, respectively, were positively influenced.

Psychiatry as a specialty choice

All surveyed trainees were asked about what had influenced them when they had considered psychiatry as a specialty choice. In terms of the factors identified to be the most positively influential for their top choice, the most positive for psychiatry was finding the patients or work interesting (64% of FY1s and 50% of FY2s). Patient contact was the next most positive factor (57% of FY1s and 49% of FY2s), with undergraduate teaching being the third most positive (52% of FY1s and 45% of FY2s). A larger proportion of FY2s than of FY1s, however, regarded undergraduate teaching as a neutral influence. Moreover, only 45% of FY1s and 40% of FY2s indicated a positive influence of aptitude in psychiatry, 30% and 35% respectively being neutral, with 26% of both FY1s and FY2s being negative. Important factors that were significantly more neutral for FY2s than for FY1s with respect to psychiatry were the influence of role-models, encouragement from seniors, team working, and morale of seniors.

Table 21.1 Numbers (%) of doctors in foundation years 1 and 2 (FY1s and FY2s) reporting influences on career choice in psychiatry

	Negative influence	No influence	Positive influence	FY1s v. FY2s (χ^2 P values)
Scientific basis of specialty				NS
FY1s	152 (44.2)	143 (41.6)	49 (14.2)	
FY2s	113 (38.2)	140 (47.3)	43 (14.5)	
Prognosis of patients				0.04
FY1s	231 (67.2)	83 (24.1)	30 (8.7)	
FY2s	170 (57.4)	91 (30.7)	35 (11.8)	
Comments by other specialists				0.002
FY1s	178 (51.7)	131 (38.1)	35 (10.2)	
FY2s	127 (42.9)	152 (51.4)	17 (5.7)	
Standing in profession				0.001
FY1s	156 (45.3)	162 (47.1)	26 (7.6)	
FY2s	93 (31.4)	173 (58.4)	30 (10.1)	
Standing among public				0.004
FY1s	137 (39.8)	184 (53.5)	23 (6.7)	
FY2s	82 (27.7)	185 (62.5)	29 (9.8)	

Table 21.2 Numbers (%) of doctors in foundation years 1 and 2 (FY1s and FY2s) without psychiatry in their programmes reporting influences

	Negative influence	No influence	Positive influence	FY1s v. FY2s (χ^2 P values)
Aptitude and skills for psychiatry				0.025
FY1s	80 (27.9)	89 (31.0)	118 (41.1)	
FY2s	67 (29.4)	92 (40.4)	69 (30.3)	
Interesting work/patients				<0.001
FY1s	74 (25.8)	40 (13.9)	173 (60.3)	
FY2s	75 (32.9)	54 (23.7)	99 (43.4)	
Role-models in psychiatry				<0.001
FY1s	85 (29.6)	111 (38.7)	91 (31.7)	
FY2s	45 (19.7)	136 (59.6)	47 (20.6)	

Of probable greater importance, however, were the factors that most trainees found were a negative influence on the possible choice of psychiatry (see Table 21.1). For both FY1s and FY2s, the most negative factors were the perceived poor prognosis of patients, comments made by other specialists, the specialty's (lack of) scientific basis and the standing of psychiatry among doctors and the public. FY1s were more negative than FY2s on all of these points; the apparently increasing neutrality among FY2s seems to indicate that work experience has a modifying influence.

Further differences became apparent when comparing FY1s with or without psychiatry against FY2s with or without psychiatry in their programmes. FY1s who would have foundation psychiatry were no different from other FY1s in terms of the influence of the patients' prognosis. However, FY2s who had done psychiatry in their programme were less negative, more neutral and more positive about patients' prognosis than FY1s who were going to have psychiatry ($\chi^2 = 5.3$, $P = 0.07$), suggesting that foundation experience of psychiatry may have reduced the influence of a negative view of psychiatric prognosis.

Table 21.2 shows some of the changes that apparently occur during the foundation years among doctors without psychiatry in their programmes. FY2s were less positive about their psychiatric aptitude and skills, were less likely to rate psychiatric work as interesting and were less positive about role-models in the specialty. This suggests that these changes arise either through distance in time from exposure to psychiatry as undergraduates or as a result of foundation experience in other specialties.

Main conclusions from the study

At the start of their foundation years, only 1.9% cited psychiatry as their first-choice career. This figure rose to 4.8% of FY2s in the fifth of their six foundations posts. Whether or not foundation doctors do psychiatry, they become more keen on the specialty during their first two postgraduate years. FY2s actually exposed to the specialty become much keener to pursue it as a career. Specific positive and negative influences on a career choice of psychiatry pertain and these are discussed below.

What influences career choice and what could be done to improve recruitment?

The predominant positively influencing factors we identified could be categorised into three loose groups:

- group A, to do with the individual's early medical school experiences (finding patients interesting, developing an aptitude for the specialty, undergraduate teaching)
- group B, to do with the influence of seniors (role-models, encouragement from seniors, morale among seniors)
- group C, to do with aspects of the working environment (patient contact, general pace of specialty, team working).

Clearly, the first two groupings are mainly related to students' undergraduate experience.

Arguably the most influential, from a recruitment point of view, is group A. Psychiatry fared reasonably well in terms of undergraduate teaching and trainees finding the patients and work interesting. However, fewer than half of all FY1s perceived that they had an aptitude for psychiatry, this being less among those who did not have psychiatry in their programme. Further, among those who did not have psychiatry in their programme, fewer FY2s than FY1s found psychiatry interesting. Unsurprisingly, these results suggest that not having psychiatric experience is associated with losing interest in, and a poorer view of aptitude for, psychiatry.

The influence of group B in career choice is also well recognised, and has been suggested as an area that could be improved within the undergraduate psychiatric experience as a way of increasing psychiatric recruitment. However, this group's influence seems more moderate, and more open to modification with general work experience – in our survey, FY2s were more neutral than were FY1s about the effect of this group of factors with regard to psychiatry.

There appear to be three specific and unique negative factors: the perceived (poor) prognosis of patients, (negative) comments made by other specialists and the perceived unscientific basis of psychiatry. Both the perceived prognosis and the scientific basis could be seen as group A factors (i.e. mainly of undergraduate origin, more influential, and less amenable to change with general postgraduate experience), with specialists' comments belonging to group B (to do with seniors, and more amenable to change with general experience). These three factors were replicated in both the FY1 and FY2 samples, suggesting validity for them, and were specific to psychiatry, being more prevalent there than for any other specialty.

Consistent with these proposed groupings is the observation that the negative influence of specialists' comments was reduced in those with general foundation experience (group B), but that perceived prognosis was rectified only among those who had psychiatric experience (group A), and was associated with a greater proportion placing psychiatry as their career of choice.

While foundation psychiatric experience seemed to reduce some of the negative influences, this was in itself insufficient entirely to reverse them; indeed, 50% of FY2s with psychiatry in their programme were still negatively influenced by perceived prognosis, and the negative influence of the perceived lack of a scientific basis to psychiatry was no different between FY1s and FY2s. Given that medical students are relatively neutral towards psychiatry at the start of their undergraduate medical training, it seems probable that these negative factors develop during the undergraduate years, and thus need to be tackled at this time.

Our survey results are consistent with the previous finding that under-graduate psychiatric clerkships improve students' attitudes to psychiatry (Singh *et al*, 1998; McParland *et al*, 2003; Eagles *et al*, 2007), in that experience of working in psychiatry seems to aid recruitment; even a brief period (4 months) is associated with increased recruitment. A suggested intervention, therefore, would be to change undergraduate psychiatric attachments so that they more closely resemble the experience of working in psychiatry (e.g. by having specific student-led clinics).

At postgraduate level, it seems highly likely that recruitment would be improved by the creation of more FY1 posts in psychiatry, given that specialty career choice is being made after only four of the six foundation posts have been completed,

Our survey is also consistent with the previous literature in terms of the negative influences upon choosing psychiatry as a career (e.g. Balon *et al*, 1999; Malhi *et al*, 2002) and it is these that perhaps need to be the focus of attention at an undergraduate level if psychiatric recruitment and psychiatry's image in medicine are to be significantly improved. We suggest that particular emphasis needs to be placed on demonstrating how different psychiatric treatments can be effective for a variety of conditions. Given that most students have a relatively brief experience of undergraduate psychiatry and the natural history of most psychiatric conditions is long, other effective ways of demonstrating the effects of psychiatric treatment need to be sought, such as showing film clips of patients before and after successful treatment. We further suggest that undergraduate curricula also need to be updated to incorporate the most recent converging scientific findings from neurobiology, neuropsychiatry and psychology, and that all of this should be introduced at an earlier stage in medical school.

References

Balon, R., Franchina, G. R., Freeman, P. S., et al (1999) Medical students' attitudes and views of psychiatry, 15 years later. *Academic Psychiatry*, **23**, 30–36.

Brown, T. M., Addie, K. & Eagles, J. M. (2007) Recruitment into psychiatry: views of consultants in Scotland. *Psychiatric Bulletin*, **31**, 411–413.

Eagles, J. M., Wilson, S., Murdoch, J. M., et al (2007) What impact do undergraduate experiences have upon recruitment into psychiatry? *Psychiatric Bulletin*, **31**, 70–72.

Goldacre, M. J. & Lambert, T. W. (2000) Stability and change in career choices of junior doctors: postal questionnaire surveys of the United Kingdom qualifiers of 1993. *Medical Education*, **34**, 700–707.

Goldacre, M. J., Turner, G., Fazel, S., et al (2005) Career choices for psychiatry: national surveys of graduates of 1974–2000 from UK medical schools. *British Journal of Psychiatry*, **186**, 158–164.

Maidment, R., Livingston, G., Katona, M., et al (2003) Carry on shrinking: career intentions and attitudes to psychiatry of prospective medical students. *Psychiatric Bulletin*, **27**, 30–32.

Malhi, G. S., Parker, G. B., Parker, K., et al (2002) Shrinking away from psychiatry? A survey of Australian medical students' interest in psychiatry. *Australian and New Zealand Journal of Psychiatry*, **26**, 416–423.

McParland, M., Noble, L. M., Livingstone, G., et al (2003) The effect of a psychiatric attachment on students' attitudes to and intention to pursue psychiatry as a career. *Medical Education*, **37**, 447–454.

Singh, S. P., Baxter, H., Standen, P., et al (1998) Changing the attitudes of 'tomorrow's doctors' towards mental illness and psychiatry: a comparison of two teaching methods. *Medical Education*, **32**, 115–120.

CHAPTER 22

Funding of the teaching of medical undergraduates

Subodh Dave & Audrey Morrison

Introduction

In this chapter, we provide an overview of the funding mechanisms for medical student education in England and the other devolved countries of the UK, the implications for undergraduate psychiatric education and recommendations for the way forward.

Traditionally, National Health Service (NHS) trusts have provided clinical training for medical students, but with many universities now offering vertically integrated courses, the division between preclinical and clinical education is blurred and it is estimated that 70% of the teaching of medical students is undertaken by NHS staff (Catto, 2000).

Tomorrow's Doctors (General Medical Council, 2003) places renewed emphasis on student-centred learning, the acquisition of clinical skills and early patient contact, all of which increase the burden of teaching medical students on NHS staff, in both hospital and primary care settings. This presents new challenges, as teaching has often not been seen as a priority and teaching done by NHS staff has traditionally been unrecognised (for example in job plans) and unrewarded (Eagles, 2005). Accountability (both clinical and financial) has been identified as the key driver for improvement in quality (Scally & Donaldson, 1998). It follows that, in the interest of accountability, funding should follow students (Eagles, 2005). The current financial pressures within the NHS make this even more important, since the expectation that better services can be delivered from current resources (Department of Health, 2008) may increase the likelihood of funds being diverted from teaching to clinical services.

The cost of educating one medical student is estimated to be in the region of £200000. Overall, in the 2005–06 cycle of funding, nearly £3.5 billion was spent on education in the NHS in England, of which a fifth (£728 million) was spent on medical student education. Efficient use of this money is of course vital, but equally important is its equitable distribution, especially as it represents a significant income stream for some trusts. Historically, the large teaching hospitals attached to universities secured the bulk of such funding at the expense of district general hospitals and primary care centres, but the latter are now increasingly offering clinical placements. An inequitable distribution of educational funding is inconsistent with the central philosophy of the modern NHS and its internal market.

Structure and flow of funding

It is recognised that NHS trusts that provide clinical placements will incur additional expenses compared with trusts that do not participate in teaching medical students. In England and Wales, these additional expenses are recompensed to the NHS through SIFT (Service Increment for Teaching). Similar funding mechanisms operate in the other nations of the UK – Additional Costs of Teaching (ACT) in Scotland and Supplement for Medical and Dental Education (SUMDE) in Northern Ireland. In Wales, the Welsh assembly funds both SIFT and the Higher Education Funding Council for Wales.

The Higher Education Funding Council for England (HEFCE) is the funding body for universities in England. Fig. 22.1 shows the source of medical education funding in England. NHS Education for Scotland (NES) and the Department of Employment and Learning, Northern Ireland (DELNI) are the bodies that fund the direct costs of medical student teaching in Scotland and Northern Ireland. Since 2001, SIFT in England has been operationally merged in a larger funding stream, MPET (Multi-Professional Education and Training), which includes funding for postgraduate medical education, dental education and non-medical healthcare education (nursing, occupational therapy, etc.). This was meant to introduce more flexibility in the funding of healthcare education within the NHS, but in practice the various funding streams within MPET have remained unchanged.

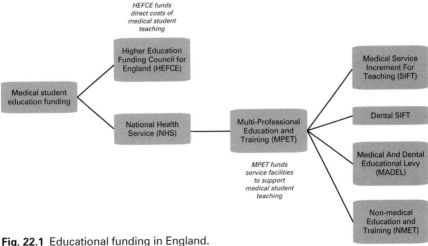

Fig. 22.1 Educational funding in England.

In England, the overall funding for medical education is held by the national budget holder, the chief medical officer, acting for the Department of Health. The responsibility for managing this budget is devolved to the strategic health authorities (SHAs), where the funding is meant to be streamed, based on national *and* local priorities, in particular taking into account the needs of the local workforce. The workforce development corporations deliver this task for the SHAs, working closely with the local NHS trusts and the local deaneries.

In Scotland, Medical ACT, supporting the additional costs of teaching undergraduates, is provided by the Scottish Government Health Directorates (SGHD) and since 2004 this has been distributed to NHS boards by NHS Education for Scotland (NES). NES is also responsible for setting policy on the use of ACT, for managing the ACT allocation model and for performance management of the processes to ensure good governance. Prior to this, funding was allocated via the Scottish Executive Health Department (SEHD) and allocated to the four Scottish teaching boards. There are now four regional ACT groups, each with an appointed chairperson and an ACT officer for each of the five Scottish medical schools, who are responsible for the planning, prioritising and approval of new developments in undergraduate education. In 2008/09 the funding amounted to nearly £70 million (NHS Education for Scotland, 2009). ACT funds are distributed by NES to all boards, based on a 'student week' calculation, and the 2008/09 allocations are shown in Table 22.1.

Previously, funding was targeted at teaching health boards/hospitals such as Lothian/University of Edinburgh and Greater Glasgow/University of

Table 22.1 Scottish Medical ACT allocation figures for 2008/09, by health board

Health board	Total allocation (£1000s)	% of total
Ayrshire & Arran	1762	3
Borders	511	1
Dumfries & Galloway	819	1
Fife	2035	3
Forth Valley	1126	2
Grampian	11627	17
Greater Glasgow	18327	26
Highland	2158	3
Lanark	2083	3
Lothian	17581	25
Orkney	21	–
Shetland	72	–
Tayside	11461	16
Western Isles	141	–
NHS Shetland	47	–
State Hospital	12	–
Total	69783	100

Glasgow, which ended up with the lion's share of teaching funding. Funding has now become more equitable with recognition of the contribution to undergraduate education provided by 'non-teaching' hospitals and health boards. However, a 'glide path' of allocation has been established to ensure that the old teaching hospitals maintain their financial stability.

Historical background to SIFT

When SIFT first came into existence in 1975, its express purpose was to improve the quality of undergraduate medical education in NHS hospitals. It also had a latent purpose, however, of compensating hospitals for the costs arising from the additional demands placed on them by the presence of medical students (Bevan, 1999). This additional funding was meant to ensure a 'level playing field' in providing teaching hospitals with resources to cover infrastructure costs associated with teaching, for example classrooms, interview rooms and lounges for students. On average, teaching hospitals were 30% more expensive per patient than non-teaching hospitals (Department of Health and Social Security, 1976) and SIFT funding was used to finance this.

Over the decades, this excess payment to these trusts persisted, irrespective of whether the facilities were currently being used for education. Various formulae were devised to calculate SIFT funding (Department of Health and Social Security, 1980; Foote *et al*, 1988), but in general they have been criticised, as the excess costs are not necessarily associated with teaching medical undergraduates (Bevan, 1999). In practice, it is difficult to separate the individual excess costs due to clinical research, postgraduate training, nursing and other non-medical training from undergraduate training. Another major criticism concerned the failure of the formulae to redress the historic inequity of the major teaching hospitals, especially those in London, being subsidised on account of their traditionally larger numbers of medical students (Sheldon, 1992). There was empirical evidence for this, as the median excess costs varied widely, from 50% higher costs in London to 12% lower costs in provincial teaching hospitals (Foote *et al*, 1988). It was felt that these significantly higher costs in London teaching hospitals meant that the whole process of calculating excess costs of teaching was a self-justifying circular exercise offering a rationale for expensive service delivery.

Readers interested in the details of the historical origins are referred to the excellent reviews by Clack *et al* (1999) and Bevan (1999).

SIFT: current system

The Winyard report (NHS Executive, 1995) reviewed the inequities in SIFT funding and recommended the current system, which has two separate budget streams: one based on student numbers, which accounts for 20% of the funding and can be calculated based on student weeks in placement; and another reflecting 'facilities costs', which accounts for the other 80% and supports training costs. The 20/80 split was not explained in the report but may have been based on the study by Foote *et al* (1988), which found that 78% of the additional SIFT funding could be attributed to indirect teaching costs.

The Winyard report advocated a move towards funding based on demonstrated costs rather than a fixed per capita funding based on student numbers. This would allow accountability and flexibility in funding. This 'demonstrated costs' model was used in the case of the funding for the four new medical schools in the UK, for which funding was based on costings determined by competitive bidding (Medical Academic Staff Committee, 2007). However, it was also recognised that suddenly withdrawing the historic funding would destabilise the finances of some trusts. The facilities costs thus maintain the historic excess funding of NHS teaching hospitals, while facilitating the move towards a model based on demonstrated costs. It was also hoped that this format of funding would promote positive changes in the delivery of medical education, with financial incentives linked to performance.

Problems with SIFT

The new funding arrangements were meant to promote accountability, innovation and quality of education, but the reality is that trusts have found it difficult to link SIFT money to specific outcomes. As indicated in the Department of Health's own accountability reports, it is not known how recipient trusts use SIFT money (Department of Health, 2003). As discussed below, this is owing to the inherent difficulty in apportioning the additional costs involved in teaching. There is, however, another systemic problem: NHS trusts have traditionally been lax in tracking SIFT money, which can disappear into general trust funds. For cash-strapped NHS trusts, SIFT moneys can offer a relatively easy way of funding NHS spending overspends (Department of Health, 2006). There have been reports of SIFT money having been used to shore up central contingency funds (Hitchen, 2007). In a tightly controlled world of clinical and corporate governance, with NHS trusts subjected to routine financial and clinical audits to ensure delivery of key targets, the relatively unsupervised SIFT funding stream can be quite vulnerable.

A 2007 survey showed that 50% of NHS trusts were unable to account for how their SIFT funding had been used (Medical Academic Staff Committee, 2007). For many, there is no mechanism to ring-fence SIFT income, as they lack an education business unit and so SIFT moneys tend to end up in one business directorate or another without any direct links to actual teaching-related expenses. This makes it difficult to differentiate between NHS clinical costs and NHS teaching costs, which allows SIFT money to be amalgamated into the NHS trusts' baseline income pot (Gutenstein, 2000). This has downstream effects. For example, there is very little correlation between SIFT allocation and 'teaching programmed activities' in consultants' job plans. Instead, many trusts seem to allocate one nominal programmed activity for teaching; this has little relationship to actual teaching activity (Medical Academic Staff Committee, 2007). The upstream effect is that there is a very tenuous link between the funding of medical education and rational development of the workforce. In the 1996–97 allocation, 90% of all SIFT money was allocated to acute teaching trusts, with the other teaching sites (including primary care clinics, community clinics and psychiatric hospitals) left to battle for the rest.

Another problem is the validity of the SIFT formula. It is difficult to calculate the costs of an out-patient clinic running more slowly because of the presence of medical students, along with the costs of the facilities (additional chairs for medical students, larger rooms, etc.). Yet trusts offering brief placements, as is the case in psychiatry, lose out on facilities funding, as the bulk of such funding goes to the larger acute trusts. Moreover, the SIFT placement costs are based on per capita costs of teaching in clinical years, calculated as student weeks. With vertical integration of curricula and the introduction of curricula centred on problem-based learning (PBL) in some schools (e.g. Derby Medical School, Liverpool Medical School), clinical teaching begins in year 1 and makes the per capita formula inaccurate, if not redundant. There are also difficulties of overlap with other funding streams such as MADEL and NMET, as the same patient may be facilitating the teaching of postgraduate trainees as well as nursing students.

Current SIFT arrangements do not support integration of teaching between disciplines. Dave *et al* (2010) have cited the difficulty in apportioning the costs of teaching students on a psychiatry placement learning about dual diagnosis in a primary care drug and alcohol clinic. It is not clear whether these costs should be paid from the mental health trust SIFT income or from the primary care trust's SIFT income. Such a flat per capita funding arrangement creates rigidity and a perverse disincentive to developing flexible teaching (e.g. teaching in a variety of settings better suited to students' learning needs and to local resources or circumstances).

The situation in Scotland, Wales and Northern Ireland

In light of all of the above problems with SIFT in England, it is perhaps not surprising that funding for student teaching varies across the UK. Before moving on to consider the other countries of the UK, it may be interesting to note funding variations in these countries (Table 22.2).

Table 22.2 Allocations for medical student education in the nations of the UK, 2008–09

Country	Funding body	Total budget (£1 000 000s)	Student numbers	Costs per student per year (£1000s)
England	SIFT	844.9	18512	27.3
Scotland	Medical ACT	69.8	3645	18.7
Wales	SIFT	50.6	1750	25.7
Northern Ireland	SUMDE	29.6	1154	25.7

Scotland

In Scotland, ACT monies also date back to the 1970s, when there was an acknowledgement that teaching hospitals were more expensive to run than non-teaching hospitals, but, historically, as with SIFT, the funding was not ring-fenced for teaching and was absorbed into other budgets without a clear system of identifying how exactly it was being used to enhance undergraduate medical education (Eagles, 2005). Initially, ACT funding had been divided into the 'direct costs' (based on the cost of delivering the curriculum in a clinical environment) of supporting medical undergraduate teaching, and the 'indirect costs' incurred by the four teaching health boards in providing a range of specialist services. When SEHD transferred the responsibility for managing the direct element of ACT funding to NES, the indirect costs (including capital charges) were redistributed to all boards, as part of their Arbuthnott formula allocation.

A report by the Standing Committee on Resource Allocation (2003) made the fundamental change that saw ACT being paid directly to boards based on activity. As a result, medical schools wrote up memoranda of understanding with partner health boards. Service-level agreements then followed, after the introduction of the new consultant contract in Scotland in 2003 (Scottish Executive Health Department, 2004) Generally, one programmed activity or 10% of a consultant's salary is assumed to be funded by ACT, but this is an approximation useful for broad, but not detailed, evaluation of departmental teaching time. This is not always reflected in individual job plans, where undergraduate and postgraduate teaching are often calculated together and/ or not reflected in a realistic way.

There is more clarity with new ACT funding, as described below, but historic funding remains hidden and difficult to extract, in a similar fashion to that described above (see 'Problems with SIFT'). Changes in 2004 brought in new, more formal and transparent mechanisms to ensure the provision of clinical teaching and the appropriate funds to support it; these funds were more insulated than previously against the resource pressures of the NHS (McKillop, 2006).

One of the key innovations when NES assumed responsibility was the use of *performance management* to achieve best value and clear accountability. The other admirable stated key aims were to deliver the highest possible quality of medical education within the NHS and to ensure a transparent and equitable approach by trying to find fairer means of distributing the ACT budget. Each regional area group appointed an ACT officer (usually university appointments, with the exception of Dundee, where the ACT officer is employed by the NHS), whose role it is to ensure accountability, and systems were put in place regarding detailed accountability criteria, by which proposals for the use of new ACT funding would be approved.

A set of guiding principles was agreed at the outset. These included an open and transparent approach, the use of one national rate for all teaching, equity of approach across Scotland, equity of funding for teaching in hospital and primary care settings, and the use of Scottish Funding Council student numbers to drive the overall allocation model. That allocation model gives total ACT funding to university medical school areas based on their total number of medical students funded by the Scottish Funding Council in that area, but the money, instead of being transferred directly, is allocated to all the health board areas delivering teaching to students from that school; for example, students from Edinburgh are placed in Forth Valley, Fife, Lanarkshire and Borders areas (see Table 22.1).

NES has developed a range of national quality standards for undergraduate teaching. The National System of Student Evaluation looks at several domains of student satisfaction, such as teaching facilities, the organisation of teaching, the delivery of scheduled teaching, opportunities for learning and clinical experience, the availability of educational and pastoral support, and the form of assessment.

There will also be a major evaluation or measurement of teaching within the NHS, looking at activity and considering what NHS teachers actually do and how much time it takes. Three categories of teaching duties are recognised (NHS Education for Scotland, 2009):

- teaching during the course of clinical service as part of clinical attachments (e.g. ward rounds, surgeries, theatre sessions)
- teaching where the student is the focus of activity (e.g. lectures, PBL sessions, project supervision)
- activities in support of teaching (e.g. administrative duties, mentoring, staff development).

Exactly how new ACT funding has been used in Scotland quite rightly varies across the country but includes new appointments (e.g. clinical teaching fellows and specialty teaching leads), payment of undergraduate travel and subsistence (to facilitate placements in more rural and remote settings, especially in primary care), funding of additional consultant teaching sessions, part funding of larger projects such as the Mathew Hay Project in Aberdeen, improved teaching facilities, and additional placements, for example in primary care (NHS Education for Scotland, 2009).

New ACT funding has also been used to promote staff development, particularly the acquisition of specific higher educational qualifications and innovations in e-learning and other technologies.

Wales

Welsh SIFT operates similarly to SIFT in England but the medical SIFT is further divided into hospital SIFT (which includes both placement and facilities SIFT) and general practice SIFT. The Welsh assembly government (WAG) oversees the entire SIFT allocation process, from setting the actual amount to the allocation to the various trusts and general practices. A hierarchical management structure ensures a chain of accountability to the WAG from the trusts receiving SIFT funds.

Northern Ireland

In Northern Ireland, SUMDE includes funding for joint university–NHS clinical academic posts as well as dental and medical SUMDE. Similar to England, medical SUMDE includes student placement funding and funding for infrastructure (facilities) (Department of Health, Social Services and Public Safety, 2008).

Funding issues specific to undergraduate psychiatric education

Mental health trusts are not immune to the financial pressures within the NHS or to the general reduction in the number of clinical academics (Department of Health, 2004). The new contract for consultants, with well-defined job plans and the creation of new specialist teams, should have created more time for supported professional activities such as teaching, but a 2008 survey suggested that medical student education, once an integral part of most consultant psychiatrists' work, has now been crowded out of an ever more pressurised job plan. Even if the time is part of the contract, heavy clinical commitments may mean teaching is still not delivered (Dogra *et al*, 2008). Under such circumstances, it is not surprising that paying attention to funding arrangements for medical education may not be top priority for clinical psychiatrists.

Mental health trusts are small players in the SIFT allocation but many trusts provide anything from 4 to 10 weeks of medical student placements (Karim *et al*, 2009). In the current funding system, most mental health trusts are not eligible for any facilities payments, as they offer placements amounting to less than 5% of the total duration of medical school teaching. However, it is not clear if all the trusts are getting even the full placement costs to which they are entitled.

Psychiatry has possibly been more affected by the recent increase in the number of medical students (House of Commons Health Select Committee, 2007). Patient contact is the cornerstone of clinical care and yet in psychiatry there is pressure on contact time with patients on account of dispersed community care and the creation of specialist teams. This has led to a reduction in the number of in-patients and in-patient facilities, where most medical student education has traditionally been delivered.

This is a difficult time for the profession, as it faces a recruitment crisis (Royal College of Psychiatrists, 2009; see also Chapters 20 and 21), with fewer medical graduates taking up psychiatry. Moreover, the stigma affecting the profession is persistent (Dogra *et al*, 2008). And yet, such threats also offer opportunities. The curricular guidelines produced by the General Medical Council (2003) clearly outline the importance of communication skills, the teaching of which psychiatrists are often best placed to deliver. The relative paucity of in-patients offers opportunities to deliver psychiatric teaching in primary care settings and to involve volunteer patients (Tew *et al*, 2004) or simulated patients (Eagles *et al*, 2007) in teaching medical students. Setting up such innovative programmes requires funding, but the current SIFT arrangements do not facilitate this. In Scotland, there is potential for medical ACT to do just this, and examples already exist.

Future directions: measurement of teaching and performance management indicators

NES has taken a lead in developing performance standards, by introducing the idea of measurement of the quantity and quality of undergraduate medical teaching, through standardised student evaluations of placement and teaching.

It is clear that the principle of funding following the student is widely accepted. However, a rigid adherence to funding by student weeks is likely to stifle innovation. The Winyard report intended to address some of the problems in SIFT funding by attempting to create a direct link between demonstrable activity and payment and by improving accountability (Department of Health, 2000). Demonstration of educational activity/ teaching requires a measure that is transparent and easily understood. Such a measure should reflect both the quantity and the quality of teaching. At present, the only measures are student weeks (one student multiplied by the number of clinical sessions), weighted student weeks (weighted by a multiple of 2 or 3 for years 1–3, in recognition of the fact that students at that stage need more supervision) and 'teaching units' (e.g. one member of staff teaching six students for one session).

While the use of these measures introduces the idea of payment by results (PbR) in teaching, there are several issues that cause concern, particularly in psychiatry. Quantifying a teaching unit in psychiatry is difficult, as a student may do a home visit with two staff members, and teaching ofen takes place in a multidisciplinary setting such as ward round or team meetings. More and more medical schools are also introducing interprofessional learning and appointing nurse educators or service user teachers. There are also inherent problems in measuring the quality of teaching in psychiatry – how can one measure effective teaching of the skills of reflection, therapeutic engagement or attitude change?

Another major concern is that the PbR model would drive funding away from universities to NHS institutions, with the risk of slanting medical training towards a technical, protocol-based training. A fixed teaching unit tariff across the board in the NHS may disadvantage medical student education *vis-à-vis* healthcare education for nurses, social workers and allied medical health professionals. This may be a real concern, especially for the newer medical schools, which have received generous SIFT funding (for facilities and placements) and may find their ring-fenced SIFT budgets being merged with the general MPET funds. This has prompted the suggestion that funding should be based on staffing costs rather than on a fixed placement or teaching unit cost (Department of Health, Social Services and Public Safety, 2008). Other concerns relate to the financial risks that some trusts may face if the new model is introduced quickly. Similar risks apply to some universities in relation to HEFCE funding if funding for the preclinical teaching years is diverted to NHS trusts.

Despite these difficulties, there is broad support for the introduction of a transparent system of costing and delivery of medical education. Introducing a demonstrated costs model does carry some risks and there are barriers to change, just as there are advantages in shoring up the status quo. These are summarised in Box 22.1.

Box 22.1 Advantages of a 'demonstrated costs' model and the barriers to change

Advantages

- Transparent
- Flexible; allows local innovation
- Linked to educational outcomes, so gives greater accountability
- Potentially greater than 'usual' income is possible, as income is linked to demonstrated costs

Barriers to change

- Fixed and assured income (although educational costs may actually outstrip income)
- Difficult to implement where there is no fresh money (e.g. if money has been disbursed among all consultants as an additional programmed activity)
- Needs resources for monitoring and administration; perceived difficulty in switching to a new system
- Lack of proactive 'bidding' may lead to mental health trusts losing out on their share
- Individual enthusiasm to teach may be lost by the 'commercialisation of teaching'

Summary

WAG in Wales and NES in Scotland have put in place educational governance structures and it is likely that similar changes will be introduced in England and Northern Ireland.

Improving accountability by linking funding to demonstrable teaching activity will allow clinical teachers to influence the funding mechanisms for medical education, which in turn will have a significant influence on the quality, organisation and delivery of teaching. There is evidence to show that good educational governance, with a transparent use of funds, can be linked to the successful delivery of education. The quantity and quality of educational provision can be monitored, and educational outcomes measured against funding (Badcock *et al*, 2006). Examples of good educational governance have been reported in psychiatry (Dave *et al*, 2010). A closer working relationship is needed between the universities and NHS trusts to recognise joint priorities, to reduce territorialism and to facilitate the creation of joint clinical academic posts with clearly defined job plans.

Robust educational leadership is vital to ensure that delivery of psychiatric education is fit for purpose, particularly in view of the challenges faced by the profession, and to ensure that psychiatry does not lose out to more technical disciplines. Awareness of the funding issues described in this chapter should strengthen the hands of teachers when negotiating for staff time and resources. Teaching psychiatric skills and attitudes to medical students is resource intensive and may involve, for example, the use of simulated patients or patient volunteers as well as the creative use of web-based and other resources. Clinical academics in psychiatry, in conjunction with professional bodies such as the Royal College of Psychiatrists, need to be involved in ensuring that the new funding mechanisms are used to the advantage of psychiatry as a profession. The integration or embedding of psychiatric teaching in curricula would be ideal, and such a strategy is supported by *No Health Without Mental Health*, which highlights that all doctors should be trained to recognise mental disorder and the links between mental and physical health (Academy of Medical Royal Colleges, 2009).

Clinical teaching of undergraduates needs to be highlighted as a priority in the NHS and with appropriate recognition and remuneration (for example in job planning and clinical excellence and distinction awards), as well as through further funded training and staff development for those who choose to teach.

References

Academy of Royal Medical Colleges (2009) *No Health Without Mental Health – The Alert Summary Report*. Academy of Medical Royal Colleges. Available at http://www.rcpsych.ac.uk/pdf/ALERT%20print%20final.pdf

Badcock, L. J., Raj, N., Gadsby, K., *et al* (2006) Meeting the needs of increasing numbers of medical students – a best practise approach. *Rheumatology*, **45**, 899–903.

Bevan, G. (1999) The medical service increment for teaching: a 400m (pounds sterling) anachronism for the English NHS? – SIFT– Education and debate. *BMJ*, **319**, 908–911.

Catto, G. R. D. (2000) Interface between university and medical school: the way ahead? *BMJ*, **328**, 1347–1352.

Clack, G. B., Bevan, G. & Eddleston, A. L. W. F. (1999) Service Increment for Teaching (SIFT): a review of its origins, development and current role in supporting undergraduate medical education in England and Wales. *Medical Education*, **33**, 350–358.

Dave, S., Dogra, N. & Leask, S. (2010) Current role of service increment for teaching funding in psychiatry. *The Psychiatrist*, **34**, 31–35.

Department of Health (2000) *Service Increment for Teaching (SIFT) Accountability Report 1999–2000.* DH. Available at http://www.dh.gov.uk/en/Publicationsandstatistics/Publications/PublicationsPolicyAndGuidance/DH_4139368

Department of Health (2003) *Funding Streams to Support Continuing the Work in Teaching PCTs.* DH. Available at http://www.dh.gov.uk/assetRoot/04/02/04/34/04020434.pdf

Department of Health (2004) *Medical Schools: Delivering Doctors of the Future.* DH. Available at http://www.dh.gov.uk/prod_consum_dh/groups/dh_digitalassets/@dh/@en/documents/digitalasset/dh_4075406.pdf

Department of Health (2006) *NHS Financial Performance – Quarter 1 2006–2007.* Available at http://www.dh.gov.uk/en/Publicationsandstatistics/Publications/PublicationsPolicyAndGuidance/DH_064747

Department of Health (2008) *High Quality Care For All. NHS Next Stage Review Final Report.* DH. Available at http://www.dh.gov.uk/en/Publicationsandstatistics/Publications/PublicationsPolicyAndGuidance/DH_085825

Department of Health and Social Security (1976) *Sharing Resources for Health in England: The Report of the Resource Allocation Working Party* (the RAWP report). HMSO.

Department of Health and Social Security (1980) *Report of the Advisory Group on Resource Allocations* (rhe AGRA report). DHSS.

Department of Health, Social Services and Public Safety (2008) *Review and Modernisation of Supplement for Undergraduate Medical and Dental Education (SUMDE).* DHSSPS Northern Ireland. Available at http://www.dhsspsni.gov.uk/consultation-document-draft-sumde-review.pdf

Dogra, N., Edwards, R., Karim, K., *et al* (2008) Current issues in undergraduate psychiatry education: the findings of a qualitative study. *Advances in Health Sciences Education*, **13**, 309–323.

Eagles, J. M. (2005) Should the NHS revise its role in medical education? *Scottish Medical Journal*, **50**, 144–147.

Eagles, J. M. Calder, S. & Wilson, S. (2007) Simulated patients in undergraduate education in psychiatry. *Psychiatric Bulletin*, **31**, 187–190.

Foote, G., Hurst, J. & Sondheimer, P. (1988) *Technical Paper on the Service Increment for Teaching (Review of the Resource Allocation Working Party Formula).* Economic Advisers' Office, DHSS.

General Medical Council (2003) *Tomorrow's Doctors* (2nd edn). GMC.

Gutenstein, M. (2000) How much? The price of medical education. *Student British Medical Journal*, **8**, 1–44.

Hitchen, L. (2007) Robbing Peter to pay Paul. *BMJ*, **334**, 388–389.

House of Commons Health Select Committee (2007) *NHS Deficits – First Report of Session 2006–07.* The Stationery Office. Available at http://www.publications.parliament.uk/pa/cm200607/cmselect/cmhealth/73/73i.pdf

Karim, K., Edwards, R., Dogra, N., *et al* (2009) A survey of the teaching and assessment of undergraduate psychiatry in the medical schools of the United Kingdom and Ireland: undergraduate psychiatry: what's going on? *Medical Teacher*, **31**, 1024–1029.

McKillop, J. H. (2006) Undergraduate medical education in Scotland, 1955 and 2005. *Scottish Medical Journal*, **51**, 23–26.

Medical Academic Staff Committee (2007) *Medical Service Increment For Teaching (SIFT) Funding Report*. British Medical Association. Available at http://www.bma.org.uk/images/Siftreport_tcm41-147112.pdf

NHS Education for Scotland (2009) *Scottish Report on Medical ACT*. NES. Available at http://www.nes.scot.nhs.uk/media/5782/mqmg04medicalactbrochure.pdf

NHS Executive (1995) *SIFT into the Future: Future Arrangements for Allocating Funds and Contracting for NHS Service Support and Facilities for Teaching Undergraduate Medical Students* (the Winyard report). NHS Executive.

Royal College of Psychiatrists (2009) *Dean's Newsletter*, May. RCPsych.

Scally, G. & Donaldson, L. J. (1998) Clinical governance and the drive for quality improvement in the new NHS in England. *BMJ*, **317**, 61–65.

Scottish Executive Health Department (2004) *Treatment of Teaching, Training and Research Under the New Consultant Contract and Development of Memoranda of Understanding Between Universities and NHS Boards* (HDL (2004) 25). Scottish executive. Available at http://www.sehd.scot.nhs.uk/mels/hdl2004_25.pdf

Sheldon, T. (1992) Service increment for teaching and research. *BMJ*, **305**, 310.

Standing Committee of Resource Allocation in NHS Scotland (2003) *Research on Additional Costs of Teaching in NHS Scotland. Final Report*. SCRA.

Tew, J., Gell, C. & Foster, S. (2004) *Learning from Experience: Involving Service Users and Carers in Mental Health Education and Training*. Mental Health in Higher Education, National Institute for Mental Health in England (West Midlands) Trent Workforce Development Confederation.

CHAPTER 23

Dealing with students in difficulty

Richard Day

Introduction

Medical students are a highly selected group. The selection criteria include intellectual ability, academic success and also, to a degree, professional qualities such as diligence and reliability. The selection process is competitive and often rigorous. Nevertheless, it is not uncommon for medical students to encounter difficulties during the course that have an impact on their academic ability, professionalism, or both. Sometimes these difficulties will also have implications for patient safety or fitness to practise.

All doctors, at whatever stage of their education and training, have a responsibility to ensure both their own professional competence and also that of their colleagues. This presents challenges, first in the identification of failing or difficult students, and second in the provision of appropriate feedback to them. Following, among others, the well publicised inquiry into children's heart surgery at Bristol (Department of Health, 2001) and the Shipman inquiry (http://www.the-shipman-inquiry.org.uk), there has been an increased focus on education and training and the need to identify poor performance. Changes in medical education at both undergraduate (General Medical Council, 2003) and postgraduate (Department of Health, 2003) levels have been made to ensure the profession is more accountable. The main driver for this is patient safety.

One of the difficulties in ensuring that poor performance is identified as early as possible is the development of a robust system of appraisal and assessment at each stage of training. In addition, the culture in which this is carried out is important to ensure relevant information on performance is available. The recognition of problem behaviours in students in a complex healthcare environment is often difficult and is influenced by the numbers of students, the length of attachments, and changes in curricular programmes and consequent expectations. In addition, the effect of personal problems on professional performance requires the judgement of the tutor or supervisor.

Good Medical Practice (General Medical Council, 2006) identifies the need for all doctors to be 'honest and objective when appraising or assessing the performance of colleagues, including locums and students. Patients will be put at risk if you describe as competent someone who has not reached or maintained a satisfactory standard of practice.'

Many tutors are often concerned with how to classify the problems identified. This can often be done using the curriculum framework on which the tutor has been asked to provide evidence of the student's performance during the attachment. One of the commonest difficulties experienced in dealing with failing or difficult students is in the collection and documentation of the relevant information. The other issue that tutors often find difficult to address is how and when to let students know that there are concerns about their performance. These are often difficult decisions to make, and although tutors should always feel able to discuss them with colleagues in the medical school, it is not always clear what the mechanism for this should be. A clinical teacher may not be familiar with medical school structures and policies, and a tutor whose role is primarily that of pastoral support may feel a conflict of interest between the support of the student and the communication of concerns to the medical school. Until recently, remediation and the provision of extra learning programmes have not been readily available.

Recognising the problem

'Problem students' can present in a number of ways. There may be evidence of academic failure, in terms of either knowledge or practical skills. The failure may be a summative failure of a whole year or of a particular module of teaching. Alternatively, it may be identified in a formative assessment or simply in formal or informal teaching activities. Other problem students may present arise from concerns about their attitudes or behaviour (General Medical Council, 2007).

Examples would be:

- non-engagement with the course – poor attendance at classes
- non-participation in tutorials, especially in any group work or other team-based activities
- non-completion of course work
- not responding to communications from the medical school
- inappropriate behaviours – discriminatory language or attitudes
- bullying
- unprofessional standards or appearance or clothing
- a lack of respect for patient confidentiality
- cheating – submission of work that is not their own, plagiarism, or cheating in examinations.

Understanding the problem

The variety of modes of presentation of 'problem students' is mirrored by a variety of different causes, with no necessary correlation of cause to presentation. There is some evidence that students who failed a final-year examination were more likely to have encountered problems, and have lower mean scores, in earlier examinations when compared with students who passed the final examination (Cleland *et al*, 2005). However, previous academic failure is not a necessary condition for current problems.

Some students, despite performing successfully enough to gain entry into medical school, nevertheless have problems with study technique or with examination technique. These problems may become apparent only later in the medical course, when the demands and expectations become greater, or when poor technique is combined with some other problem or stress. Poor study techniques often involve an overemphasis on rote knowledge, poor focus on the objectives or outcomes required by the course, poor time management with consequent failure to cover all that is required, or an inability to limit the depth of study in one area, with associated failure to study another area in enough depth. Sometimes students attempt to use study methods that do not complement their strongly preferred learning style, for example when a kinaesthetic learner tries to study by writing and rewriting notes (Burns, 2006).

Health problems are a frequent difficulty and mental health problems especially so. Rates of depressive symptoms in medical students have been measured using a variety of self-report instruments (Stecker, 2004; Dahlin *et al*, 2005; Tjia *et al*, 2005; Levine *et al*, 2006; Goebert *et al*, 2009), with estimates of moderate to severe depression ranging from 5–10% up to 25% of students reporting depressive symptoms. Rates of depression in medical students are typically found to be higher than in other student populations. The effects of significant depression on motivation, concentration and other cognitive functions are likely to lead to poor performance at medical school.

Other mental health conditions tend to be less frequently a problem but can have specific effects on the way a student presents with problems. For example, students with significant obsessive symptoms may be unable to hand in written course work for fear that it is not good enough or may feel that they have to know everything about each subject and therefore be unable to cover the breadth of knowledge required.

It is also clear that students with mental health problems are reluctant to notify the medical faculty of this. The stigmatisation of mental health problems is exacerbated in medical students, as many worry that it will count against them in some way (Givens & Tjia, 2002; Chew-Graham *et al*, 2003). For medical students with depression, for example, specific worries (if it became known they had the condition) include: that they will not be allowed to continue to study medicine; that it will be recorded on their academic record; that they will be perceived as being weak; that they will not be successful in getting jobs in the future; and, importantly, that it will not be kept confidential.

Aside from health problems, failing students often have a variety of other stressors in their lives. This may include ill health in a family member or friend. If that person is geographically distant, the student may feel very concerned but ultimately helpless; on the other hand, if that person is close enough, the student may spend a considerable time in travel and visits, and may even provide care. All this affects their ability to study. Bereavements will have a marked and sustained effect on a student's ability to study and perform (Dyrbye *et al*, 2006; Dunn *et al*, 2008).

Interpersonal friction can also be a factor – whether between the student and parents, the student and flatmates, or with the student as the third party affected by friction between others.

Financial and debt concerns can have a considerable affect (Ross *et al*, 2006). This may be in terms of worry as to where finances will be found for course fees or subsistence; or may be the effect of trying to study medicine while working almost full time as well.

As with mental health problems, students who present as 'problems' have often not sought appropriate help or support from family or faculty and have instead allowed a problem to develop and grow until it causes significant academic problems, rather than seek help at an earlier stage.

Communicating the problem

If concerns are identified about a student's academic or clinical performance, or attitudes and behaviour, it is important to communicate this to the student in as helpful and therefore effective a way as possible. The provision of this constructive, albeit negative, feedback is important, whether the issue is of poor performance on a clinical attachment, or failure in final summative examinations. There can be a reluctance to give this

---

Box 23.1 Pendleton's rules

After a specific activity that the student has performed and the tutor has observed, or at the end of a clinical attachment or module of teaching:

- students are asked to comment on what they thought they did well
- the tutor adds comments on what else was done well
- students are asked what they would want to do differently next time (i.e. what they didn't do so well)
- the tutor suggests and discusses what the student may wish to change on the next occasion

---

Box 23.2 The SET-GO framework

- *What the student **saw***. This should be descriptive, specific and non-judgemental. (The tutor may then prompt if necessary with either or both of the next two steps.)
- *What **else** the student saw* (e.g. 'What happened next?'). Again, this should be in descriptive terms.
- *What does the student **think**?* Reflection by the student, who is then given an opportunity to acknowledge and problem solve.
- *Clarify the **goal** to be achieved*. An outcome-based approach should be used.
- *Any **offers** of help or advice on how to achieve the goal* (suggestions and alternatives).

---

type of negative feedback. There may be a concern that this information will prove harmful rather than helpful, that it will upset the student or be rejected as unfair (Brown & Cooke, 2009). Without this kind of feedback, though, the problems are unlikely to be addressed.

There are various models that can provide a useful framework for the giving of feedback. Pendleton's rules (Pendleton *et al*, 2003) focus on a four-stage structure (Box 23.1). An alternative structure that has been suggested is the SET-GO framework (Silverman *et al*, 1997) (Box 23.2).

Other suggestions on how to give feedback (particularly feedback that is essentially negative) emphasise some of the qualities of effective feedback rather than simply the process. Thus, feedback should be given on the basis of what has been observed by the tutor (rather than being entirely based on what someone else has observed). It should be given soon after the event rather than after a delay, during which memories become less clear. Feedback should be clear and unambiguous so that it cannot be misunderstood or avoided. Also, it should be as specific as possible – give examples rather than speaking in generalisations: 'You would have done better to ask an open question when you asked about sleep disturbance' rather than 'You ask too may closed questions'. It is also suggested that feedback be 'owned' and personalised, in that the tutor should say 'I think … you would have done

---

Box 23.3 CORBS

- Clear – don't be vague
- Owned – in giving feedback, give your own perception
- Regular – give soon after the event, so students can use the feedback to make changes
- Balanced – discuss strengths as well as weaknesses
- Specific – generalisations are never very helpful, so always give examples

---

better to ask an open question when you asked about sleep disturbance' rather than to speak in absolutes.

As in the two models of the structure of giving feedback, it is suggested that it is helpful to ask students what they think first of all, before giving your opinion; and also that it is good to be balanced (i.e. cover strengths as well as weaknesses). Much of this is summarised in the CORBS acronym (Box 23.3).

Addressing the problem

Given the wide variety of potential problems, it is important, with any 'problem student', specifically to look for background causative factors. Whether with academic failure or unprofessional behaviour, there may be mitigating factors that affect the response given to the student.

Decisions need to be made about the extent of the problem and thus the extent of the response. Some students need merely to be directed to suitable sources of help and support. Others may need to resubmit course work, repeat modules of teaching or resit examinations. Less frequently the best option is for a student to take temporary withdrawal from studies (for example to recover from illness) and even less frequently it may be necessary to suspend students from their studies.

Medical students are often initially resistant to the suggestion of these measures. As mentioned above, there is a feeling of having not to appear 'weak' or in need of 'help' and a fear that a career in medicine will be jeopardised. Students need to be allowed time to consider the options but may well agree, for example, to take temporary withdrawal on health grounds. If, however, students lack insight into their problems, then, occasionally, suspension of studies, with or without fitness-to-practise procedures, is necessary.

There are likely to be a number of supports available to students that they may either be unaware of or have intentionally avoided. If there are health problems, then they should be directed to their general practitioner or student health services. For mental health problems, the accreditation standards of the US Liaison Committee on Medical Education (2008) state that 'The health professionals who provide psychiatric/psychological counseling or other sensitive health services to medical students must have no involvement in the academic evaluation or promotion of the students receiving those services'. This should reduce student concerns about confidentiality and academic progress and also reduce the potential for a conflict of interest in the psychiatrist. However, there is an argument that psychiatrists involved in the curriculum are in a better position to help the student and also that to follow this guidance may simply increase the stigma of psychiatric illness by its identification as 'sensitive' and the requirement for it to be handled differently to other 'non-sensitive' illnesses (Kavan *et al*, 2008).

Various support services are usually available within universities and medical schools, such as student counselling services, financial guidance, academic support and study skills, and disability services. Often as well, a medical school will have a student support or pastoral care scheme, whereby a tutor or teacher will offer academic or non-academic support to a small number of students. These systems do not always work very effectively, but in circumstances where a student is identified as having difficulties, the arrangement of specific academic or pastoral support can be of benefit.

Additionally, a medical school may have an identified committee whose remit is to monitor, in a supportive way, the progress of students who have been identified as having problems or who are in need of specific support. This committee would also be in a position to make decisions about referral to fitness-to-practise procedures (General Medical Council, 2007).

Summary

It is important to acknowledge that a significant minority of medical students do encounter problems during the course of their studies. These problems arise from the usual combination of academic, relationship, social, financial and health pressures, and can often have an impact on a student's academic performance or professional behaviour. There is an expectation that these behaviours will be recognised and that struggling students will be provided with support (General Medical Council, 2009, domain 6). Medical schools therefore have a responsibility to develop clear processes to deal with students with problems.

Those who are involved in teaching students need to be aware of the ways in which problems present and the variety of factors behind them. They also need to develop the skills, in terms of giving useful and effective feedback, to be able to help students identify the ways in which they are struggling and to formulate a plan to change or improve.

References

Brown, N. & Cooke, L. (2009) Giving effective feedback to psychiatric trainees. *Advances in Psychiatric Treatment*, **15**, 123–128.

Burns, E. R. (2006) Learning syndromes afflicting beginning medical students: identification and treatment – reflections after forty years of teaching. *Medical Teacher*, **28**, 230–233.

Chew-Graham, C. A., Rogers, A. & Yassin, N. (2003) 'I wouldn't want it on my CV or their records': medical students' experiences of help-seeking for mental health problems. *Medical Education*, **37**, 873–880.

Cleland, J., Arnold R. & Chesser, A. (2005) Failing finals is often a surprise for the student but not the teacher: identifying difficulties and supporting students with academic difficulties. *Medical Teacher*, **27**, 504–508.

Dahlin, M., Joneborg, N. & Runeson, B. (2005) Stress and depression among medical students: a cross-sectional study. *Medical Education*, **39**, 594–604.

Department of Health (2001) *The Report of the Public Inquiry into Children's Heart Surgery at the Bristol Royal Infirmary 1984–1995: Learning from Bristol* (CM 5207(I)). DH.

Department of Health (2003) *Modernising Medical Careers. The Response of the Four UK Health Ministers to the Consultation on Unfinished Business: Proposals for Reform of the Senior House Officer Grade.* DH.

Dunn, L. B., Iglewicz, A. & Moutier, C. (2008) A conceptual model of medical student well-being: promoting resilience and preventing burnout. *Academic Psychiatry*, **32**, 44–53.

Dyrbye, L. N., Thomas, M. R., Huntington, J. L., *et al* (2006) Personal life events and medical student burnout: a multicenter study. *Academic Medicine*, **81**, 374–384.

General Medical Council (2003) *Tomorrow's Doctors* (2dn edn). GMC.

General Medical Council (2006) *Good Medical Practice*. GMC.

General Medical Council (2007) *Medical Students: Professional Behaviour and Fitness to Practise.* GMC.

General Medical Council (2009) *Tomorrow's Doctors* (3rd edn). GMC.

Givens, J. L. & Tjia, J.(2002) Depressed medical students' use of mental health services and barriers to use. *Academic Medicine*, **77**, 918–921.

Goebert, D., Thompson, D., Takeshita, J., *et al* (2009) Depressive symptoms in medical students and residents: a multischool study. *Academic Medicine*, **84**, 236–241.

Kavan, M. G., Malin, P. J. & Wilson, D. R. (2008) The role of academic psychiatry faculty in the treatment and subsequent evaluation and promotion of medical students: an ethical conundrum. *Academic Psychiatry*, **32**, 3–7.

Levine, R. E., Litwins, S. D. & Frye, A. W. (2006) An Evaluation of depressed mood in two classes of medical students. *Academic Psychiatry*, **30**, 235–237.

Liaison Committee on Medical Education (2008) *Functions and Structure of a Medical School: Standards for Accreditation of Medical Education Programs Leading to the M.D. Degree.* Association of American Medical Colleges.

Pendleton, D., Schofield, T., Tate, P., *et al* (2003) *The Consultation: An Approach to Learning and Teaching.* Oxford University Press.

Ross, S., Cleland, J. & Macleod, M. J. (2006) Stress, debt and undergraduate medical student performance. *Medical Education*, **40**, 584–589.

Silverman, J., Draper, J., Kurtz, S. M., *et al* (1997) The Calgary–Cambridge approach to communication skills teaching II: the SET-GO method. *Education for General Practice*, **8**, 16–23.

Stecker, T. (2004) Well-being in an academic environment. *Medical Education*, **38**, 465–478.

Tjia, J., Givens, J. L. & Shea, J. A. (2005) Factors associated with undertreatment of medical student depression. *Journal of the American College of Health*, **53**, 219–224.

CHAPTER 24

Training medical students to promote good mental health in secondary schools

Peter Sloan, Maggie McGurgan, Holly Greer
& Róinin McNally

Introduction

This chapter describes the creation of a mental health educational intervention, its delivery in secondary schools and its development into a module within the undergraduate medical curriculum.

Background to educational interventions in schools

Stigmatisation of psychiatric illness has been evident for as long as illness has existed (Bhugra, 1989). It has long been recognised that a great deal of fear and misunderstanding surround mental illness (Byrne, 1997; Link *et al*, 1997; Jorm *et al*, 1999). Even today, stigmatising attitudes are widespread and people with mental health problems such as schizophrenia, alcoholism or substance misuse are often perceived as violent and unpredictable (Crisp *et al*, 2000). These attitudes prevail in the general population but are also known to be present within the medical profession. More than half of the medical students and doctors surveyed by Mukherjee *et al* (2002) shared such beliefs. Negative opinions appear to lessen as a doctor's career progresses, which suggests that improved education at an earlier stage of medical training, and exposure to psychiatry in practice, may lead to the adoption of more reasonable attitudes.

Stigmatising attitudes and negative stereotypes form at an early age (Wahl *et al*, 2002). Evaluation of school programmes suggests that education is an effective tool in improving understanding of mental health. This is particularly evident if the intervention incorporates contact with people suffering from mental health problems (Esters *et al*, 1998; Pinfold *et al*, 2003; Shulze *et al*, 2003).

Adults with a better understanding of mental illness are less likely to endorse stigma and discrimination (Roman & Floyd 1981; Link & Cullen, 1986; Link *et al*, 1987; Brockington *et al*, 1993). It can therefore be postulated that enhancing understanding in children may prevent the development of such prejudice. In light of this evidence, a group of senior trainees on the Public Education Committee of the Royal College of Psychiatrists in Northern Ireland sought to develop a mental health educational intervention for school students.

Origins of the mental health workshop project

Significant planning and discussion took place before delivery of the intervention. The initial objective was to create a 2-hour workshop that would use a variety of media to address mental illness and stigma, and promote good mental health. It was decided that two pilot workshops would be presented and evaluated before a final version was developed and delivered to schools.

The pastoral care teachers of the two pilot schools were contacted for practical advice on content and procedures. There were differing opinions on subject matter according to topical issues in the area and the school ethos. Schools also had policies on the information that can be imparted to children about issues such as alcohol, drugs and self-harm, thus a certain amount of flexibility was required. The relevant child protection guidelines were adhered to and parental consent was obtained. Each pilot workshop was presented to approximately 40 children aged 14–15 years.

It is difficult to write health education material that is to appeal to, and benefit, a younger generation of individuals, as they have different levels of knowledge and points of reference. However, coordinators came to view the pilot as an opportunity to experiment with different formats, which could then be rated by the students and teachers using feedback questionnaires. The students themselves would thus mould the content of the final version. A range of approaches was used, including drama, poetry, didactic methods, interactive tasks and the use of celebrity images. All students and teachers attending the workshop completed an evaluation form. They were asked to rank formats in order of preference and also commented on duration, relevance and overall quality of the presentation.

The three most favoured methods of delivery were: dramatic presentation, celebrity images and multimedia didactic education.

Qualitative feedback included the following comments:

Students with shorter attention spans were unable to fully concentrate for 2 hours. [Teacher]

The mental health talk was interesting. Would have liked to hear more about drugs and eating disorders. [Student]

The media/film images really went down well; however, a couple of those used were too old to be relevant to the pupils. [Teacher]

This feedback was used to modify the educational component of the presentation. To aid attention and engagement, the duration was reduced to 75 minutes.

Current workshop outline

The workshop is designed to cater for six pupils per facilitator. It is divided into core components as follows.

Introduction

The workshop begins with a brief introduction to mental health. Differences between mental health and physical health are discussed. The role of the psychiatrist within the healthcare system is defined and a series of celebrity images is used to introduce the concept of mental health problems. Students are asked to identify pictures of celebrities who have spoken openly about their mental health difficulties to the media, and describe problems they may have encountered. This particular format engages the pupils and promotes audience participation.

Dramatic presentation

The focal part of the workshop is a dramatic presentation called *The Most Popular Boy in School*. This is a short sketch that describes a lunchtime encounter between two characters, Molly, and the most popular boy in school, Paul. On the outside they are very different. Paul appears to lead a carefree existence, captains the school rugby team and fends off the attentions of the girls in his class. Molly, on the other hand, is traumatised by her parents' recent divorce and spends much time at school by herself. We go on to learn, however, that they are both quite similar under the surface. Paul is experiencing family problems as well but is better at concealing these. The central message deals with the healthy and unhealthy coping mechanisms utilised by the two characters. The drama is conducted against a backdrop of images projected onto a screen that have relevance to the story line and reinforce the underlying themes.

Didactic presentation

This section uses a traditional lecture-style approach to impart factual information on a range of mental health conditions. The concept of stigma is introduced by discussing images of psychiatry that the media portrays and the misconceptions society holds.

Poetry is used to illustrate the derogatory way in which language can depict people with mental health problems and the marginalisation that can result (Box 24.1).

A number of mental health conditions particularly relevant to teenagers are then covered in more detail. Rather than simply listing symptoms and signs, this segment has a positive focus and emphasises the treatments available for each condition and ways of accessing help.

> **Box 24.1** Poem used in the educational workshop
>
> **Just Words?**
> Schizo, psycho, nutter, freak;
> Crazy, loser, loner, geek.
> Mental, oddball, spacer, mad;
> Loony, bonkers, dangerous, bad.
> Wacko, threat, capable of killing;
> Insane, scary, not the full shilling.
> Animal, maniac, wrong in the head;
> Violent, evil ... better off dead.
>
> Reproduced with permission © M. McGurgan 2009

Facilitated small-group work

The audience is then broken into groups of six to eight pupils, each facilitated by a doctor. Groups are given the task of examining a particular topic in more detail. Pre-prepared information packs are provided for facilitators. These contain resources to aid in generating discussion. Ideas are recorded in the form of a poster, which is then presented to the group as a whole, by nominated pupils, at the end of the session.

Summary

The workshop concludes with a summary of local sources of help and pertinent information on methods of access. Each pupil is provided with a copy of the *Headstuff* mental health information leaflet published by the Royal College of Psychiatrists.

Adaptation of the original format for special schools

It is well documented that young people with intellectual disability have limited access to mental health education resources (http://www.mencap.org.uk). In the spirit of *Equal Lives* (Bamford Review of Mental Health and Learning Disability, 2005) and *Valuing People* (Department of Health, 2001), the expansion of the project into special schools was explored. Given the increased prevalence of mental health problems among people with intellectual disabilities (Smiley, 2005), it was believed that the intervention would be valuable to this group.

Learning disability speech and language therapists gave advice on necessary adaptations to workshop format and communication style.

A special school was selected and agreed to participate. Following an information-sharing session, a pilot workshop was developed. This adapted version was then delivered to a class of pupils aged 16–19 years. Individual pupils' needs were taken into consideration and content was adapted accordingly. Key messages were retained, but adjustments to methods of delivery were required to ensure understanding. Wording, text size, font and imagery were optimised, as advised by the Good Information Group (Belfast Health and Social Care Trust). This is a local initiative that aims to improve communication between people with intellectual disabilities and healthcare professionals.

The special-school version focuses more on the recognition of emotions and identification of problems. Relevant mental illnesses are introduced but factual information is simplified and unnecessary detail avoided. More visual aids and interactive activities are incorporated, to facilitate engagement. For example, in one task students are asked to help create recipes for good and bad mental health. Ingredients such as 'good diet', 'exercise' and 'alcohol' are placed in the appropriate mixing bowls, each represented by a visual prop.

Similar celebrity images are used as a method of introduction, as these individuals are subjected to the same media influence as their mainstream peers. The drama from the mainstream version is also used without amendment.

Smaller numbers are used in group-work tasks, to enable more attention to be given to individual pupils. Posters are created by each facilitator and presented to the group as a whole.

Positive responses to the special-school version led to the delivery of this workshop across Northern Ireland, despite the absence of formal advertising.

Sustainability concerns

The intervention is a labour-intensive resource. Owing to the importance placed on small-group teaching within the workshop, one doctor is required for every six pupils present. The running and management of the project therefore require a sizeable workforce. Furthermore, the project was created and is delivered entirely by a small group of psychiatric trainees. Reliance solely on this finite group would ultimately compromise the long-term sustainability of the venture. The use of novel resourcing methods was therefore discussed.

Management of the project by the local health promotion agency was considered. Despite enthusiasm, limited funding prevented the allocation of protected resources to further its development.

In line with the College's 'action plan' on recruitment into psychiatry (Pidd, 2004), it was recognised that the project promoted a positive image of psychiatry and psychiatrists. Delegation to other healthcare professions

---

Box 24.2 Potential benefits and drawbacks of involving medical students in the delivery of mental health educational interventions

Benefits
- Promotion of positive image of psychiatry and psychiatrists
- Exposure to clinical practice in mental health may increase recruitment into the specialty
- The less pronounced student–pupil age difference may enhance rapport
- All medical students in the UK have undergone appropriate child protection checks
- Protected time is available to embark on such a project within the mandatory student-selected component within the undergraduate medical programme

Drawbacks
- Close supervision is required with regard to information imparted, owing to the lower level of expertise
- More support has to be provided for the development and delivery of the intervention, which is in any case labour intensive

---

would potentially lose this valuable recruitment opportunity. It was thus considered vital that control be retained by doctors.

The large untapped resource of the medical student body was acknowledged. Numbers, and therefore enthusiasm, would be replenished annually, and influence over content and format would be possible. The potential benefits and drawbacks of involving medical students in the delivery of mental health educational interventions are presented in Box 24.2. It was clear that the benefits of using medical students to further this resource outweighed any potential drawbacks and provided an exciting new direction on which efforts could be focused. It was believed that the workshop could be further developed through the programme of student-selected components (SSCs) at the local medical school.

The SSC programme

The current version of *Tomorrow's Doctors* (General Medical Council, 2009) states that the curriculum must have both core and SSCs. In a standard 5-year curriculum it is stipulated that a minimum of 10% of total time must be available for SSCs. They provide students with an opportunity to explore subjects of particular interest in greater depth than the core curriculum allows. SSCs also encourage the development of self-directed learning skills and the consideration of future career paths (see Chapter 15).

Modules within the SSC programme are available in a variety of formats – that is, based around work in the library, laboratory, clinical specialty or community. Locally, the SSC programme is delivered during years 2 and 3 of the undergraduate medical curriculum in parallel with the core teaching programme. In year 2, a maximum of 72 hours of contact time per semester is timetabled.

Liaison with the university

The deputy director of the Centre for Medical Education at the local university was contacted and a meeting was set up with the SSC management committee. It was initially suggested that a mental health component could be introduced to an existing SSC module entitled 'Medics in primary schools', which until then had focused entirely on physical health promotion and education. It was recognised that the existing body of work was too large to incorporate into an established SSC and thus warranted the development of a separate module.

For the initial module, a decision was made to focus solely on the special-school format of the workshop. This was largely for logistical reasons, such as well-established links with two schools close to the university, smaller class sizes and increased numbers of classroom assistants. It was believed that these factors increased opportunity for the medical students to access optimal support from experienced teachers and maximised constructive contact with the students. It was anticipated that the module would, after it had been properly established within the special schools, be brought to a wider range of schools, including mainstream schools.

The structure and content of such a module was discussed. It was agreed that an appropriate format would be the division of the 12-week module into three sections:

- development of expertise through formal teaching on mental health and a range of mental illnesses
- the development of a mental health workshop by the students
- delivery and assessment of the student workshops.

All contact beyond this point was with the SSC coordinator for year 2, who advised on further steps in the process of module development. At the local university, students are given the opportunity to choose SSCs from a booklet that describes around 40 modules. This booklet is distributed to all year 2 medical students and three preferences are ranked in order. A module descriptor was developed in accordance with university guidelines, to include information on module content, potential learning outcomes, teaching methods and assessment procedures. The module title, 'Heads above the rest', was chosen to acknowledge the significance of mental well-being in the maintenance of health.

There was a large amount of interest from the year group; however, for practical reasons only 12 students could take the module, divided into two groups of six.

Module development

The next step was to develop content of the three components of the module, in line with its delivery as a 12-week educational programme, as per university semester structure.

Learning objectives

The learning objectives describe what the students are expected to achieve by the end of the module. By the end of the module, the medical students should be able:

- to describe common mental health problems, in particular those affecting teenagers
- to identify ways of optimising good mental health
- to understand the psychological and social problems affecting people with intellectual disabilities
- to interact with young people who have an intellectual disability and their teachers
- to demonstrate how teaching skills must be adapted to enable effective communication with young people who have an intellectual disability
- to deliver a workshop to promote good mental health using methods such as didactic teaching, drama and group work
- to promote positive images of mental health services.

These objectives were divided into three sections and individual lesson plans were devised for achievement of all learning objectives by the end of the module.

Development of student knowledge base

The first section of the module utilised a combination of didactic teaching methods and interaction with professionals, patients, school students, family members and carers to impart a broad knowledge base.
Seminars covered:

- concepts of health and introduction to mental health
- the biopsychosocial model (Engel, 1977)
- the classification and description of common mental disorders
- intellectual disability and mental disorders affecting this group
- stigma in mental health and intellectual disability.

Students had the opportunity to visit a hospital for people with intellectual disabilities and to speak to staff and patients in both acute in-patient and day care settings. This enabled consideration to be given to the potential challenges of communicating with a person with intellectual disability.

The impact of intellectual disability upon the family unit was demonstrated to students through attendance at a workshop facilitated by the mother of a child with Down syndrome. Students were given the opportunity to ask questions to contextualise prior learning.

Students spent an afternoon at the school where they would present their workshop. They were encouraged to discuss structure and content with the relevant pastoral care teachers and received information about the specific mental health needs of the class.

Development of the student workshop

This section focused on small-group teaching and was largely interactive. Students participated in a series of facilitated discussions aimed at developing a final version of their workshop. Module coordinators were available at each session but students were encouraged to generate and build upon their own ideas.

Three formal facilitated workshops discussed the following:

- mental health information relevant to teenagers with intellectual disability and appropriate methods of delivery
- the use of drama as an educational tool
- the development of practical small-group tasks to illustrate the application of acquired knowledge.

Sessions were allocated within the timetable for private study and completion of each component. Workshops were rehearsed with module coordinators prior to delivery within the schools. This allowed for correction of inaccuracies in factual content and supported the development of student confidence.

Delivery of workshop and module assessment

The final version of each workshop was delivered to an audience of approximately 20 pupils at each school. Teaching staff had the opportunity to review subject matter before it was delivered, to ensure that all material was appropriate. The four module coordinators were silent observers, assessing overall content and structure (see 'Creating a marking scheme', below).

Following workshop delivery, time was allocated for completion of the reflective portfolio (discussed below). This was submitted for assessment as per university guidelines.

Students were then given the task of designing an original poster to promote ways of attaining good mental health using knowledge and experience gained throughout the module. These were produced in collaboration with the illustration department of the university and presented to the module coordinators for assessment. Posters were then given to each school, where they remain on permanent display.

The final session of the module was timetabled to allow for feedback of the assessed components and student evaluation of the module.

Development of a student study guide

A study guide was produced to function as a reference manual for students. It described the structure of the module, and broke it down into manageable components to facilitate successful navigation. An overview of each session was given and the individual weekly learning objectives were included.

The mental health information leaflets on the Royal College of Psychiatrists' website (http://www.rcpsych.ac.uk) were recommended to students as an essential learning resource. Additional reading material included the undergraduate core text for psychiatry and a variety of mental health education websites.

Documentation of student guidance and university regulations was included as stipulated. This contained advice about plagiarism, attendance, late submission of work and information regarding student support networks.

Assessment procedures were described and marking schemes ratified by the university were included as appendices to the study guide. A standardised student module evaluation form gave students the opportunity to provide feedback.

Assessment procedure

General assessment guidelines

In keeping with the ethos of the acquisition and assessment of key transferable skills, examinations are not normally used to assess student competence at the end of an SSC module. The following assessment techniques are commonly used to assess knowledge and skills:

- essay/dissertation
- oral presentation
- reflective portfolio
- clinical project
- literature review
- practical skills.

Coordinators are instructed to select at least two assessment techniques for any module. It is obviously important to ensure that assessment methods match the learning outcomes of the module. The SSC management committee of the local university is welcoming of innovative methods of assessment; however, these must be approved in advance of study guide publication.

SSC module assessment

Students spend the majority of the semester working towards presentation of the mental health education workshop. It is therefore appropriate that both content and delivery of this intervention are evaluated. Three methods of assessment are used:

- Module coordinators observe delivery of each workshop and award an overall group mark. Consideration is given to individual contribution relative to the group as a whole and assessors are given the opportunity to adjust individual marks accordingly.
- The poster, which serves as a written record of the accomplishments of the group, is presented to module coordinators and a further group mark awarded.
- Students are required to produce individual reflective portfolios (see below) that outline their experiences and progression through the module. This is awarded an individual score and functions to discriminate between students.

The three components are weighted for their contribution to the overall award for the module, as follows:

- workshop delivery, 30%
- reflective portfolio, 50%
- poster presentation, 20%.

Student guidance on assessment

Information on each assessed component was provided in the study guide, as follows.

Reflective portfolio

It was explained that the portfolio was to function as a record of progress through the module and that it should include reflections at the completion of each stage. Students were advised that there were no fixed rules on how it should be compiled and were encouraged to be as creative as possible. The following framework was provided as a guide:

- *Beginning*
  - Introduction, including aspirations for the module.
- *Middle*
  - Planning
  - Consideration of the needs of the audience
  - Explanation of decisions regarding the content and structure of the workshop
  - Outline of resources used
  - Description of delivery of the workshop
  - Personal reflections on group performance
- *End*
  - Balanced evaluation of successes and failings
  - Identification of potential improvements
  - Summary of learning outcomes achieved

General guidance was given on layout, standardised formatting, word count and referencing. Notification was given on penalties for the late submission of course work.

Educational workshop

The purpose of the intervention was explained to students in detail during the introductory lectures.

Poster presentation

It was outlined in the study guide that the poster should promote ways of attaining good mental health. Students were advised to consider who would read the poster and how the format should be tailored accordingly.

Posters (prepared using Microsoft PowerPoint software) were printed by the university illustration department. Students were instructed to submit an e-copy of their poster to the module coordinator on disk or by email to facilitate review by the external examiner.

Creating a marking scheme

To ensure consistency in marking across modules, criterion-referenced pro forma have been developed by the SSC management committee for each of the approved SSC assessment techniques. It is mandatory that coordinators, when assessing student work, use these standardised templates. Minor modifications can be made, however, to suit the specific module. It is advised that, wherever possible, students' work should be double marked and that all fail and borderline work *must* be double marked.

Coordinators must keep copies of student assessments and any written feedback distributed, as these are required for external examiners and inspection visits from the General Medical Council.

Reflective portfolio

Marks were awarded for:

- reflections at the outset of the module
- accurate and relevant content with evidence of active learning
- coherence and continuity
- description of the module's impact on personal development
- reflections on the impact on future professional practice
- evidence that learning objectives were met.

Overall marks were weighted in favour of content and impact on personal development.

Workshop

Marks were awarded for:

- evidence of preparation and planning
- appropriate factual content
- innovative use of resources and originality of approach
- quality of drama, group work and delivery.

Module coordinators were given the opportunity to moderate the mark for an individual student based upon that individual's contribution (see above).

Poster presentation

Marks were awarded for:

- appropriate use of source materials
- design and layout
- oral presentation.

Again, the opportunity was given to moderate individual marks based on student contribution.

Evaluation and development of the SCC module

The inaugural module proved to be a great success and we received resoundingly positive feedback from both the medical students and the special schools involved. The following themes emerged from the analysis of student feedback forms.

- Students requested that more time be allocated to formal didactic teaching, with a more in-depth coverage of pertinent mental health issues.
- With limited clinical contact in Year 2, students appreciated the opportunity to spend time in both clinical and day care settings. More emphasis will therefore be placed on such contact in future modules.
- Students suggested that they would benefit from observing a mental health workshop at the beginning of the module to clarify desired content and format.

Students especially enjoyed delivering their work in the special school setting. Having highlighted the time and effort required to develop each workshop, they requested further opportunities to deliver it in other schools.

As anticipated, coordinators aim to expand the initiative, to involve more medical students and more schools. This process ought to be straightforward now that the model is established and proving popular with the students.

Summary

The opportunity to bring innovative and much needed mental health education to schoolchildren in Northern Ireland has been exceptionally rewarding, shaping the experimental pilot workshop into a popular SSC module.

While development of the module within the local university advances, invaluable support from local trainees has enabled the continuation of the original workshop project within mainstream schools across Northern Ireland.

The four course coordinators look forward to supporting UK-wide expansion of this type of intervention, particularly via the SSC programme within medical schools in collaboration with the Royal College of Psychiatrists.

Acknowledgements

We wish to express our thanks to the Public Education Committee of the Royal College of Psychiatrists in Northern Ireland, and indeed to the many consultants and peers who have supported and assisted us. We would also like to thank the two special schools involved in the first SSC module.

References

Bamford Review of Mental Health and Learning Disability (2005) *Equal Lives: Review of Policy and Services for People with a Learning Disability in Northern Ireland.* Department of Health, Social Services and Public Safety. Available at http://www.dhsspsni.gov.uk/index/bamford/published-reports/learning-disability-report.htm

Bhugra, D. (1989) Attitudes towards mental illness: a review of the literature. *Acta Psychiatrica Scandinavica*, **80**, 1–12.

Brockington, I. F., Hall, P., Levings, J. *et al.* (1993) The community's tolerance of the mentally ill. *British Journal of Psychiatry*, **162**, 93–99.

Byrne, P. (1997) Psychiatric stigma: past, passing and to come. *Journal of the Royal Society of Medicine*, **90**, 618–621.

Crisp, A. H., Gelder, M. G., Rix, S., *et al.* (2000) Stigmatisation of people with mental illness. *British Journal of Psychiatry*, **177**, 4–7.

Department of Health (2001) *Valuing People: A New Strategy for Learning Disability for the 21st Century* (CM 5086). The Stationary Office.

Engel, G. L. (1977) The need for a new medical model: a challenge for biomedicine. *Science*, **196**, 129–136.

Esters, I. G., Cooker, P. G. & Ittenbach, R. F. (1998) Effects of a unit of instruction in mental health on rural adolescents' concepts of mental illness and attitudes about seeking help. *Adolescence*, **22**, 469–476.

General Medical Council (2009) *Tomorrow's Doctors. Outcomes and Standards for Undergraduate Medical Education.* GMC.

Jorm, A. F., Jacomb, P. A. & Christensen, H. (1999) Attitudes towards people with a mental disorder: a survey of the Australian public and health professionals. *Australian and New Zealand Journal of Psychiatry*, **33**, 77–83.

Link, B. G. & Cullen, F. T. (1986) Contact with the mentally ill and perceptions of how dangerous they are. *Journal of Health and Social Behaviour*, **27**, 289–302.

Link, B .G., Cullen, F. T., Frank, J., *et al* (1987) The social rejection of former mental patients: understanding why labels matter. *American Journal of Sociology*, **92**, 1461–1500.

Link, B. G., Striening, E. L. & Rahav, M. (1997) On stigma and its consequences: evidence from a longitudinal study of men with dual diagnosis of mental illness and substance abuse. *Journal of Health and Social Behaviour*, **38**, 177–190.

Mukherjee, R., Fialho, A., Wijetunge, A., *et al* (2002) The stigmatisation of psychiatric illness: the attitudes of medical students and doctors in a London teaching hospital. *Psychiatric Bulletin*, **26**, 178–181.

Pidd, S. (2004) *Revised Action Plan on Recruitment and Retention of Psychiatrists.* Royal College of Psychiatrists. Available at http://www.rcpsych.ac.uk/pdf/Revised%20Action%20Plan%20on%20Recruitment%20and%20Retention%20of%20Psychiatrists2.pdf

Pinfold, V., Toulmin, H., Thornicroft, G., *et al* (2003) Reducing psychiatric stigma and discrimination: evaluation of educational interventions in UK secondary schools. *British Journal of Psychiatry*, **182**, 342–346.

Roman, P. M. & Floyd, H. (1981) Social acceptance of psychiatric illness and psychiatric treatment. *Social Psychiatry*, **16**, 21–29.

Shulze, B., Richter-Werling, M., Matschinger, H., *et al* (2003) Crazy? So what! Effects of a school project on students' attitudes toward people with schizophrenia. *Acta Psychiatrica Scandinavica*, **107**, 142–150.

Smiley, E. (2005) Epidemiology of mental health problems in adults with a learning disability: an update. *Advances in Psychiatric Treatment*, **11**, 214–222.

Wahl, O. F., Wood, A. & Richards, R. (2002) Newspaper coverage of mental illness: is it changing? *Psychiatric Rehabilitation Skills*, **6**, 9–31.

CHAPTER 25

Women in medicine

Rosalind Ramsay & Sheila Hollins

Introduction

The relevance of this chapter, in a book which is primarily about teaching students and secondarily about recruitment into psychiatry, may not be immediately obvious. There are, however, several salient reasons for its inclusion. The number of newly qualified doctors who are women has grown significantly over recent years, and the number of women psychiatrists is likely to grow to an even greater extent, since women preferentially select psychiatry as a medical career. We thus predict a higher number of female readers than male readers of this book but, we hope, it will be helpful for all readers to have an understanding of the broader issues relating to women in medicine. More specifically, issues relating to women in medicine will pervade both teaching and recruitment strategies. More female psychiatrists will be teaching more female students with the expectation that identification and role-modelling will be of benefit to teaching, recruitment and career progression in the specialty.

Historical background

In ancient civilisations such as Egypt and Greece, women played a role in the healing professions, while in England in the Middle Ages nuns would provide care within convents and for their surrounding communities. A few women gained formal qualifications, for example at the famous medical school in Bologna. However, as medical training became defined through formal education and qualifications rather than apprenticeship, a professional medical monopoly developed and women were excluded. The female Scottish surgeon James Miranda Barry (1792–1865) qualified and worked in the Army Medical Service, in disguise as a man. During the 19th century there were demands that women be able to gain admission to the medical profession but medical schools and examining bodies refused to accept them.

Elizabeth Garrett Anderson (1836–1917) was inspired by the example of the first female American medical graduate, Elizabeth Blackwell (1821–1910), and eventually succeeded in joining the medical register in 1866, via the Society of Apothecaries, after her father threatened to take the Society to court. Some British women obtained a medical education at universities on the Continent. Garrett Anderson and other pioneering women along with some male allies set up the London Medical School for Women in 1874. By the early 20th century, women had established their right to a medical education and employment but they faced restrictions in pursuit of their profession. In 1915 the War Office gave a group of women doctors some premises for a military hospital in Endell Street in London, and they treated 26000 patients in the years up to 1919 (Hall, 2004).

In the inter-war period, many teaching hospitals – with notable exceptions such as the Royal Free and Edinburgh Medical School – were reluctant to admit women and qualified women doctors found it difficult to develop their careers. A recommendation in the Goodenough report (Goodenough, 1944) that all medical schools should be required to admit women was implemented through the National Health Act in 1948, but many medical schools retained a maximum quota of 10–15% women until the mid-1960s.

Since then the number of women medical students and women working as doctors in different grades has increased very substantially. Numbers appear to have stabilised at just less than 60%; in 2007, 59% of UK medical graduates were female, this being the same percentage of women who entered UK medical schools in 2007/08.

Issues facing women in medicine

Although the numbers of women going to medical school and qualifying as doctors have increased significantly, there was a perception that women were not progressing in their careers in the same way as their male colleagues. To facilitate medical workforce planning, the British Medical Association's Health and Policy Research Unit started a longitudinal study of 1995 medical graduates, to gain some understanding of the career aspirations and choices of newly qualified doctors. The study followed up the sample of 609 doctors every 10 years to investigate career trends and the reasons behind them. The British Medical Association (2006) found that 30% of the mixed-sex cohort were currently working less than full time and a further 40% would consider doing so in the future. Among the women graduates, 94% were working less than full time or would consider doing so in the future. Some respondents expressed difficulties with less than full-time work, for example 'I'm trying to do a full-time job in part-time hours, but I'm perceived by others as being a hobby doctor.' Women were twice as likely as men to want to become general practitioners (GPs) but were less interested in hospital specialties such as surgery, radiology and anaesthetics.

A longer-term study of the career progression of more than 7000 doctors who graduated in 1977, 1988 and 1993 from all UK medical schools (Taylor *et al*, 2009) found that women who had worked full time during training achieved principal status in general practice or consultant status slightly quicker than men. Women who had always worked full time were underrepresented in general practice and in surgical specialties. The authors concluded that women who progressed more slowly than men had not worked full time throughout their training. They found no evidence of direct discrimination but suggested that indirect discrimination may influence career choice, for example because of the lack of part-time training opportunities. Interestingly, their analysis of career choices found that women, both those who had always worked full time and part-timers, were overrepresented in psychiatry (8% compared with 5% of men in the three cohorts) and part-time men were significantly more likely to choose psychiatry (8%, compared with 5% of men who worked full time) than any other specialty apart from general practice. This suggests that psychiatry is an attractive specialty for those who may wish to work part time at some point in their career. Taylor *et al* (2009) attributed the overall slower progression of women to the higher proportion of women who worked part time. Men who worked part time had a similar career trajectory to women who worked part time. Having children did not affect the speed of career progression of women.

Isobel Allen, emeritus professor of health and social policy at the Policy Studies Institute, has carried out research on doctors and their careers since the 1980s, when the Department of Health commissioned her to assess the implications of the increasing number of women medical graduates. She found that men and women experienced similar problems and constraints in their careers, suffering from what they regarded as a rigid and conservative career structure; they wanted more flexible working patterns that would allow all doctors to lead a normal family life (Allen, 2005). She records some changes in culture, with the more outrageous questions at interviews disappearing and a less powerful 'old boy' network, but overall she believes the medical profession has been slow to adapt to the fact that women have accounted for over a half of medical students since the mid-1990s. Young women continue to find achieving a work–life balance more stressful than their male peers. Allen's work also highlights the difference between men's and women's career paths, with an M-shaped distribution to many women's careers: a peak in the early years, a dip in the middle and the potential for a peak in the later years.

More information about the issues women may have in developing their careers in medicine comes from analysing the success of women compared with men in receiving employer-based awards (EBAs) and national clinical excellence awards from the Advisory Committee on Clinical Excellence Awards (ACCEA). The 2008 ACCEA report stated:

We have again analysed this year's awards by level, specialty, regional subcommittee, age, gender, ethnicity and time to award. In relation to specialty and gender, the analysis indicates that apparent disparities are due to small numbers of applicants from under-represented groups rather than applications being less successful.

The report commented that, allowing for the small numbers available for analysis, there was no evidence of gender bias in terms of the awards made, but ACCEA did express concerns about the low number of eligible women applying for bronze awards. Compared with men, those women who do apply for a bronze award are more likely to get an award on their first application but women who are turned down at their first application are less likely to reapply than their male colleagues. However, the number of women holding an EBA is reported to be consistent with the numbers of women consultants, with women in some regions holding a higher proportion of awards than men.

Women in academic medicine

Two recent reports, *Women in Academic Medicine: Challenges and Issues* (British Medical Association, 2004) and *Women in Academic Medicine: Developing Equality and Governance and Management for Career Progression* (British Medical Association, 2007), have highlighted the particular difficulties women doctors face in academic posts. The 2004 report refers to the glass ceiling women in academic medicine experience, which seems to prevent promotion to the more senior posts. This is illustrated by the relatively low number of women professors. At professorial level, only 11% of clinical academics are women and two UK medical schools still have no female professors. Only two of the 33 heads of UK medical schools are women (British Medical Association, 2007).

The 2007 report aims to help raise awareness of current gender disparities. Women were less likely to have regular appraisal and also reported a lack of role-models, an important factor in career progression. Fewer women were on editorial boards for journals or grant-giving panels or achieved an editorship. More women than men saw working conditions as influential in their current choice of employment. For those who saw working conditions as influential, both men and women considered flexible working as the most important factor. The report concluded that the problems men and women face are similar but they do not appear to have the same impact on ultimate achievement for men as they do for women.

Killaspy *et al* (2003), looking at the issues for women in academic psychiatry, commented, 'We are not attracting and retaining women into senior academic posts.' Their research found that women were significantly less likely than men to pursue an academic career and, within academic posts, women were much less likely to occupy a professorial position than men.

Women in leadership positions in medicine

Twenty medical royal colleges and faculties in the UK and Ireland – including the Royal College of Psychiatrists – belong to the Academy of Medical Royal Colleges. Many colleges have never had a woman President and as of 2009 only one of the 20 was female. For example, to date there has been one woman President of the Royal College of Anaesthetists, two of the Royal College of Psychiatrists, two of the Royal College of Physicians and one of the Royal College of Radiologists. Professor Dame Carol Black was the second woman to chair the Academy, the first being Dame Fiona Caldicott, the first woman President of the Royal College of Psychiatrists. Within the Royal College of Psychiatrists at one point while the second female President was in post, the Registrar and Treasurer were also women.

Dr Patricia Hamilton is the first Medical Director of Medical Education, England, and Dr Elizabeth Paice is the chair of the Conference of Postgraduate Medical Deans. Seven of the 21 postgraduate deans in the UK are currently women.

Gender pay gap

Using data from the Women in Academic Medicine cohort of the Athena Survey of Science, Engineering and Technology 2006, Connolly & Holdcroft (2009) found that female doctors earn 19% less than male doctors. This cohort includes trainees and consultants on National Health Service (NHS) and academic contracts. The gender difference is greater in the NHS (22%) than in academia (16%). Factors influencing the pay gap include grade, hours worked, experience, administrative roles and specialty. The authors comment, 'overall, gender pay gaps are lower for doctors starting their careers but quite sizeable gaps emerge even among similarly successful men and women'.

Feminisation of medicine

Despite the increase in the numbers of female medical students and trainees, with notable exceptions, there remains a relative dearth of women in senior positions. In 2004, Professor Dame Carol Black, while President of the Royal College of Physicians, raised questions about the consequence of more women going into medicine. 'The women admitted to medical school do well, they work well and they graduate well. The distinctions go to the women. But then, they start to make choices to balance their family and their lifestyle' (Laurance, 2004). Women were not reaching the top of the profession. Dame Carol warned that within a decade women doctors would outnumber men and that this 'feminisation' of medicine would lead

305

to the profession losing status, influence and ultimately remuneration (Laurance, 2004). Dame Carol also expressed concern that there would be an insufficient number of women doctors willing to work in particularly demanding specialties that have unsocial hours or to participate in all the activities that made up the professional life of a senior doctor.

Roberts (2005) also explored the implications of more women entering medicine. She too pointed out the gender differences in choice of specialty, with better-remunerated specialties that require a higher degree of technical skill attracting men, while there are more women in the lower-paid, less technically focused specialties. She described the underrepresentation of women in academic posts, particularly at a higher level, although she noted that the number of female vice-chancellors was increasing. There have also been relatively few women involved in medical politics, with no female President of the General Medical Council and only six of the 19 elected doctors on the Council's governing council at that time were women (Roberts, 2005).

Women doctors, however, have been continuing to try to establish themselves across the different specialties. Surgery, which epitomised the high-earning technical specialty favoured by men, has seen the establishment of a Women in Surgery department and Opportunities in Surgery department to support and promote surgery as a career for a wider range of applicants, including women. In 2009 the President of the Royal College of Surgeons commented on a new report published by the Royal College of Physicians on the career choices of women, saying 'Managing surgical cases is both highly unpredictable and technical, going some way to explain why there are fewer women going into surgery' (Black, 2009). His suggestion that women might lack certain skills and attributes illustrates the attitudes still held towards women in medicine among some medical leaders, mitigated to only a limited extent by the President's retort that his comments had been taken out of context.

Possible solutions

Some governmental perspectives on women and medicine are indicated in Box 25.1

Within the medical profession: patterns of work

The move towards shorter working hours (see Box 25.2) should be helpful to women doctors.

Medical Women's Federation (MWF)

Women doctors have been looking at ways to help themselves and develop their careers. The Medical Women's Federation has represented the

Box 25.1 International and government perspectives on women in medicine

The World Health Organization's plan of action for women and health
The World Health Organization advocates gender equality in health. It aims to increase knowledge and to strengthen the health sector response by gathering evidence and supporting gender mainstreaming in health policies and programmes.

European Union and gender equality
The Treaty of Rome (1957) introduced the basic principle of equal pay. Subsequently the European Union has supported equal rights at work, protection from indirect discrimination and harassment at work and equal rights outside the workplace. The Union applies the principle of gender mainstreaming to all policies and activities.

UK Government Equalities Office (GEO)
The GEO is responsible for equalities legislation and policy in the UK. It also leads on the government's international obligations to implement the Convention on the Elimination of All Forms of Discrimination Against Women (CEDAW), the Bejing Declaration and Platform for Action, and the European Union's Roadmap for Equality between Women and Men. The Equality and Human Rights Commission provides advice and guidance and works to implement an effective legislative framework and raise awareness of individual's rights (http://www.equalityhumanrights.com).

Box 25.2 Changes in working pattern (McNally, 2008)

There have been a number of changes in recent years that have promoted shorter working hours for all doctors and more managed timetables. These include:

- the European Working Time Directive, which allows a maximum of 48 hours work per week
- national selection programmes and the allocation of a national training number, leading to a completion of the Specialist Training Certificate, which means that if you take a career break you will have a training post to return to afterwards
- organisation of less than full-time training (flexible training) through the deaneries
- the new consultant contract, with specified programmed activities in the job plan
- the new general practitioner contract, which removed the necessity to do on-call work

---

interests of women doctors in the UK since 1917 and aims to advance the personal and professional development of women in medicine as well as to improve the health of women and their families. The federation has 13 local groups to support women doctors; it helps them to network with other women for help and advice. It also has formal and invited representation on a number of national committees and charitable organisations, including the NHS Employers Medical Workforce (Equality and Diversity) Reference Group and various committees of the British Medical Association. It is recognised as a national nominating body by the Advisory Committee on Clinical Excellence Awards (De Souza & Ramsay, 2008).

Improving Working Lives for Doctors

The Department of Health launched the Improving Working Lives (IWL) initiative (2001) to make the NHS a better place to work in. It was underpinned by six standards addressing issues around employment services, work–life balance, flexible working, valuing staff, training and personal development for staff.

Improving Working Lives for Doctors (Department of Health, 2002) described a number of individual examples of flexible working, including on the Flexible Careers Scheme (FCS), flexible training and flexible retirement. It illustrated some of the other ways of working flexibly, including as a locum, in a job share, or as a part-time doctor, and with different patterns of hours, for example in school term time only. *Improving Working Lives for Doctors* saw the IWL initiative as achieving improvements in the recruitment and retention of doctors, professional confidence and job satisfaction, the day-to-day working environment, and to services. The *Making Part-time Work* report (Medical Women's Federation, 2008) pointed to the changes that need to happen to accommodate the changing workforce and suggested how to overcome the barriers to part-time working, which included attitudes. The report also explored how to support career development for part-time doctors.

In the wake of Carol Black's comments to the *Independent* in 2004 about her concerns that the profession was becoming female dominated (see Laurance, 2004), the Royal College of Physicians invested in a 2-year research exercise by a sociologist which led to the publication of *Women and Medicine: The Future* (Royal College of Physicians, 2009). The report comments that two findings are of central importance: first, the preference of women doctors for part-time or other forms of flexible working; and second, the comparative preference of women for working in specialties that offer more 'plannable' working hours and more patient contact. It comments that 'these will affect the future organisation and delivery of patient care'. Preserving the highest quality of care with an increasingly part-time workforce will be challenging, and will need innovative workforce planning and financial modelling.

The report makes a number of recommendations to policy makers (Royal College of Physicians, 2009):

- The organisational implications of changing workforce patterns and preferences with respect to working hours and specialty choices should be urgently examined so that the effective delivery and continuity of patient care are not compromised.

- The economic impact of changing work patterns and their interaction with policy initiatives needs to be evaluated.
- To gain timely, rigorous and systematic insights into the implications of the new workforce trends, critical information gaps must be filled with some urgency.
- The scope and detailed coverage of workforce planning need to be extended and its analytic methods upgraded to take full account of the demographic shifts now underway.
- Individual doctors at each stage in their career – and especially at the point of selecting their preferred specialty – should be provided with far more extensive information, guidance and feedback on their career choices and aspirations.

The Chief Medical Officer, Sir Liam Donaldson, in his annual report for 2006 included a chapter 'Women in medicine' with the subtitle 'Opportunity blocks' (Chief Medical Officer, 2007). 'Key facts' from the report are shown in Box 25.3. He acknowledged that 'Today the problem is not access to medical school but rather how we ensure the female medical workforce is able to fulfil its potential once in employment'. He concluded with three recommendations for change:

- The number of flexible training places for doctors should be expanded.
- A national working group should be established.
- In surgery and other specialties where the proportion of women is low, mentorship schemes should be reinforced.

Box 25.3 Five key facts about women working (Chief Medical Officer, 2007)

- Two-thirds of new medical students are women, yet less than 30% of consultants, 11% of professors and 36% of senior lecturers are female.
- Studies of women doctors' attitudes and experiences show that many regret entering the profession because of the barriers to career progression that they encounter.
- European Union data identify the main obstacles to maintaining women in the general workforce as inflexible working hours, poor child-care provision and an absence of tax incentives.
- Similar obstacles confront women doctors, exacerbated by the work patterns in modern medicine (particularly the need for 24-hour cover); the hurdles in academic medicine appear particularly unfriendly to women.
- While the National Health Service was a pioneer in flexible working and child care in the workplace, these measures have not been developed sufficiently to address the fundamental problems that impede women doctors' careers.

The national working group established in line with the second recommendation was chaired by Baroness Ruth Deech and its report was launched in October 2008. Its recommendations were targeted in three areas (Deech, 2009):

- improving existing structures to improve career advancement at critical points
- ensuring that new processes (e.g. revalidation) have the flexibility and capacity to accommodate doctors with different working patterns
- providing more support for the practical realities of caring for a child or dependent relative.

Women in psychiatry

Over 10 years ago the Women in Psychiatry Special Interest Group (WIPSIG) was set up at the Royal College of Psychiatrists (Ramsay, 2005). The founding chair had identified the need for a Special Interest Group for women psychiatrists and also women patients. She had had four children under the age of 6 while working in a full-time consultant post. There were already 878 women consultants in the UK but little thought was given to ways of working part time and flexible training was a relatively new concept. Women in-patients were admitted to mixed wards and the particular needs of women with a mental illness were generally not considered. The newly formed WIPSIG had the dual aims of addressing the needs of women psychiatrists and also of women patients in mental health services. During its first 10 years, membership of WIPSIG grew to 1277, including 83 men.

It has worked to achieve its aims in a number of ways (Ramsay, 2004). In terms of career development, these have included:

- focus on training needs of psychiatrists, including gender awareness and the mental health needs of women
- raise the profile of women in academic psychiatry through an annual prize on a theme related to women's mental health
- promote networking, training and support for WIPSIG members through sessions at the College annual meeting and other conferences
- facilitate flexible working patterns by organising a job-share register
- raise issues around gender discrimination within the College (see below).

WIPSIG was interested in the findings of an external review of College structures commissioned in 2001 to identify any discriminatory practices. This review, conducted by the Centre for Ethnicity and Health at the University of Central Lancashire, highlighted issues around gender equality that the College should address. The College President at that time invited Sheila Hollins to set up a gender equality scoping group. This group

Table 25.1 Royal College of Psychiatrists data on proportions of women in psychiatric roles

	Percentage women
Members, 2008	45
Fellows, 2008	24
Total trainees	46
Affiliates and Specialist Associates	42
Membership of Council	69
Editorial boards of College journals:	
British Journal of Psychiatry	21
Advances in Psychiatric Treatment	25
Psychiatric Bulletin/The Psychiatrist	20
MRCPsych applications	34
Successful applicants	39

developed a gender equality statement of intent and a gender equality action plan (Royal College of Psychiatrists, 2005). The plan was adopted by the College Council as College policy in 2005. It requires the monitoring (and reporting to the College Council) of the gender breakdown of College committees, journal editorial boards, candidates entering and passing the MRCPsych examination, and those nominated for awards or positions. Women doctors are in fact achieving particularly well in psychiatry, as shown in Table 25.1.

Other required actions include:

- having a policy of zero tolerance regarding gender harassment, intimidation, bullying, victimisation or unjustified discrimination by or between members, associates, trainees and staff
- ensuring that core training and education of members, associates and trainees include capability in gender issues
- ensuring that all members, trainees and associates have access to and are able to fully benefit from all functions of the College, regardless of gender.

This work was in line with the then current edition of *Good Psychiatric Practice* (Royal College of Psychiatrists, 2004), which highlighted equality issues, stating that the core attributes required for good psychiatric practice include 'being sensitive to gender', with a commitment to equality, anti-discriminatory practice and working with diversity. The subsequent third edition of *Good Psychiatric Practice* (2009) takes this further in saying 'A psychiatrist must provide care that does not discriminate and is sensitive to gender' (p. 12) and 'You must treat your colleagues fairly and with respect. You must not bully or harass them, or unfairly discriminate against them.... You should challenge your colleagues if their behaviour does not comply with this guidance' (p. 27).

Two (male) psychiatrists have tried to evaluate the impact on the specialty of the growing numbers of female psychiatrists (Wilson & Eagles, 2006). They concluded that the overall effect was likely to be positive. Women tend to be more empathic than men (in general) and, partly for this reason, may conduct better mental state examinations (Fabrega *et al*, 1994). There is consistent evidence that female medical students start with more positive attitudes to psychiatry than do their male colleagues, giving rise to the hope that a snowball effect may occur of women attracting women into the specialty.

Summary

Women are continuing to choose medicine as a career and more particularly continuing to choose psychiatry. Although many women achieve leadership positions within the profession, many others give more weight to having a reasonable work–life balance. This throws up very real questions about how best to support women to achieve their potential as medical leaders without undermining their other important roles as mothers and carers. Themes running through many recent reports on women in medicine, as summarised in this chapter, underlie the need to promote flexible working and to identify role-models with whom women can identify at different stages of their careers, alongside the ready availability of mentoring. Groups such as the MWF, or within psychiatry the WIPSIG, recognise the dilemmas and issues women doctors face and can take an organisational approach to bringing about necessary change in the profession. The authors of this chapter recognise that many men also aspire to work in more flexible services and look forward to the day when flexible working patterns are the norm, to allow all doctors to achieve a healthy work–life balance.

References

Advisory Committee on Clinical Excellence Awards (2008) *Annual Report*. Department of Health. Available at http://www.dh.gov.uk/prod_consum_dh/groups/dh_digitalassets/@dh/@en/documents/digitalasset/dh_092421.pdf

Allen, I. (2005) Women doctors and their careers: what now? *BMJ*, **331**, 569–572.

Black, J. (2009) Female medics 'to outnumber male'. *BBC News*, 2 June.

British Medical Association (2004) *Women in Academic Medicine: Challenges and Issues*. BMA.

British Medical Association (2006) *The BMA Cohort Study of 1995 Medical Graduates, 10th Report*. BMA. Available at http://www.bma.org.uk/healthcare_policy/cohort_studies

British Medical Association (2007) *Women in Academic Medicine: Developing Equality in Governance and Management for Career Progression. Executive Summary and Recommendations*. BMA.

Chief Medical Officer (2007) Women in medicine: opportunity blocks. In *On the State of Public Health: Annual Report of the Chief Medical Officer 2006*. Department of Health.

Connolly, S. & Holdcroft, A. (2009) *The Pay Gap for Women in Medicine and Academic Medicine*. British Medical Association.

Deech, R. (2009) *Women Doctors: Making a Difference. Report of the National Working Group on Women in Medicine for the Chief Medical Officer*. Department of Health.

Department of Health (2001) *Improving Working Lives Standard*. Department of Health.

Department of Health (2002) *Improving Working Lives for Doctors*. Department of Health.

De Souza, B. & Ramsay, R. (2008) Medical Women's Federation celebrates its long history. *BMJ Careers*, 4 March.

Goodenough, W. (1944) *Report of the Interdepartmental Committee on Medical Schools*. Ministry of Health and Department of Health for Scotland.

Fabrega, H., Ulrich, R. & Keshavan, M. (1994) Gender differences in how medical students learn to rate psychopathology. *Journal of Nervous and Mental Disease*, **182**, 471–475.

Hall, L. A. (2004) Women and the medical professions. Online article at http://www.lesleyahall.net/wmdrs.htm

Killaspy, H., Johnson, S., Livingston, G., *et al* (2003) Women in academic psychiatry in the United Kingdom. *Psychiatric Bulletin*, **27**, 323–326.

Laurance, J. (2004) The medical time bomb: too many women doctors. *Independent*, 2 August.

McNally, S. A. (2008) Women in medicine. In *So You Want to be a Brain Surgeon?* (eds S. Eccles & S. Sanders) (3rd edn), pp. 86–88. Oxford University Press.

Medical Women's Federation (2008) *Making Part-time Work*. Medical Women's Federation. Available at http://www.medicalwomensfederation.org.uk/files/Part-time%20full%20report%20final.pdf

Ramsay, R. (2004) Women in Psychiatry Special Interest Group. *BMJ Career Focus*, **328**, 116.

Ramsay, R. (2005) Women in psychiatry: ten years of a special interest group. *Advances in Psychiatric Treatment*, **11**, 383–384.

Roberts, J. (2005) The feminisation of medicine. *BMJ Careers*, 8 January, p. 1315.

Royal College of Physicians (2009) *Women and Medicine: The Future*. Royal College of Physicians.

Royal College of Psychiatrists (2004) *Good Psychiatric Practice* (2nd edn) (CR125). RCPsych.

Royal College of Psychiatrists (2005) *Gender Equality Action Plan*. RCPsych.

Royal College of Psychiatrists (2009) *Good Psychiatric Practice* (3rd edn) (CR154). RCPsych.

Taylor, K., Lambert, T. & Goldacre, M. (2009) Career progression and destinations, comparing men and women in the NHS: postal questionnaire surveys. *BMJ*, **338**, 1735.

Wilson, S. & Eagles, J. M. (2006) The feminisation of psychiatry: changing gender balance in the psychiatric workforce. *Psychiatric Bulletin*, **30**, 321–323.

Index

Compiled by Linda English